# FRONTIERS IN IMMUNOGENETICS

# FRONTIERS IN IMMUNOGENETICS

Proceedings of a Symposium
in Honor of Professor Ray D. Owen with contributions from
former students and colleagues held at
the California Institute of Technology,
Pasadena, California, June 2 and 3, 1980

*Editor:*

WILLIAM H. HILDEMANN, Ph.D.
*University of California School of Medicine*
*Center for the Health Sciences*
*Los Angeles, California*

ELSEVIER/NORTH-HOLLAND
NEW YORK • AMSTERDAM • OXFORD

Published by:

Elsevier North Holland Inc.
52 Vanderbilt Avenue, New York, New York 10017

Sole distributors outside the U.S.A. and Canada:

Elsevier/North-Holland Biomedical Press
335 Jan van Galenstraat, P. O. Box 211
Amsterdam, The Netherlands

Library of Congress Cataloging in Publication Data

International Symposium for Immunogenetics (1980 :
California Institute of Technology)
Frontiers in immunogenetics.

Bibliography: p.
Includes index.
Contents: Immunophylogeny, from sponges to hagfish to mice / W.H. Hildemann -- Current status of the rat major histocompatibility complex / Elizabeth P. Blankenhorn -- The B and C systems of cattle revisited / Clyde Stormont -- [etc.]
1. Immunogenetics--Congresses. 2. Immunology, Developmental--Congresses. 3. Owen, Ray David, 1915- I. Owen, Ray David, 1915- . II. Hildemann, W. H., 1927- [DNLM: 1. Immunogenetics--Congresses.
QW 541 I61f 1980]
QR184.I5 1980 616.7'9 81-5516
ISBN 0-444-00624-9 AACR2

Manufactured in the United States of America

# Contents

# Biographical Preface

Life for Ray David Owen began on a dairy farm in Wisconsin in 1915—a close-to-nature environment he remembers was a great place to grow up. Owen's father was not only a dairy farmer, but also a cattle fancier who sparked Ray's early interest in genetics with discussions of blood lines and pedigrees. The farm formed an important part of Ray's life with chores to be done before and after attendance at the Genesse State Graded School (two teachers, 8 grades) and Waukesha High School. He and his future wife, June, both entered Carroll College, a Presbyterian Church-connected liberal arts college in Waukesha, during the Great Depression in 1933. Ray Owen majored in biology and minored in chemistry, math, English and French. Professors Nanz and Ray, each being a one-man department of biology and of chemistry in this small college, both encouraged Owen to become a biological scientist. In 1937, Ray Owen became a Ph.D. student at the University of Wisconsin in Madison, where his major professor was L.J. Cole. His graduate research focused on the biochemical and developmental genetics of birds. He also studied hybrid sterility among different species of pigeons, guinea fowl and chickens. Because behavioral differences among species preclude natural interspecific mating, he developed a method of artificial insemination of small birds. Although Ray has since researched many species ranging from protozoans and sponges to mice and people, he has never overcome his early fondness for pigeons.

On completion of his Ph.D. in Genetics in 1941, Owen began work on blood group inheritance in dairy cattle. This research was to shape not only his career but also those of others in the fields of immunology and genetics. As a postdoctoral fellow, Ray became associated with the laboratory of Professor M.R. Irwin at Wisconsin. Irwin is believed to have coined the term "immunogenetics" and in a sense is a founder of modern immunogenetics. Owen, in collaboration with graduate

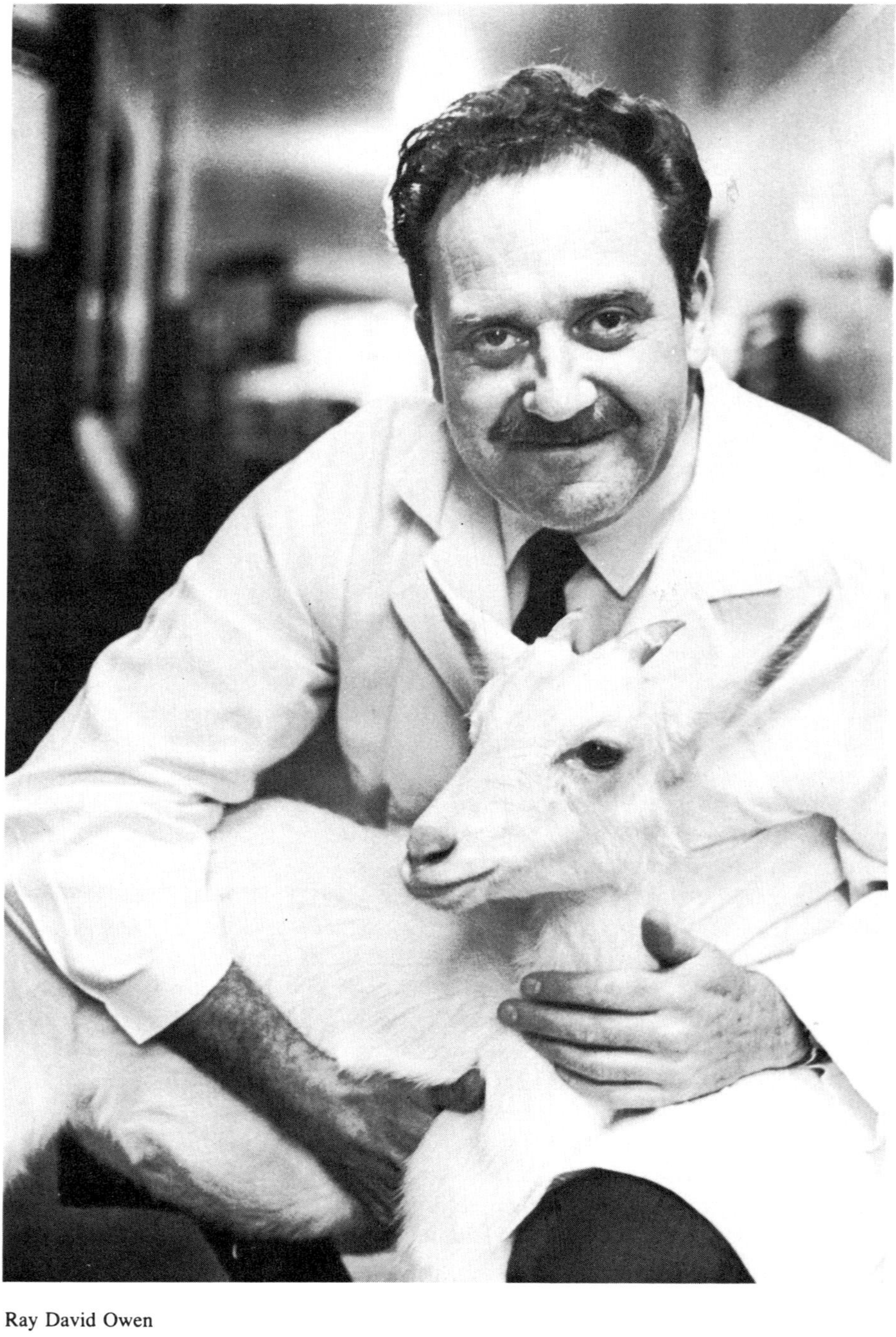

Ray David Owen

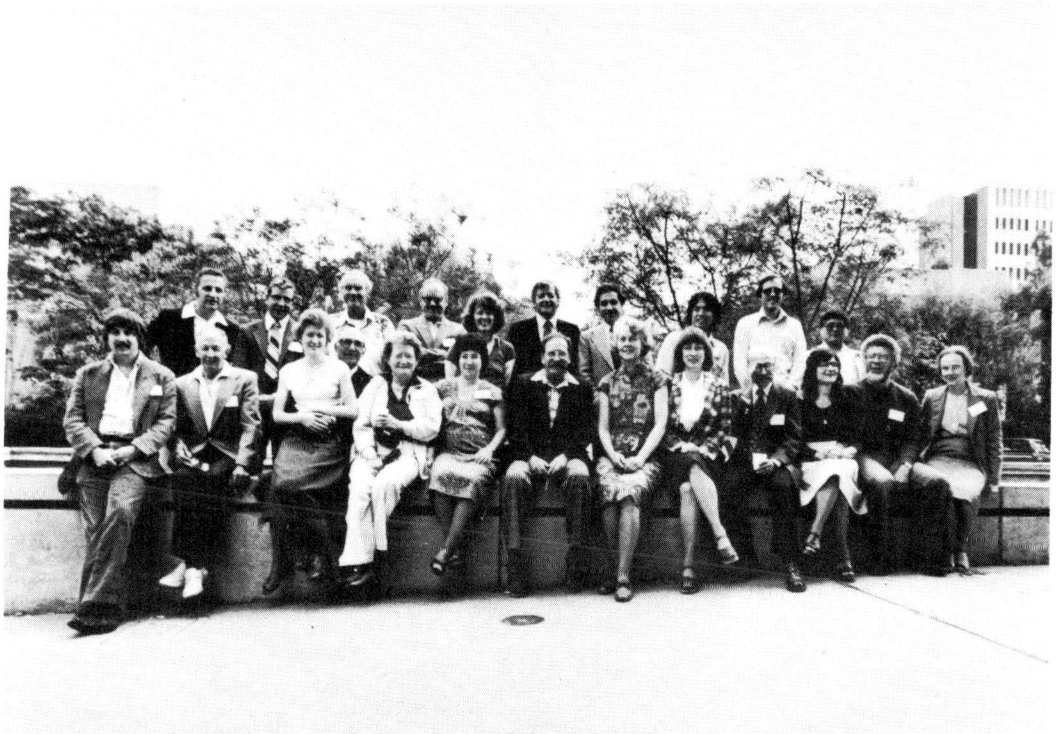

**Front row, left to right:** J. Frelinger, C. Stormont, S. Melvin, W. Stone, E. Russell, S. Rosenberg, R. Owen, E. Christensen, L. Blankenhorn, I. Rappaport, Lee Herzenberg, Len Herzenberg, G. Rosenquist.

**Back row, left to right:** R. Gilden, D. Shreffler, W. Hildemann, D. Nanney, J. Klotz, B. Sanders, V. Marinkovich, D. Asai, T. Douglas, S. Tokuda.

student Clyde Stormont, did much of the early work on the genetics of red-cell antigens in cattle. During the course of these studies, Owen made a classic discovery that subsequently revolutionized immunology. By use of blood group markers, he found that vascular anastomoses between bovine twin embryos result in reciprocal transplantation of hematopoietic tissues between the embryos. The transplanted cell lineages persist throughout the animal's life. Such acquired tolerance represents a major evasion of graft rejection that would occur if tissue were exchanged between immunologically competent individuals rather than embryos. This phenomenon of immunological tolerance, later explored in depth by Owen and his friend Peter Medawar among others, remains an important area in contemporary immunobiology and in studies of immunoregulation.

In 1946, Owen, already an assistant professor at the University of Wisconsin, came to Caltech as a Gosney Fellow, and in 1947, he accepted appointment as an associate professor of biology at Caltech. In California, Ray decided to switch the focus of his research from cattle to laboratory animals. Owen realized that he could not pursue cattle studies in urban Pasadena, and that there were many approaches using small laboratory animals which were impossible in cattle. He began an intensive study of laboratory rats and soon developed immunogenetic markers for studies of parabiotic exchange in rats. His postulation that immunosuppressive treatments such as X-radiation might permit establishment of otherwise incompatible transplants came to fruition, in collaboration with Odell and Lindsley at Oak Ridge National Laboratory, in the first successful bone marrow transplants to irradiated recipients. During the 50's, Owen extended his interests to human subjects focusing on heterogeneous antibodies to human blood groups in normal and immune serum, and what appeared to be evidence for actively acquired tolerance to Rh antigens. His mammalian studies culminated in a classic paper on tolerance published in the Proceedings of the Royal Society. He also took advantage of opportunities for collaboration with people at Caltech, working on tobacco mosaic virus serology with Sam Wildman, the immunogenetics of enzymes with Clem Markert, and antigenic variations in *Tetrahymena* with John Loefer, David Nanney, and Jean-Marie Dubert. His highly successful textbook, *General Genetics,* written with Adrian Srb of Cornell University, appeared in first edition in 1952, and was revised in 1965. This book was a bestseller and for many years was the most-used text in the field. Ray Owen's lecture and laboratory course in Immunology was undoubtedly one of the best and most demanding in the United States. Those of us who were privileged to be exposed to Ray's inspired teaching remember the experience as one of the high points at Caltech. Incidentally, the original anti-mouse Ss serum, now known to be anti-C4, was produced for the immunology laboratory course at Caltech.

Owen's remarkable breadth of immunogenetic interests emerged in numerous frontier fields. As Ray's first Ph.D. student in the early 50's, Irving Rappaport completed a series of immunochemical studies of albumin molecules. Owen, with wife June and young sons, David and Griffith, spent the summer of 1954 at the

Friday Harbor Marine Laboratory studying the specificity of cell aggregation reactions in sponges in cooperation with Dixie Lee Ray (now Governor of Washington). About this time, Ray became increasingly interested in phylogeny and encouraged graduate student Bill Hildemann to investigate the transplantation genetics and immunology of fishes, because practically nothing was then known about the immunogenetics of lower vertebrates. This led to pioneering publications concerning transplantation immunity and allogeneic polymorphism in fishes. During the 50's, Henry Gershowitz intensively studied blood group inheritance in pigeons. The late Jim Berrian and Leslie Brent pursued extensive research on transplantation immunogenetics in mice. The far-reaching concept of the "uniqueness of the individual," in Medawar's phrase, emerged in the late 50's, partly as a result of diverse studies from Owen's laboratory. With another graduate student, Don Shreffler, Owen studied the histocompatibility genetics of the mouse. Their identification of the *Ss* locus in the early 60's, found by Shreffler to subdivide the major immunogene complex, played a key role in the ultimate dissection of the *H-2* complex.

During most of the decade of the 1960's, Ray Owen served as the third Chairman of the Division of Biology at Caltech. In this demanding position he was successor to the illustrious George Beadle who in turn had assumed the leadership role from Thomas Hunt Morgan. At this juncture, Owen decided to omit his name from research contributions coming out of his laboratory, reporting work done mainly by younger people. Yet he remained intimately involved in the day-to-day working of the laboratory, the design of experiments, and the support of research. Students of this time will never forget standing at the coffee room chalkboard describing to Ray the design of a complex experiment—on asking Ray if it would be worth doing, he would lean back in his chair, puff his pipe and ask, "What do *you* think?"

During this period, Bob Sanders, a postdoctoral fellow, became particularly interested in the developmental immunogenetics of blood cell antigen in chickens. He discovered a strong correlation between one erythrocyte antigen and hematogenous tumors. This became an early example of an onco-fetal antigen. In the late 60's, a new wave of graduate students appeared on the horizon. This group was if anything more eclectic than previous ones. Susan Melvin worked to define differentiation antigens of the thymus and bursa in pigeons, as well as the effect of immunosuppression on the generation of spontaneous tumors in mice. Tommy Douglas worked extensively on characterization of the rat Thy-1 antigen. Suzanne Rosenberg, who originally came to the laboratory to study rotifer immunogenetics, ended by working on the topology of cattle blood group antigens expressed on lymphocytes and red cells. Jeff Frelinger studied transferrins in pigeons, and worked to define a rational selective mechanism for the maintenance of transferrin polymorphism in feral pigeon populations. During most of this time, Libby Blankenhorn was a technician in the laboratory, but became transmutated into a graduate student and ultimately finished a study of the strucuture of rat Ia alloantigens. The discovery of Ia antigens in the mouse was earlier made by two former graduate students, Shreffler and Frelinger, working with Chella David. The postdoctoral fellows in the laboratory during this time were equally diverse. Although David Dusenberry came to work on rotifers, he finally settled on behavioral genetics of a free living soil nematode. Ron Acton apparently did everything during his postdoc, from autoimmune disease to tumor immunobiology to protein chemistry. Joan Klotz studied extensively the possible polymorphisms of alpha feto-protein.

Ray Owen's record of institute and community service during the 60's and 70's was exceptional if not unparalleled. His wife, June, recalls that Ray was on 22 major committees at one time and accordingly travelled to Washington, D.C. at least 16 times per year. Here we only sample the impressive array of organizations Owen has served, often as an Officer or Chairman of key committees. These include the United Nations, World Health Organization, National Research Council, National Academy of Science, National Institutes of Health, Genetics Society of America, American Cancer Society, National Science Foundation, and Oak Ridge National Laboratory. He served as President of the Genetics Society of America, as a member of the Board of Directors of the American Society of Human Genetics, and as a member of the Editorial Board of the Annual Review of Genetics. For three years, Owen was the "Scientist-Member" of the three-person President's Cancer Panel. During this time, he provided strong leadership on the panel and affirmed the need for basic biological research as the cornerstone for the national cancer program. Those of us in the laboratory then regarded his service as an inconvenience, since Ray was away so often. Viewed from a later vantage point, we can only be awed by his energy.

If Ray Owen were to single out one particular activity he remembers with pride, it would probably be his chairmanship of an ad hoc faculty committee on the freshman year at Caltech, whose work led to three historic changes. These were the inauguration of pass-fail grading to make adjustment to Caltech less traumatic for its freshmen, the introduction of electives into a previously rigid freshman curriculum, and, especially, the admission of women to Caltech's freshman class. Ray's unusual sensitivity to student needs evolved from many years of undergraduate teaching and service on the critical Admissions Committee. He still teaches a freshman course, Current Research in Biology, which meets, as always, in his home in the evenings during the first quarter. He also continues to teach the laboratory course in Immunology. Beginning in 1975, Owen became Dean of Students and Vice President for Student Affairs, while continuing as Professor of Biology. We are aware that he really knows most of the nearly 800 Caltech undergraduates, recognizes their problems, and cares for them deeply. They clearly reciprocate such recognition and concern with great appreciation.

Among numerous honors, Ray Owen received the Gregor Mendel Medal on the occasion of the Mendel Centennial in Czechoslovakia in 1966. He has been awarded honorary Doctor of Science degrees from Carroll College (1963), University of the Pacific (1966), and the University of Wisconsin (1979).

Ray Owen, the person, has changed little since his immigration from Madison to Pasadena. The aspects of his life which have given him the most pleasure include his family, his home, his garden (we remember especially the camellias and chrysanthemums), his friends in the international community of scientists, his research, and his teaching. We, his students, owe much to his guidance, and we like to believe he found part of his fulfillment in us. On the occasion of his 65th birthday, we, students and colleagues alike, salute Ray Owen.

Bill Hildemann

Jeff Frelinger

*June, 1980*

FRONTIERS IN IMMUNOGENETICS

# SECTION I:

# Allogenic Polymorphism and Immunophylogeny

Hildemann, ed. Frontiers in Immunogenetics

# Immunophylogeny: From Sponges to Hagfish to Mice

W.H. Hildemann

*Immunogenetics Group, UCLA School of Medicine, and Dental Research Institute, Los Angeles, California*

## Introduction

When I first had the privilege of joining Ray Owen as a Ph.D. student at Caltech in the summer of 1953, the new field of immunogenetics involved few investigators, and they were mostly pursuing blood group studies in which immunological methodology was used to explore genetic variation. Immunology then was restricted to mammals and birds with emphasis on serum antibodies and their reactivities. Apart from a few forward-looking people, immunology was regarded merely as a technical resource for blood grouping and microbiological studies rather than a basic discipline in its own right. At this juncture, Ray Owen was eager to encourage graduate students and postdocs to explore new areas. Moreover, he argued for combinations of whole animal, cellular, and molecular experiments rather than narrowly focused research. Although he himself is a bird lover, he soon recognized that I had a predilection for aquatic creatures and especially fishes. Thus, my Ph.D. thesis problem became the immunology and immunogenetics of goldfish.

Teleost fishes were already known to produce humoral antibodies to xenogeneic antigens, more rapidly at higher water temperatures (Cushing 1942). Allograft rejection had been observed in lower vertebrates (Goodrich and Nichols 1933; Vogel 1940), but its immunologic basis was unknown. Most immunologists in the early 50's gratuitously assumed that "lower animals" would lack the subtly discriminating immunorecognition capacities of mammals. There was therefore considerable surprise at our finding of alloantibody production and inherited individual differences in cellular antigens in goldfish (Hildemann 1956). The existence of tissue transplantation immunity with a memory component in this fish (Hildemann 1957, 1958), also shown to have a complex immunogenetic basis (Hildemann and Owen 1956), led to recognition of the "uniqueness of the individual" as a broad biological principle (Medawar 1957). By 1960, we had shown that both alloantigenic individuality and exquisite immunocompetence were characteristic of diverse teleost fishes and anuran amphibians (Hildemann and Haas 1959, 1960). The time was not yet ripe to suspect immunocompetence underlaid by allogeneic polymorphism in invertebrates. Spiegel (1955), then a postdoctoral fellow at Caltech, had extended classic studies showing species specificity in sponge cell aggregation or fusion, but otherwise nonspecific phagocytosis a la Metchnikoff (1893) was assumed to meet the immunologic needs of lower metazoans.

With the discovery of acquired tolerance by Owen (1945) confirmed and extended by Billingham et al. (1956), immunogenetic attention remained concentrated on birds and mammals. Ease of tolerance induction was shown to depend not only on recipient immaturity but on the strength of the histocompatibility barriers involved. With increasing definition of the genetic rules of transplantation (Snell 1948), inbred lines of mice became the animals of first choice for most studies. It soon emerged that allogeneic polymorphism in mice, and higher vertebrates generally, was so great that tissue compatibility could be expected only among isogeneic animals. This was of course a depressing realization for clinical transplanters. However, the finding of specific immunosuppression under certain circumstances by antigen-induced tolerance, by immunoblocking antibodies, and by suppressor cells has opened the difficult field of dynamic immunoregulation. Although the same immunogenetic rules were found to apply to higher and lower vertebrates (Hildemann 1972), their immunoregulatory circuits appear substantially different. Certainly the cytoarchitecture of the immune system and the molecular classes of immunoglobulins inducible become progressively more complex from primitive fishes to mammals. In the pursuit of evolutionary insight and underlying mechanisms, I and my students have studied in turn bony fishes, amphibians, primitive fishes, annelids, echinoderms, corals, and sponges. Now our emphasis is on the latter three phylums of invertebrates, though we maintain a continuing research program in the "bread-and-butter" realm of mouse immunogenetics. My romance with the reluctant Pacific hagfish has had its ups and downs—alternatively gratifying and frustrating (literally sticky). Tropical corals and sponges are at least beautiful to behold. Also, I can blame Ray Owen for my interest in invertebrate immunogenetics which began at Caltech with studies of hemoglobin synthesis in *Daphnia* (Hildemann and Keighley 1955). In this overview, I shall cite major new insights that have emerged especially during the decade of the 1970's. These are summarized with emphasis on key transitional phylums of lower metazoans and primitive vertebrates, ending with much studied mice.

## Immunocompetence in Sponges and Coelenterates

Until recently, the prevailing paradigm considered invertebrate defenses, often equated with phagocytosis and encapsulation of foreign entities, as lacking in sharp discrimination. The notion that specific recognition in invertebrates is restricted to self-constituents and that only vertebrates recognize foreignness in a discriminating manner still persists (Marchalonis 1977). Certainly, the extensive allogeneic polymorphism of ciliary antigens and other cell-surface molecules displayed by protozoan species is recognized in an immune sense by multicellular "host" animals. Protozoan nucleocytoplasmic alloincompatibility, when demonstrable, appears to be intracellular and enzymatic rather than immunological in character (Tartar 1970). If essential immunocompetence is defined in terms of adaptive defense of the integrity of the body (individual), only three functional components need be invoked: (1) antagonistic or cytotoxic reaction following intimate contact, (2) selective or specific reactivity, and (3) inducible memory or selectively altered reactivity on secondary contact. These criteria appear minimal in the sense that specificity and incompatibility alone describe cell recognition reactions in protozoan (Preer 1968) and plant reproduction (Heslop-Harrison 1978). A plant-oriented reader may pause to note the curious reversal of incompatibility in angiosperms, namely, that self pollen is actively rejected whereas non-self pollen with appropriate cell-surface markers is accepted by the stigma. Specificity and memory in concert clearly apply to the central nervous system and are therefore insufficient benchmarks of immune reactivity.

To our initial surprise, immunocompetence as defined above has been found in two species of tropical sponges under controlled laboratory conditions. In the most studied *Callyspongia diffusa* from Hawaii (Hildemann et al. 1979, 1980), very extensive polymorphism of histocompatibility (H) molecules was revealed by incompatibility among 480 different allogenei pairings without exception. This represents some 960 individual clones utilized as alloparabionts or sources of fitted allografts. Compatible intracolony fusions in this ramose species are abundant in nature, but intercolony or allogeneic fusion has not been observed, even where separate colonies are in close proximity. Isogeneic parabionts invariably fuse compatibly within one to two days, whereas a similarly early but morphologically different tissue fusion between alloparabionts is followed by cytotoxic rejection. *Callyspongia* exhibit a uniform purple pigmentation throughout their soft tissues; their skeletal framework, consisting of brown horny fibers, is resistant to decomposition in sea water. Thus, any soft tissue death is promptly quantifiable by disappearance of purple-colored tissue from the skeletal framework. Allogeneic cytotoxicity can be objectively scored as definitive when soft tissue destruction extends 1.0 mm or more to either side of a parabiotic interface. Consistent cytotoxic reactivity provoked by allogeneic cell-surface contact in *Callyspongia* is manifest in a continuum of strong to weak histoincompatibilities; however, strong reactions are most frequent at normal temperatures of 23°–27°C. First-set (1°) median reaction times ranged from 7 to 9 days at 27°C. Second-set (2°) but not third-party alloparabionts consistently displayed accelerated rejection when repeat graftings were performed soon after maturation of first-set reactions. Heightened transplantation immunity or memory persists for at least 2–3 weeks after contact sensitization.

The directionality, vigor, and timing of alloparabiotic rejection in this species all depend mainly on the genetic constitutions of the interacting clones. This is perhaps most persuasively evident from the essentially identical rejection reactions observed in replicate interclonal combinations. Moreover, given interclonal combinations display predictably strong, moderate, or weak incompatibilities that are not influenced by graft dosage. Interclonal reciprocity in graft dosage achieved at 8:1 size ratios by parabiosis of large pieces (48 $cm^2$) to small pieces (6 $cm^2$) of about the same thickness revealed that both the degree of incompatibility and direction of cytotoxicity depended on clonal genotypes and not graft dosage (Hildemann et al. 1980). Alloreaction times are inversely proportional to the strength of the H barrier. In other words, strong or extensive killing reactions begin earlier than weak ones in both 1° and 2° responses. Tissue bridges become conspicuous early, especially between interclonal combinations that are strong reactors. The bridges, exhibiting a whitish hyperplasia, contain an abundance of mesohyl or leukocyte-type cells which are probably responsible for subsequent allogeneic killing. Allocytotoxic reactions are usually restricted to the immediate contact zone extending 2 to 5 mm from the interface.

Given the long-standing, negative attitude concerning immunocompetence in invertebrates, many have remained skeptical, especially about the existence of specific memory in sponges. Because the essence of immunologic memory remains mysterious even in mammals, we have been particularly interested in its characteristics in lower invertebrates. How soon does early "memory" (i.e., heightened alloimmunity) develop and how long does it persist in the absence of further stimulation? Diverse interclonal combinations of *Callyspongia* were set up in quadruplicate and replicate pairs were disjoined after 1, 2, 4, or 8 days of contact. Thus the same genotype combinations were being compared at each of four time intervals. The sponges were rejoined at new interfaces as second-set parabionts 3 days after initial separation. Maximal allosensitization indicated by accelerated second-set reactivity was gradually achieved after 2 to 8 days of primary contact as a function of the interclonal combination. Although induction of alloimmunity as such requires at least 2 days of contact, allorecognition in initial tissue fusion is visually evident within one day. Similar allorecognition in mammalian mixed skin cell-lymphocyte culture reactions also requires less than one day (Tanaka and Sakai 1979). When primary and secondary alloparabiotic reactions of the same clones were compared concurrently under identical experimental conditions, it soon became evident that 2° reactions occurred more rapidly and with much greater severity than 1° reactions (Hildemann et al. 1980). Although potent immunity persists for at least 2–3 weeks after primary separation in *Callyspongia,* we have yet to test successfully for possible long-term memory in this species.

Specific transplantation immunity has also been demonstrated in the marine sponges *Hymeniacidon perleve* from Scotland (Evans and Curtis 1980) and *Xestospongia exigua* from Palau in the western Caroline Islands (Hildemann and Linthicum, in preparation). Both of these species exhibit discriminating alloimmunity and selectively accelerated rejection of second-set grafts. Several other species of sponges have shown allogeneic incompatibilities revealed by consistent parabiotic nonfusion or cytotoxic reactions, but these have yet to be examined in immunologic perspective (Hildemann et al. 1979; Van de Vyver 1980).

Convincing evidence of allogeneic incompatibility under controlled testing in the phylum Coelenterata has been reported for representatives of two of the three classes, Hydrozoa and Anthozoa, but not Scyphozoa (jellyfishes). In the hydroid, *Hydractinia echinata*, clones obtained asexually from single colonies fuse compatibly, whereas allogeneic colonies usually fail to fuse when grown in contact. Breeding experiments suggest that alloincompatibility is governed mainly by multiple *H*-alleles of one locus (Ivker 1972). However, a more complicated genetic basis is suggested by the hierarchy of histoincompatibilities affecting the intensity of "hyperplastic overgrowth" reactions observed. The impressive polymorphism of histocompatibility markers found in the coral *Montipora* (Hildemann et al. 1980) and in the gorgonian (sea fan) *Eunicella* (Theodor 1976) suggests that each separate clone or colony has a distinctive array of immunorecognition molecules. We found parabiotic incompatibility among 890 different pairings of clones of *Montipora verrucosa* without exception. More than 1400 reciprocal histoincompatibilities were actually recorded. As in *Callyspongia,* the directionality, severity and rate of rejection in *Montipora* were mainly determined by the genetic constitutions of the interclonal parabionts. Allograft reaction times were inversely related to the strength of the H barrier and were closely temperature dependent. Among 1479 alloparabiotic combinations of *Eunicella,* Theodor observed only 11 or 0.7% compatible fusions, whereas 99.3% were incompatible. Even the few compatible gorgonians could have come from the same clones, since all animals were tested from the same area. Among the sea anemones *Anthopleura elegantissima* and *A. krebsi,* isogenic individuals comprising separate clones produced by asexual reproduction live in compatible contact. Whenever allogeneic nonclonemates touch, an antagonistic behavior pattern is initiated that results in tissue damage to one or both anemones. Physical contact between tentacles or acrorhagi of genetically different anemones, not mere proximity, is required to evoke a cytotoxic response (Bigger and Hildemann 1980). Obviously, no single *H*-locus, even with a large number of alleles, could account for these remarkable results. Rather, the "uniqueness of the individual" principle (Medawar 1957), no doubt reflecting a multiplicity of separate gene products, applies to multicellular invertebrates as well as vertebrates.

In parabiosis experiments between nonclonal plates of *Montipora,* contact avoidance reactions in zones of soft tissue proximity were seen early, a week or more before any allogeneic cytotoxicity appeared where contact was fixed. Cell-surface recognition of foreignness visually precedes any tissue destruction which requires a sensitization period of a week or more, even at elevated temperatures. In a typical large series, allograft reactions led to localized bilateral necrosis with a primary MRT of 22.0 (19.2 to 25.3) days at 25°C (Hildemann et al. 1977). After 40 days in contact, parabiosis between the same pairs at new interfaces yielded accelerated rejection with an MRT of 11.6 (9.4 to 14.4) days. Third-party allografting from a quite separate population, following completion of first-set interfacial reactions, showed definitive reactions either at 7–16 days, characteristic of heightened 2° responses, or at 19–35 days, typical of 1° reactions. The disparity between accelerated and non-accelerated reactions supports the assumption of immunogenetic specificity underlying this memory. Vigorous alloimmune memory persisted in other experiments for 4 weeks after primary separation, but disappeared after 8–16 weeks. Immunologic primitiveness in corals may therefore be reflected in the lack of long-lived memory as found among vertebrates.

## Immune Reactivities of Higher Invertebrates

Here my overview shifts to annelid worms, echinoderms and protochordates. I shall be citing mostly work by my own students and former students who have made key contributions in an early, but ongoing stream of studies. Beginning in the mid-sixties, studies by Cooper and Duprat pointed to the existence of specific transplantation immunity with concomitant immunologic memory in earthworms (Cooper 1970). Orthotopic integumentary allografts and control autografts of modest size were observed in a large series of earthworms (*Lumbricus terrestris*) maintained at an optimal 15°C by Cooper. Allografts showed moderate to weak incompatibility whereas autografts survived permanently. Although prolonged rejection from 38 to 153 days occurred in tests among Oregon worms or Canadian worms and in tests between these populations, most 1° allografts in all combinations were intact or partly viable even after 8 months. Second-set transplants made about a week after 1° grafting yielded some accelerated, some equal, and some prolonged responses in comparison to first-set survival times. Such erratic manifestation of incompatibility and "memory" has raised doubts about the specificity of adaptive immunity in annelids (Dales 1978).

Experiments with nemertean worms have also suggested a lack of sharply discriminating immunocompetence at the helminth level of phylogeny, because allogeneic "patchwork chimeras" of contrasting color phenotypes survive compatibly for many months (Bierne 1980). However, this could result from low experimental temperature, massive tissue exchange, and consequent tolerance. Xenograft incompatibilities between species of earthworms tend to be stronger and evident earlier. Leukocyte-type cells called coelomocytes appear chiefly responsible for rejection of foreign grafts in annelids. These cells, including both granulocytes and lymphocyte-like cells, on adaptive transfer to naive *Lumbricus* 5 days after placement of an *Eisenia* graft caused accelerated rejection of new *Eisenia* grafts (Linthicum et al. 1977). The immunologic specificity of xenograft reactions remains doubtful because of uncontrolled genetic and metabolic variables inherent in such experiments. Cellular immunity inherent in circulating leukocytes appears responsible for transplantation immunity in annelids and is accompanied by short-term, though erratic, immune-type memory. This cell-mediated immunity evidently functions in the absence of immunoglobulin-type antibodies. Attempts to detect production of humoral antibodies in annelids have given uniformly negative results. Hemagglutinins, a hemolysin, a ciliate lysin, and a ciliate-immobilizing factor of separate specificities are demonstrable in sipunculid coelomic fluid, but these reactivities do not reside in immunoglobulins, nor do they appear to be specifically inducible (Cooper 1976).

Because of technical problems and lack of investigative effort, the immunopotentialities of arthropods and of mollusks remain unsettled. However, unequivocal immunorecognition at the allogeneic level has been described among the higher invertebrate phylums of echinoderms and tunicates. Phylogenetic characteristics of these two groups put them just below the vertebrates. Evidence of specific allograft immunity was first obtained with a sea cucumber (*Cucumaria tricolor*) and a sea star (*Protoreaster nodosus*), both from the tropical Pacific (Hildemann and Dix 1972). Integumentary allografts in *Cucumaria* invariably exhibited slow rejection with survival times of 129 to 185 days at 22°–26°C, whereas early repeat grafts survived 60 days or less. Slow rejection of initial allografts was also found to be typical of *Protoreaster*. The California sea star *Dermasterius* maintained at a maximum but near optimal temperature of 15°–16°C yielded median survival times of 213 (170 to 266) days for first-set integumentary allografts and 44.2 (17.7 to 110.5) days for second-sets (Karp and Hildemann 1976). Allograft rejection in all instances was marked by infiltration with granular leukocytes and lymphocyte-like cells.

Unrelated California sea urchins (*Lytechinus*) at 15 to 16°C surprisingly reject primary integumentary allografts in about 30 days and secondary grafts in only 12 days (Coffaro and Hindgardner 1977). This early responsiveness at low temperature suggests strong histoincompatibility in contrast to the findings with other echinoderms. Accelerated memory reactions appeared to be more specific in the sea stars than in the sea urchins based on survival times of third-party grafts. Because the extent of polymorphism of H molecules in the test populations is unknown, the issue of specific versus wide-ranging memory in these species is unsettled. Cross-reactions suggestive of limited specificity of immune memory may be frequent whenever successive antigens are allogeneic or derived from similar sources. Use of chemically-defined antigens and haptens in invertebrates could circumvent this problem, provided of course a suitable immunoassay is available. Limited attempts to detect immune reactions toward xenogeneic cells and proteins in echinoderms have not been decisive. Although discriminating cell-mediated immunity obviously exists in echinoderms, governing mechanisms remain unknown.

Solitary tunicates and colonial tunicates both exhibit allograft incompatibility leading to slow rejection. We found progressive primary rejection of tunic allografts in solitary *Ciona intestinalis* associated with invasion by lymphocytes, granulocytes and macrophages—an outcome similar to that found among vertebrae species (Reddy et al. 1975). In colonial species of the family Perophoridae, isogeneic pieces always fused to share a common vascular system, whereas random colonies were rarely compatible in parabiosis (Freeman 1970). All colonies obtained by sexual reproduction were reported to fuse with either parent colony. Although allogeneic parabiosis experiments in various colonial ascidians have revealed extensive H polymorphism under complex genetic control, colony specificity in *Botryllus primigenus* has been ascribed to a single gene complex with multiple alleles (Tanaka

1975). Mating of AB × CD incompatible colonies yielded progeny of supposed types AC, AD, BC, and BD, all able to fuse compatibly with both parents. However, compatible parabiosis among F1 and F2 progeny colonies occurred only when at least one postulated allele was common. In other words, putative AC colonies could fuse with AD colonies but not with BD. If each postulated allele produced an antigen in the usual codominant manner, Parent ⇌ F1 combinations in the *Botryllus* example cited should be mutually incompatible. The interpretation of these findings proposed by the Japanese investigators is obviously in conflict with the immunogenetic rules of transplantation applicable to most if not all vertebrates. Testing of progenies derived from interpopulation matings of *Botryllus* should be revealing in this connection.

In *Amaroecium* species, parabiosis of tunic-free zooids of two potentially histoincompatible, larval colonies is reported to produce reciprocal tolerance. Two separate zooids cut into pieces and then grafted result in viable chimeras with organs composed of cells of each genotype as shown by $^{3}$H-thymidine labeling (Scott and Shuh 1963). This mutual tolerance achievable by allogeneic parabiosis of young tunicates may account for the inconsistency of allograft rejection found in colonial species. Neither leukocyte mobilization nor a possible memory component has been reported in the alloimmune responses of colonial tunicates. These information gaps surely invite investigative efforts. From a genetic standpoint, there is a striking paucity of evidence from matings and progeny testing of immunopotentialities among invertebrates generally.

A current summary of immunopotentialities known in invertebrates circa 1980 is given in Table 1. Extensive allogeneic polymorphism of cell-surface macromolecules is characteristic of all animals including protozoans. Immunorecognition of subtle differences among allogeneic markers is the rule among most phylums of multicellular animals. Arthropods and mollusks could represent notable exceptions, though I myself would bet otherwise. The discriminating alloimmune competence found even in sponges and coelenterates becomes less surprising as one realizes that this capacity persists throughout metazoan phylogeny.

## The Hagfish Story

Hagfish and lampreys, the most primitive living vertebrates, probably evolved from the Ostracoderm group of jawless Devonian fishes which are regarded as the first chordates. Although hagfish lack jaws, paired fins, stomach, thymus and bone marrow, their extensive gut is endowed with abundant lymphoid tissue and their blood carries an array of lymphocyes and granulocytes. We have looked repeatedly, but in vain, for a thymus in juvenile and adult Pacific hagfish (Riviere et al. 1975). Nevertheless, hagfish (*Eptatretus stoutii*) invariably reject skin allografts. Slow reactions are typical with median survival times for first-set grafts about 72 days and second-sets only 28 days at 18°–19°C (Hildemann and Thoenes 1969). The observed sequence of lymphocyte/granulocyte infiltration, capillary hemorrhage and pigment cell destruction is typical of reactions toward skin allografts described in

**Table 1.** Immunopotentialities Known in Invertebrates Circa 1980.[a]

| Phylum or subphylum | Immunocytes or defensive cells demonstrable | Allogeneic cell-surface polymorphism evident | Specific allograft rejection[b] | Immunologic memory demonstrable[c] | |
|---|---|---|---|---|---|
| | | | | Short-term | Long-term |
| Protozoans | No | Yes | No | No | No |
| Sponges | Yes | Yes | Yes | Yes | ? |
| Coelenterates | Yes | Yes | Yes | Yes | No |
| Annelids | Yes | Yes | Yes | Yes | ? |
| Arthropods | Yes | Yes | ? | ? | ? |
| Mollusks | Yes | Yes | ? | ? | ? |
| Echinoderms | Yes | Yes | Yes | Yes | ? |
| Tunicates (Protochordates) | Yes | Yes | Yes | ? | ? |

[a]Vertebrate-type immunoglobulin antibodies have *not* been demonstrated in any invertebrate species; inducible circulating "antibodies" found in annelids and arthropods are mainly bactericidins and are not strictly specific.

[b]Xenograft rejection is characteristic of *all* invertebrates, including protozoans, but this probably involves biochemical or enzyme-substrate incompatibilities.

[c]Short-term memory is meant to indicate specifically heightened reactivity for up to 8 weeks after a primary reaction; long-term memory implies heightened allogeneic reactivity persisting for >8 weeks.

higher vertebrates. Survival times of third-party grafts in lieu of second-set grafts on sensitized hagfish ranged from 19 to 85 days. These results within one large population (Point Dume, California) reveal multifarious transplantation antigens with many of frequent occurrence in this species. Progeny analyses have been thwarted because only sterile eggs are obtained in captivity. Lampreys also exhibit moderate histocompatibility barriers as indicated by prolonged allograft rejection times at 20°C.

Pacific hagfish and lampreys can produce specific serum antibodies to diverse xenogeneic antigens (Raison et al. 1978a). Repeated immunization of hagfish with sheep erythrocytes, keyhold limpet hemocyanin or group A streptococcal carbohydrate has yielded IgM-type antibodies in high titer. Sugar inhibition studies indicated that rhamnose was the immunodominant sugar recognized in the streptococcal A carbohydrate by hagfish antibody, whereas N-acetylglucosamine is the major determinant recognized by antibodies from mammalian species. Molecular properties of hagfish immunoglobulins, including carbohydrate content, are similar to those described for lampreys and elasmobranchs. Purified hagfish antibodies have an intact weight of about 160,000 daltons. This low molecular weight form is found mostly in a noncovalently associated polymer of high molecular weight. After sodium dodecyl sulfate gel electrophoresis under reducing conditions, heavy chains of mobility identical to mouse $\mu$ chains and light chains of significantly slower mobility than mouse $\lambda$ chains are obtained (Raison et al. 1978b). This antibody appears to have an unstable tertiary structure because it dissociates at low concentrations of reducing agents. Although both hagfish and lampreys possess heavy chains similar to mammalian μ chains with light chains of higher weight than the mammalian counterpart, the lability of the antibodies of both species suggests a lack of disulfide bonding of the polypeptide chains.

In contrast to an impressive system of cell-mediated immunity, hagfish exhibit a minimal system of humoral antibody production. Poor development of a system of circulating antibodies in cyclostomes is suggested by the following: (a) low levels of immunoglobulin in hagfish and lamprey serum (Marchalonis and Edelman 1968, Raison et al. 1978b); (b) the apparent lack of a thymus gland and of plasma cells (Riviere et al. 1975; Linthicum 1975); (c) the prolonged immunization required to evoke detectable serum antibody to potent antigens even at elevated temperatures (Thoenes and Hildeman 1970; Linthicum and Hildemann 1970); and (d) failure to detect induced serum alloantibodies under any conditions. This last limitation may apply to all primitive fishes below teleosts. In any event, Milton Tam and I tried repeatedly, to no avail, to elicit alloantibodies in both hagfish and sharks. However, sharks do possess a definitive thymus, a discrete spleen and some plasma cells. Elasmobranchs also are excellent producers of antibodies to xenogeneic antigens (Johnston et al. 1971; Clem et al. 1975) and they display discriminating transplantation alloimmunity (Borysenko and Hildemann 1970). Raison et al. (1978b) have proposed that hagfish (cyclostomes) may be unique among vertebrates in lacking a separate humoral antibody system equivalent to the B lymphocyte-plasmacyte system. On this basis, the serum IgM of immunized hagfish could result from late shedding of lymphocyte-bound immunoglobulin rather than active secretion. No evidence for divergence of cyclostome lymphocytes into separate T- and B-cell systems has yet been discerned.

That IgM, the structurally most elaborate of antibody classes, should occur in hagfish at the apparent beginning of immunoglobulin phylogeny remains surprising. The finding of homology regions or domains of about 110 amino acids within the light and heavy Ig chains has led to the supposition that the ancestral immunoglobulin gene coded for such units (Marchalonis 1977). Thus the variable (V) region of the H chain extends 110 to 115 residues from the amino terminus, while the constant (C) domains, each extending some 107 residues, are homologous in sequence to one another as well as to similar domains in the light chain. The IgM-type antibodies of all vertebrates are comprised of some 5 different C domains and 2 V domains. Hence, repeated ancestral gene duplication concomitant with diversification and adaptive selection were required to achieve the first functional IgM. Even this is of course an oversimplification, because IgM requires additional genes for J-chain synthesis and for glycosyl transferases to attach requisite carbohydrate to specific positions on the H- and L-chains. Identification of IgM as the "original antibody" is accordingly doubtful. Functional precursors are therefore being sought among the invertebrates.

Hagfish, as well as certain annelids, arthropods, and higher vertebrates including mammals, give bactericidin responses to diverse Gram-negative bacteria. This nonimmunoglobulin reactivity is detectable as early as 2 days after injection and yields short-lived memory, but its specificity is rather broad (Acton et al. 1969). Such primeval, humoral immunoresponsiveness evidently evolved in invertebrates and persisted despite subsequent evolution of more discriminating immunoglobulins. The genetic control of bactericidin responses has yet to be analyzed in any species. The serum complement system characteristic of higher vertebrates is not required for bactericidin activity. Primitive fishes and invertebrates may not even possess a complement system.

## Higher Vertebrates: From Fishes to Mammals

Depending on the species and class of vertebrates, IgM antibodies may occur as dimers (rays), tetramers (bony fish), pentamers (sharks and mammals), and hexamers (anuran amphibians). The adaptive value of such variation in polymerization is unknown. Bony fishes regularly give excellent IgM-type antibody responses to cellular, viral and protein antigens (Clem and McLean 1975; Litman and Kehoe 1978). Like cyclostomes and elasmobranchs, many teleosts produce only high- and low-molecular weight IgM, but others, exemplified by lungfishes of both African and Australian species and the giant grouper, produce a second major class of Ig designated IgN (N for new) because of its distinctive heavy chain structure. Urodele amphibians, similar to most fishes, produce only IgM-type antibodies, whereas anurans can synthesize both IgM and IgG-like antibodies. Reptiles possess three distinct classes of immunoglobulins: a high-molecular weight IgM form (17S-19S); an IgG or IgY (7.5S) analogous to that found in birds; and a small 5-6S class designated IgN because of its similarity to lungfish IgN. In addition, a cell-bound IgD has recently been reported in turtles. The existence of five major classes of immunoglobulins in birds, though not all apparently in a single species, is evident (Table 2). IgE may have evolved only in higher mammals as a distinctive sixth molecular class helpful in resistance to animal parasites.

**Table 2.** Progressive Evolution of Immunoglobulin Antibody Complexity Among Classes of Vertebrates.

| | Types of immunoglobulin antibodies[a] | | | | | |
|---|---|---|---|---|---|---|
| **Class or group** | **IgM** | **IgN** | **IgG/IgY** | **IgA** | **IgD** | **IgE** |
| Hagfish and lampreys | + | 0 | 0 | 0 | 0 | 0 |
| Sharks and rays | + | 0 | 0 | 0 | 0 | 0 |
| Bony fishes | + | 0/+ | 0 | 0 | 0 | 0 |
| Amphibians | + | 0 | 0/+ | 0 | ? | 0 |
| Reptiles | + | + | + | 0 | +? | 0 |
| Birds | + | + | + | + | + | 0? |
| Mammals | + | + | + | + | + | + |

[a] + indicates presence of Ig class, while 0 indicates its absence; 0/+ indicates some species within this vertebrate class produce the corresponding type of antibodies while other species do not.

Immunophylogenetic progression among vertebrates is revealed by increasing diversification of immunocytes and of immunoglobulin classes/subclasses. The stepwise appearance of specialized tissues as the thymus (elasmobranchs), bone marrow (bony fishes), and lymph nodes (anuran amphibians) indicates a parallel increase in cytoarchitectural complexity (Table 3). However, the first appearance of three or more molecular classes of immunoglobulins in reptiles and birds has no obvious correlates at the level of immunocyte differentiation. Very little is known about the multipartite integration of macrophage, T- and B-cell functions in non-mammalian vertebrates. All vertebrates possess cell-mediated immunity with memory and are capable of IgM antibody production. Moreover, all vertebrates possess gut-associated lymphoid tissue plus blood lymphocytes, granulocytes, and macrophages. Beyond these common denominator traits, all else may be regarded as adaptive specialization.

The phylogeny of immunity, including the major immunogene complex (*MIC*), has been reviewed from several perspectives (Hildemann 1972; Borysenko 1976; Cohen 1980). An evolutionary transition or progression in both transplantation immunity and serum antibody production is first evident in the bony fishes. Quantitative studies of transplantation reactions in diverse genera of advanced bony fishes have invariably revealed strong alloimmune reactions among genetically disparate individuals (Leeloy and Hildemann 1977). In the context of transplantation immunity, the transition from weak or slow to strong or rapid responsiveness recurs within each of the classes of bony fishes, amphibians, and reptiles. Thus, frogs exhibit acute allograft rejection, strong mixed lymphocyte culture reactions and lethal graft-vs-host reactions (GVHR), whereas salamanders, lower on the amphibian branch of the phylogenetic tree, are weak reactors in all of these categories (Cohen 1980). If the *MIC* were defined solely in terms of these histocompatibility criteria then the *MIC* is evident only in advanced bony fishes, anuran amphibians, birds, and mammals. However, the *MIC*, at least at the mammalian level, now appears to represent a spectrum of closely-linked genes broadly involved in immunorecognition and immunoregulation. In the best studied species of mice and people, three or four distinctive classes of genes have been identified with the *MIC:* (1) *H* genes coding for membrane-bound glycoproteins involved in allogeneic immunorecognition, (2) *Ia* genes coding for membrane-bound glycoproteins involved in activation of T-lymphocytes, (3) *Ir* genes involved in macrophage or helper T-cell regulation of antibody responses to diverse antigens, and (4) complement genes governing synthesis of certain serum complement components. *MIC* products apparently promote cooperative interactions between macrophages and lymphocytes, between subsets of T-cells, between T-cells and B-cells, and between killer cells and their specific targets.

My own immunogenetics group at UCLA has recently focused on the actions of *I*-region genes within the *MIC*. A decisive effect of the interallelic combination of *H-2 IC* region-induced GVHR was found with *H-2* congenic and recombinant C57BL/10 mouse strains (Clark and Hildemann 1977a,b). $IC^{d}$ recipients showed GVH responses running the gamut from none to moderate to strong, depending on

**Table 3.** Increasing Cytoarchitectural Complexity of the Immune System from Primitive Fishes to Mammals.[a]

| Class or group | Thymus | Bone marrow | Lymph glands or nodes | Blood granulocytes and lymphocytes | Reactions to primary tissue allografts (cell-mediated immunity[b]) | |
|---|---|---|---|---|---|---|
| | | | | | Moderate | Strong |
| Hagfish and lampreys | 0? | 0 | 0 | + | + | 0 |
| Sharks and rays | + | 0 | 0 | + | + | 0 |
| Bony fishes | + | + | 0 | + | + | + |
| Amphibians | + | + | + | + | + | + |
| Reptiles | + | + | + | + | + | 0 |
| Birds | + | + | + | + | + | + |
| Mammals | + | + | + | + | + | + |

[a] + indicates presence of corresponding types of cells or reactivity.

[b] Moderate histocompatiblity barriers are found in animals representing all vertebrate classes, but strong barriers are the rule in advanced bony fishes, anuran amphibians, and most (?) birds and mammals.

the donor *IC* allele of the inoculated (i.e., responding) lymph node cells. The severity of the allogeneic reactions induced also varied as a function of the *IC* alleles in other strain combinations. Disparities at the *I-B* or *I-J* regions did not evoke detectable GVHR. Similar differences in immune responsiveness have been repeatedly found for other individual regions within the *H-2* complex. Although *H-2K* and *H-2IA* region donor-recipient differences usually cause acute allograft reactions, other *H-2* region (*H-2D, IB, IC,* and *S*) differences yield alloincompatibilities ranging from weak to strong depending on the allelic combination. Evidently the uniqueness of the *MIC* resides in its multigenic totality, rather than in properties peculiar to individual loci. Both gene dosage and gene product interactions can be decisive.

*Ir* genes linked to the mouse *MIC* control the immune response to a variety of haptens and macromolecular antigens. We have recently characterized the *I*-region genes that regulate specific immune responses of mice to the hapten 2,4,6-trinitrophenyl conjugated to autogenous mouse serum albumin (TNP-MSA) (Urba and Hildemann 1979; Wicker et al. 1980, 1981). Among C57BL/10 congenic lines, $H\text{-}2^b$ and $H\text{-}2^d$ strains are high responders, whereas $H\text{-}2^a$, $H\text{-}2^k$ and $H\text{-}2^{y2}$ strains produce low levels of IgG antibodies in tests for indirect TNP-specific plaque forming cells (PFC) and serum antigen-binding capacity. High responsiveness controlled by $H\text{-}2^d$ is inherited dominantly, but high responsiveness controlled by $H\text{-}2^b$ is inherited recessively. The high responsiveness controlled by $H\text{-}2^b$ is only partially recessive on C3H and A strain backgrounds. Thus $H\text{-}2^b/H\text{-}2^a$ F1 mice yield 20–40% of the PFC produced by $H\text{-}2^b$ homozygotes. However, high responsiveness associated with the $H\text{-}2^d$ haplotype remains dominant on the C3H background. Although graded regulation of responsiveness to TNP-MSA is attributable to both *H-2* and non-*H-2* genes, a hierarchy of haplotypes in order of decreasing immune responsiveness is evident as follows: $H\text{-}2^d > H\text{-}2^b > H\text{-}2^k$, $H\text{-}2^a$ or $H\text{-}2^{y2}$.

The high immune responses of both $H\text{-}2^d$ and $H\text{-}2^b$ mice have now been mapped to the *I-A* (K) region of the major immunogene complex (Wicker et al. 1981). No modifying effects were observed from *MIC* genes to the right of *I-A* in either responder haplotype. Whether high responsiveness controlled by $H\text{-}2^b$ or $I\text{-}A^b$ is inherited with complete or partial recessivity depends on strain background, sex of the responder, and route of immunization. Early events in TNP-MSA responsiveness were also examined using an antigen-specific, T-cell dependent proliferation assay *in vitro* with lymph node cells obtained from primed high or low responder animals. Genetic mapping and mode of inheritance in this assay corresponded with the findings in the PFC assay measuring later IgG antibody production. Both early and late responses therefore appear to be under the same *Ir* gene control. Both intralocus gene dosage effects and *Ir* gene product interaction may account for low responsiveness in certain *H-2* heterozygotes. Interaction between antigen-presenting cells and T-cells may be the critical, early step in the immune response controlled by our *I-A*(*Ir-6*) locus. Much work of course remains to be done on the effects of individual immunogenes of the major complex on immunorecognition and immunoregulation. We should also like to know when and how the *MIC* evolved from invertebrates or primitive vertebrates.

ACKNOWLEDGMENTS
Much of the recent research cited in this overview has involved active collaboration among numerous co-workers, including postdoctoral fellows and Ph.D. students as follows: Charles Bigger, Edward Clark, Ian Johnston, Paul Jokiel, Scott Linthicum, Robert Raison, Walter Urba, and Linda Wicker. It is a pleasure to acknowledge their salutary contributions and critical judgment. This work was supported by National Institutes of Health Grants CA 23025 and AI 15705.

# References

Acton, R.T., Weinheimer, P.F., Hildemann, W.H., and Evans, E.E. 1969. Induced bactericidal response in hagfish. J. Bacteriology 2:626–628.

Bierne, J. 1980. Viable animals obtained by grafting pieces from several nemertean adults. Transplantation 29:74–75.

Billingham, R.E., Brent, L., and Medawar, P.B. 1956. Quantitative studies on tissue transplantation immunity. III. Actively acquired tolerance. Philos. Trans. Roy. Soc. London (Ser. B.) 239:357–414.

Bigger, C.H. and Hildemann, W.H. 1980. Cellular defense systems of the coelenterata. In Ontogeny and Phylogeny of the Reticuloendothelial System. M. Sigel and N. Cohen, eds. New York: Plenum Press, in press.

Borysenko, M. 1976. Phylogeny of immunity. Immunogenetics 3:305–326.

Borysenko, M. and Hildemann, W.H. 1970. Reactions to skin allografts in the horn shark, *Heterodontis francisci*. Transplantation 6:545–551.

Clark, E.A. and Hildemann, W.H. 1977a. Genetics of graft-versus-host reactions. I. Production of splenomegaly and mortality in mice disparate at *H-2I* subregions. Immunogenetics 4:281–293.

Clark, E.A. and Hildemann, W.H. 1977b. Genetics of graft-versus-host reactions. II. Interallelic effects and regulation of GVHR by antirecipient alloantibodies. Immunogenetics 5:309–324.

Clem, L.W. and McLean, W.E., 1975. Phylogeny of immunoglobulin structure and function. VII. Monomeric and tetrameric immunoglobulins of the margate: A marine teleost fish. Immunology 29:791–799.

Clem, L.W., McLean, W.E., and Shankey, V. 1975. In Immunologic Phylogeny. W.H. Hildemann and A.A. Benedict, eds. New York: Plenum Press.

Coffaro, K.A. and Hindgardner, R.T. 1977 Immune response in the sea urchin, *Lytechinus pictus*. Science 197:1389–1390.

Cohen, N. 1980. Salamanders and the evolution of the major histocompatibility complex. In Contemporary Topics in Immunobiology. Vol. 9. J.J. Marchalonis and N. Cohen, eds. New York: Plenum Press.

Cooper, E.L. 1970. Transplantation immunity in helminths and annelids. Transplantation Proc. 2:216–221.

Cooper, E.L. 1976. Comparative Immunology. Englewood Cliffs, New Jersey: Prentice-Hall, Inc., chap. 11, pp. 197–202.

Cushing, J.E. 1942. An effect of temperature upon antibody production in fish. J. Immunol. 45:123–126.

Dales, R.P. 1978. Second-set graft rejections do they occur in invertebrates? In Cell-Cell Recognition. A.S.G. Curtis, ed. London: Cambridge University Press.

Evans, C.W. and Curtis, A.S.G. 1980. Graft rejection and cytotoxicity in marine sponges. In Phylogeny of Immunological Memory. M.J. Manning, ed. New York: Elsevier North Holland, pp. 15–26.

Freeman, G. 1970. Transplantation specificity in echinoderms and lower chordates. Transplant. Proc. 2:236–239.

Goodrich, H.B. and Nichols, R. 1933. Scale transplantation in the goldfish, *Carrasius auratus*. Biol. Bull. 56:253–265.

Heslop-Harrison, J. 1978. Cellular Recognition Systems in Plants. Baltimore: University Park Press. p. 60.

Hildemann, W.H. 1956. Goldfish erythrocyte antigens and serology. Science 124:315–316.

Hildemann, W.H. 1957. Scale homotransplantation in goldfish (*Carrasius auratus*). Ann. N.Y. Acad. Sci. 64:775–790.

Hildemann, W.H. 1958. Tissue transplantation immunity in goldfish. Immunology 1:46–53.

Hildemann, W.H. 1972. Phylogeny of transplantation reactivity. In Transplantation Antigens, Markers of Biological Individuality. B.D. Kahan and R.A. Reisfeld, eds. New York: Academic Press.

Hildemann, W.H., Bigger, C.H., Johnston, I.S., and Jokiel, P.L. 1980. Characteristics of transplantation immunity in the sponge *Callyspongia diffusa*. Transplantation 30:362–367.

Hildemann, W.H. and Dix, T.G. 1972. Transplantation reactions of tropical Australian echinoderms. Transplantation 2:624–633.

Hildemann, W.H. and Haas, R. 1959. Homotransplantation immunity and tolerance in the bullfrog. J. Immunol. 83:478–485.

Hildemann, W.H. and Haas, R. 1960. Comparative studies of homotransplantation in fishes. J. Cell. and Comp. Physiol. 55:227–234.

Hildemann, W.H., Johnston, I.S., and Jokiel, P.L. 1979. Immunocompetence in the lowest metazoan phylum: Transplantation immunity in sponges. Science 204:420–422.

Hildemann, W.H., Jokiel, P.L., Bigger, C.H., and Johnston, I.S. 1980. Allogeneic polymorphism and alloimmune memory in the coral, *Montipora verrucosa*. Transplantation 30:297–301.

Hildemann, W.H. and Keighley, G. 1955. Techniques for studies of hemoglobin synthesis in daphnia. Amer. Naturalist 846:169–174.

Hildemann, W.H. and Owen, R.D. 1956. Histocompatibility genetics of scale transplantation. Transplant. Bull. 4:132–134.

Hildemann, W.H., Raison, R.L., Cheung, G. et al. 1977. Immunological specificity and memory in a scleractinian coral. Nature 270:219–223.

Hildemann, W.H. and Thoenes, G.H. 1969. Immunological responses of Pacific hagfish. I. Skin transplantation immunity. Transplantation 6:506–521.

Ivker, F.B. 1972. A hierarchy of histoincompatibility in *Hydractinia echinata*. Biol. Bull. 143:162–174.

Johnston, W.H., Jr., Acton, R.T., Weinheimer, P.F. et al. 1971. Isolation and physicochemical characterization of the IgM-like immunoglobulin from the stingray *Dasyatis americana J. Immunol. 107:782–793*.

Karp, R.D. and Hildemann, W.H. 1976. Specific allograft reactivity in the sea star *Dermasterias imbricata*. Transplantation 22:434–439.

Leeloy, H.K. and Hildemann, W.H. 1977. Tissue transplantation immunity in Hawaiian mullet (*Mugil cephalus*). Transplantation 23:109–111.

Linthicum, D.S. 1975. Ultrastructure of hagfish blood leukocytes. In Immunologic Phylogeny. W.H. Hildemann and A.A. Benedict, eds. New York: Plenum Press.

Linthicum, D.S. and Hildemann, W.H. 1970. Immunologic responses of Pacific hagfish. III. Serum antibodies to cellular antigens. J. Immunol. 4:912–918.

Linthicum, D.S., Marks, D.H., Stein, E.A., and Cooper, E.L. 1977. Graft destruction in earthworms: An electron microscopic study. Europ. J. Immunol. 7:871–876.

Litman, G.W. and Kehoe, J.M. 1978. The phylogenic origins of immunoglobulin structure. In Comprehensive Immunology. 5. Immunoglobulins. G.W. Litman and R.A. Good, eds. New York: Plenum Press.

Marchalonis, J.J. 1977. Immunity in Evolution. London: Edward Arnold, Ltd., pp. 316.

Marchalonis, J.J. and Edelman, G.M. 1968. Phylogenetic origins of antibody structure. III. Antibodies in the primary immune response of the sea lamprey, *Petromyzon marinus*. J. Exp. Med. 127:891–914.

Medawar, P.B. 1957. The Uniqueness of the Individual. London: Methuen & Co., pp. 191.

Metchnikoff, E. 1893. Comparative Pathology of Inflammation. New York: Dover Publ. Inc. (Republished in 1968), pp. 224.

Owen, R.D. 1945. Immunogenetic consequences of vascular anastomoses between bovine twins. Science 102:400–402.

Preer, J.R. 1968. Genetics of Protozoa. In Research in Protozoology, Vol. 3. T.T. Chen, ed. New York: Pergamon Press.

Raison, R.L., Hull, C.J., and Hildemann, W.H. 1978a. Production and specificity of antibodies to streptococci in the Pacific hagfish, *Eptatretus stoutii*. Develop. and Compar. Immunol. 2:253–262.

Raison, R.L., Hull, C.J., and Hildemann, W.H. 1978b. Characterization of immunoglobulin from the Pacific hagfish, a primitive vertebrate. Proc. Natl. Acad. Sci. 11:5679–5682.

Reddy, A.L., Bryan, B., and Hildemann, W.H. 1975. Integumentary allograft versus autograft reactions in *Ciona intestinalis:* A protochordate species of solitary tunicate. Immunogenetics 1:584–590.

Riviere, H.B., Cooper, E.L., Reddy, A.L., and Hildemann, W.H. 1975. In search of the hagfish thymus. Amer. Zool. 15:39–49.

Scott, F.M. and Schuh, J.E. 1963. Intraspecific reaggregation in *Amaroecium constellatum* labeled with tritiated thymidine. Acta Emb. Morph. Exp. 6:39–54.

Snell, G.D. 1948. Methods for the study of histocompatibility genes. J. Genet. 49:87–108.

Spiegel, M. 1955. The reaggregation of dissociated sponge cells. Ann. N.Y. Acad. Sci. 60:1056–1078.

Tanaka, K. 1975. Allogenic distinction in *Botryllus primigenus* and in other colonial ascidians. In Immunologic Phylogeny. W.H. Hildemann and A.A. Benedict, eds. New York: Plenum Press.

Tanaka, S. and Sakai, A. 1979. Minimum length of time required for alloantigen recognition. Transplantation 27:260–264.

Theodor, J.L. 1976. Histoincompatibility in a natural population of gorgonians. Zool. J. Linnean Soc. 58:173–178.

Thoenes, G.H. and Hildemann, W.H. 1970. Immunological responses to Pacific hagfish II. Serum antibody production to soluble antigen. In Developmental Aspects of Antibody Formation and Structure. J. Sterzl and I. Riha, eds. Prague: Academia Pub. House of Czechoslovakia.

Urba, W.J. and Hildemann, W.H. 1979. Functional analysis of *H-2* linked genetic control of immune responsiveness to TNP-MSA. J. Immunol. 123:209–215.

Van de Vyver, G. 1980. Second-set grafts in fresh-water sponges. In Phylogeny of Immunologic Memory. M.J. Manning, ed. New York: Elsevier-North Holland, pp. 27–34.

Vogel, H.H., Jr. 1940. Transplantation of autogenous and homologenous skin in adult *Rana pipiens*. J. Exptl. Zool. 85:437–474.

Wicker, L.S. and Hildemann, W.H. 1980a. Two distinct high responder phenotypes are both controlled by *H-2* genes mapping in *K* or *I-A*. Immunogenetics, in press.

Wicker, L.S., Urba, W.J., and Hildemann, W.H. 1980b. Hierarchy of *H-2* haplotypes governs inheritance of immune responsiveness to TNP-MSA. Immunogenetics 10:235–246.

Hildemann, ed. Frontiers in Immunogenetics

# Current Status of the Rat Major Histocompatibility Complex

Elizabeth P. Blankenhorn

*Department of Pathology, School of Medicine, University of Pennsylvania, Philadelphia, Pennsylvania*

The rat major histocompatibility or immunogene complex *(MHC)* has been the subject of several recent and good reviews (Günther and Štark 1977; Gasser 1977), so I will confine this discussion of the serology and genetics of this region to information collected from a number of laboratories since 1977. I will start with a brief introduction for this audience on a little rat history.

In the beginning, immunologists were looking at the rat red blood cell for hemagglutinins and hemolytic antigen-antibody reactions. Early studies on rat blood groups was summarized by Ray Owen (1962) in a paper describing his own contributions to the field. Owen was interested in the development of rat immunogenetic markers for studies of parabiotic exchange in this species, and began his studies in 1946. Two antigens were defined in these experiments, called C and D, detected by the use of rabbit heteroantiserum. Also included in this work was the retesting of *AgA*, first described by Burhoe (1947). Ray also characterized antigens E and F on rat red cells, although the reagents used to detect these hemagglutinins were weak, and the genetic markers that they revealed have essentially been lost to rat immunogenetics. It was in this context that Aptekman and Bogden discovered an antigen on rat tumor cells in 1955 (Aptekman and Bogden 1955), and also on rat red blood cells (Bogden and Aptekman 1960). They designated this antigen R-1, but it was later known as *AgB*. In 1962 other rat strains were being tested for *AgB* (Palm 1962), and the segregation analysis indicated that a single gene (Bogden and Aptekman 1962) with a series of different alleles was responsible for the trait. In 1966 the earliest work was done to establish that *AgB* was the dominant antigen responsible for the local graft-versus-host reaction (Elkins and Palm 1966) and therefore was the prime candidate for the "major" histocompatibility antigen of the 14 or so proposed to distinguish one rat strain from another (Billingham et al.

1962). This distinction for *AgB* in the rat paralleled that for *H-2* as the immunodominant cell surface antigen in the mouse, and similarities between the two antigens have been recognized ever since. Like *H-2*, the rat AgB antigens are serologically complex (Günther and Štark 1977). Furthermore, following the demonstration of immune response genes *(IR)* linked to *H-2* in the mouse, *IR* genes were discovered in rats, likewise linked to *AgB* (reviewed in Gasser 1977). Much work has gone into the development of congenic and recombinant inbred strains of mice, and the number of informative genetic crossovers within the *H-2* complex that have become available is much greater than the number of similar crossovers in the rat *AgB* region. It is for this reason that alternative approaches have been undertaken for the study of rat *MHC* antigens. With this basic introduction, then, I would like to discuss some of these new methods and the reapplication of some old ones, the results obtained, and the implications they have provided about the nature of the rat *MHC*. We must now switch, however, to the correct terminology for the rest of the discussion. The old name *AgB* of Palm and her co-workers in Philadelphia, and the alternate name *H-1*, used for at least ten years by Štark and Günther and others, have both made way for the new designation, *RT-1*. The classical transplantation antigens found on red blood cells, lymphocytes, and skin, are called *RT-1A* antigens, and the antigens associated with the mixed lymphocyte reactivity and the immune response genes (*Ia* antigens) are known as *RT-1B* antigens.

One approach has been the deliberate identification and maintenance of rats bearing chromosomal recombinations between the *RT-1A* and *RT-1B* genes. This effort has been made by several laboratories (Butcher and Howard 1977; Štark et al. 1977) and a list of eight of the nine available recombinants has recently been published (Howard 1979). It has been recognized for some time that there are laboratory rats that are "natural" recombinants, including the MNR, MR, BDVII, B3, and KGH strains among others. Furthermore, many wild rats tested (Shonnard et al. 1976; Cramer et al. 1978a) have chromosomes with combinations of *RT-1* genes not normally found in inbred rats. A number of interesting observations have been made on wild rat populations. For example, the wild rats demonstrate quite clearly that the degree of polymorphism of *MHC* alleles is very different between rats and mice. Of all the rats isolated from the wild (more than 200 as of this writing), even those from very different geographic locations, most were found to have *RT-1A* and *RT-1B* antigens that were similar or identical to those of the eight common inbred strains (Cramer et al. 1978a). This result has been confirmed in Germany by Günther as well (Günther 1979). This is in sharp contrast to the results of Jan Klein and others (Klein 1975), in whose study wild mice were demonstrated to have very highly polymorphic *H-2K* and *H-2D* antigens. The experiments with rats therefore reveal that extensive polymorphism is a feature that is often, but not always or necessarily, found in the *MHC* of mammals. Furthermore, the University of Pittsburgh group demonstrated that the immune responsiveness of the wild rats and their progeny to a synthetic polypeptide antigen was closely linked to but separable from the MLR determinant (Cramer et al. 1978b). Recent studies from these investigators have shown that the MLR determinants are also distinct from certain *Ia* antigens in inbred strains (Cramer et al. 1978b). In similar work with this group of wild animals, it was found that very strong linkage disequilibrium existed between certain alleles at the *RT-1A* and *RT-1B* loci. Interestingly, the combinations selected for were different from the combinations of *RT-1A* and *RT-1B* alleles that are found in common inbred strains of rats. Tests of other markers in the wild rat group showed that the rats were not extensively inbred, and an estimate of the disequilibrium that would be produced only by close linkage of the two *RT-1* loci is one-third of that observed. These authors suggest that the disequilibria are due to selective pressure (Wagener et al. 1979). In summary, studies on the *RT-1* antigens and *RT-1*-linked immune responsiveness of wild rats have demonstrated at least two *RT-1B* products, a restricted polymorphism of both *RT-1A* and *RT-1B* alleles, and the possibility of strong selective pressures favoring the expression of certain combinations of *MHC* gene products. Work to discover other wild and inbred recombinant chromosomes proceeds in several laboratories at present.

The second part of this chapter is devoted to a subject on which my own research has touched, and that is the characterization of rat *MHC* antigens by immunochemical methods. I started my work on this topic while I was a graduate student with Ray Owen, and received considerable support in my efforts from Lee Hood. I have indicated in the preceding section that the rat *MHC*, as studied by serological and functional assays, has for some time been divided into at least two segments—one containing the gene(s) for *RT-1A* products, and one containing the genes for one and probably two *RT-1B* products. Concurrently with these studies, we and several other investigators (Blankenhorn et al. 1978; Cecka et al. 1980; Shinohara et al. 1977; McMaster and Williams 1979) have compiled results about the chemical nature of *RT-1A* and *RT-1B* molecules (for a recent review, see Howard 1978). Very briefly, because this work was discussed thoroughly at my thesis seminar at Caltech nearly two years ago, our analysis was performed as follows. Radiolabeled *RT-1A* molecules were prepared from lymphocytes by immunoprecipitation and separation on SDS-polyacrylamide gels. When these preparations were submitted to N-terminal sequencing analysis, we found two molecules, distinguished only by one substitution of isoleucine for leucine at amino acid position five (Blankenhorn et al. 1978). These molecules closely resembled similarly prepared *MHC* antigens from mouse, human, and guinea pig. Three of the four rat *RT-1A* antigens revealed two sequences each, also distinguished by isoleucine and leucine substitutions. Each of the four sequences is unique.

Results from Götze and Sporer (Götze 1978; Sporer et al. 1978) confirmed our own and showed that DA (and other) rats have two separable *RT-1A* antigens detectable serologically using rat alloantisera to private and public determinants. These authors also provided evidence for two different *RT-1B (Ia)* antigens in three rat strains. This was not unexpected: Early work by David Sachs and his colleagues (Shinohara et al. 1977) had suggested that two *I*-region genes would be present in rats, and more recent studies on the wild rats had indicated the same conclusions. In fact, in 1975, Eberhard Günther demonstrated complementation between inbred rats in the immune response to HGAL, which indicated that 2 *IR* genes were present (Günther and Rüde 1975). At Caltech, we decided to isolate the rat *Ia* antigens by employing a panel of cross-reactive mouse anti-*Ia* alloantisera (Cecka et al. 1980; Blankenhorn et al. 1980). We submitted the resulting molecules to microsequencing and to analysis by two-dimensional gel electrophoresis. Our results demonstrated unequivocally that two classes of *RT-1B* antigens exist in the rat: the *Ia* antigens cross-reactive with the mouse *I-E* antigens, and those cross-reactive with the mouse *I-A* antigens. Thus, in inbred strains where no clear genetic recombinants existed at the time to separate these two regions, we were able to define and distinguish the two gene products. Our study included an analysis of the molecules by peptide mapping, a sensitive technique that demonstrated the close relatedness of each rat *Ia* polypeptide to its mouse *Ia* homologue. This demonstration of two rat *Ia* antigens was also confirmed by analysis of mouse antirat *Ia* monoclonal antibodies (McMaster and Williams 1979). I will return to the general topic of monoclonal antibodies in the last part of this discussion.

In summary, we now have a better, but still incomplete, picture of the rat *MHC* genes. It is not known to which *RT-1B* class of antigens the MLR or separable immune response genes belong, but information on that question should be forthcoming. I will mention briefly that a third *MHC*-linked, *RT-1C* region has been studied by several investigators. *RT-1C* was originally identified as causing a histocompatibility effect (Kohoutová et al. 1978; Stock and Günther 1979) and is presumed to be situated nearer *RT-1B* than *RT-1A*. This region also encodes an antigen or series of antigens that are recognized by cytotoxic T-cells (Marshak et al. 1977; Sieck et al. 1979). The mutual identity of the *RT-1C* antigens defined by three different groups has not been established, and I will report primarily on the "CT" antigen studies that are being done in our department at the University of Pennsylvania Medical School. For example, it has been found (Marshak et al. 1977) that immunization of Lewis rats with lymphocytes from the $RT\text{-}1^{1}$-compatible Fischer strain results in the generation of cytotoxic T-cells to Fischer target lymphocytes which also kill cells from three $RT\text{-}1^{1}$ rats and cross-react on target cells from five other *RT-1* haplotypes, including DA. The killing response to CT determinants is not always *MHC* restricted, although CT antigens themselves are *MHC*-linked. Experiments done with PVG.1R targets show that the CT genes are found to the "right" of the *RT.1B* region. To date, no antibodies to CT have been detected in tests of appropriate sera, although deliberate immunizations by others (Stock and Günther 1979) between rats essentially congeneic for *RT-1C* have resulted in cytotoxic antibodies to antigens that may be identical to CT. Like CT, these *RT-1C* antigens are represented on rat T and B-lymphocytes, and are distinct from *RT-1A* and *B*. Recent work in our department has shown that immunization of DA rats with cells from the $RT\text{-}1^{a}$ congenic strain, L.AVN, results in the detection of another CT antigen. Cytotoxic lymphocytes from DA anti-L.AVN donors are able to kill certain mouse lymphocyte targets, and the gene(s) controlling the mouse target antigen is linked to *H-2* (T. Sieck, personal communication). Experiments defining these mouse and rat CT antigens are in progress. A representation of the current genetic map of *RT-1* is given in Figure 1.

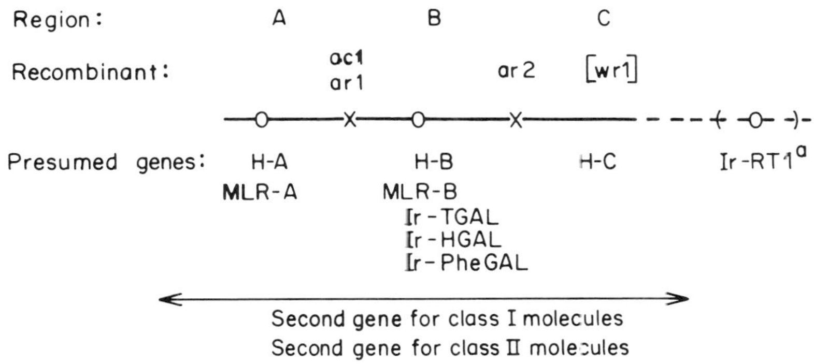


**Figure 1.** The rat major histocompatibility gene complex (adapted directly from Günther and Štark 1979). Regions A, B, and C control the expression of genes for *RT-1A, RT-1B,* and *RT-1C,* respectively. *H-A, H-B,* and *H-C* designate reported histocompatibility effects which map to each region, and MLR-A and MLR-B represent minor and major mixed lymphocyte responses, respectively. The immune response *(IR)* genes to several synthetic polypeptide antigens are located in the *RT-1B* region. *Ir-RT-1*$^a$ is an immune response gene to the *RT-1a*$^a$ antigen, thought to be linked to the rat *MHC*. Positions of recombination are given for the ac1, ar1, ar2, and wr1 recombinants.

The third part of this overview on recent developments in rat *MHC* immunogenetics will be devoted to a discussion of monoclonal antibody reagents to the *RT-1* gene products. For several reasons, described in detail by McKearn and his colleagues (McKearn et al. 1979) and by Howard and his (Howard et al. 1978), homogeneous antibody reagents prepared to specific rat *MHC* antigens provide a very powerful probe for investigation of both the biological and chemical aspects of the major histocompatibility complex. The rat is an especially interesting species for study in this regard—while the *MHC* of rats is not as well defined as *H-2* in mice, strong homologies are found between *RT-1* and *HL-A* or *H-2* at both the molecular (Blankenhorn et al. 1978; Cecka et al. 1980) and the functional levels. The *RT-1* complex is important in a number of immunological phenomena. For example, alloantisera to graft donor *RT-1* antigens are remarkable in their ability to affect the immune response of the recipient animal, resulting in both humoral and cellular suppression. The use of monoclonal antibodies (mcAbs) can elucidate which specific target antigens are involved in such suppression. Furthermore, mcAbs to rat *MHC* antigens are comparatively easy to make. Typically, between 10% and 50% of the tissue culture wells assayed after a given hybridization are positive for antibody to *RT-1*, whereas one recent report on anti-*H-2* mcAbs cites an antibody production efficiency of less than 1% (Ozato et al. 1980). Monoclonal reagents from McKearn's laboratory (and similarly from Howard's) have been employed in several different studies.

The functional analysis of allograft suppression has been repeated with monoclonal reagents (McKearn et al. 1979). In one experiment, several mcAbs were tested for their enhancement of survival of (Lewis × BN)$F_1$ renal allografts into

Lewis rat hosts. Some, but not all, of the monoclonal Lewis anti-BN (anti $RT\text{-}1A^{n}$) antibodies were able to induce a state of specific graft enhancement as profound and as long-lasting as treatment with an appropriate alloantiserum. This type of experiment demonstrates that Abs directed to transplantation antigens, as well as antibodies in *Ia* alloantiserum (Davies and Alkins 1974; Soulillou et al. 1976), are able to suppress completely the immune response to foreign allografts. The ability of hybridoma supernatants to depress rat *in vitro* immune responses has been reported as well (McKearn et al. 1979).

A second area in which the role of monoclonal antibodies has been useful is in their cross-reactivity with *MHC* antigens of other species (Smilek et al. 1980). Like some of the mouse alloantisera we used for our rat *Ia* antigen isolations (see above), the mcAbs can show a paradoxical ability to detect antigens that are polymorphic in the homologous (rat) species, but are monomorphic in other species. For example, the Lewis anti-BN mcAb D4.37 detects $RT\text{-}1^{n,a,u}$ and $RT\text{-}1^{b}$ but not $RT\text{-}1^{l}$ or $RT\text{-}1^{c}$. This same antibody, in the presence of complement, kills all human, mouse, and rabbit targets tested. This conservation of determinants between two species has provided discussion in the past (Bodmer 1973; Sachs et al. 1977; Blankenhorn et al. 1980) and will no doubt continue to do so when the results from monoclonal antibody analysis are collected. These studies do prove, however, that the cross-reactions that occur are not explicable merely by presuming that different antibodies within an alloantiserum are responsible for the cross-reacting activity. Perhaps more striking is the result that in some cases the affinities of these mcAbs for rat or human targets appear to be identical. Given that mcAbs to man and mouse may be difficult to prepare, strongly cross-reactive rat antirat mcAbs, especially when they do detect polymorphic determinants (Smilek et al. 1980), may be very useful for the elucidation of the *MHC* antigen structure of these other species.

The number and expression of rat *RT-1* antigens and antigenic determinants are also being studied with mcAbs. Certain mcAbs detect gene dosage effects with great sensitivity (Howard et al. 1978) and these reagents also distinguish differences in the homozygous expression of, for example, $RT\text{-}1A^{a}$, on red blood cells from rats with different genetic backgrounds. This provides a useful tool for examining genetic control of expression of *RT-1A* antigens and, in fact, one such gene may be linked to *RT-1* itself. In other cases, mcAbs have been seen to discriminate between the levels of expression of *RT-1A* on lymphocytes and on erythrocytes (Smilek, in preparation). The binding of certain mcAbs to cross-reacting lymphocytes is much stronger than the binding of the same antibody to red blood cells of the same cross-reacting strain. The influence of "background" genes on the red blood cell expression of cross-reacting *RT-1A* antigens is under investigation.

The several groups of immunologists studying mcAbs are all interested in discovering the number of antigens and antigenic sites that make up the total MHC product. Although earlier work, reported above, including my own, has indicated that there are at least two *RT-1A* molecules, we have never really seen any trace of the second molecule in more conventional serological assays. In wild rat populations, where, as I have mentioned, "rearrangements" of the *RT-1* complex are

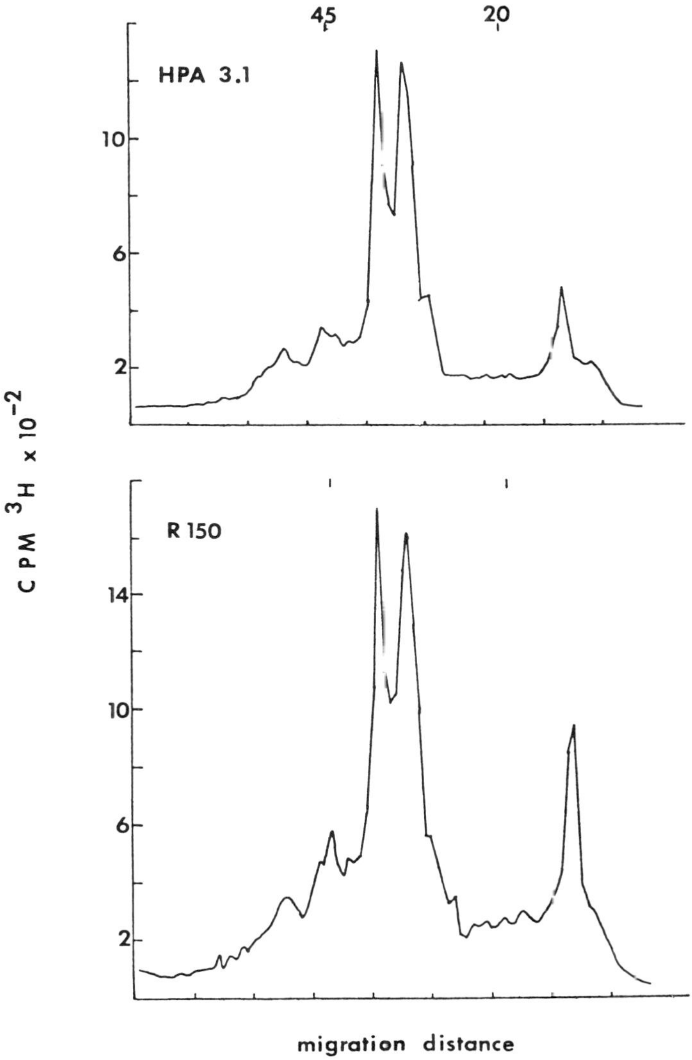


**Figure 2.** *RT-1B* antigens from BN rats. Radiolabeled BN spleen antigens were precipitated either with HPA 3.1 (top), an anti-*RT-B*$^{n}$ monoclonal antibody, or with R150 (bottom), an alloantiserum made to BN lymphocytes. Precipitates were run on 11% SDS polyacrylamide gels. Gels were sliced into 1 mm sections, and each slice was monitored for radioactivity by liquid scintillation counting. The two characteristic *Ia* peaks are found between the 45,000 and 20,000 molecular weight markers.

common, a recombinant dividing two *RT-1A* antigens has never yet been found. The possibilities exist, as pointed out by Cramer and his colleagues (Cramer et al. 1978b), that the two putative *RT-1A* genes are so tightly linked, or are under such strong selective pressure, that two discernable products never result from crossovers in this region. Alternatively, the second molecule may display no "private" antigenic specificities. It is also possible that conventional alloantisera cannot be expected to detect only one molecule. The use of mcAbs may help to clear up this confusion. Radiolabeled RT-1A antigens might routinely be discriminated from one another with these highly specific reagents, which represent a broad range of host reactivities to the donor immunogen. This approach has been attempted by Howard and his colleagues with combinations of two different mcAbs (Howard et al. 1979); in this study, however, the mcAbs were directed to determinants either on the same molecule or to determinants which cross-reacted with two molecules. Similar reagents were reported by Günther and colleagues (Elsässer-Beile and Günther 1979). Nevertheless, we are currently testing other pairs of mcAbs to prove the universal existence of the elusive second *RT-1A* molecule. One problem has been that some of the mcAbs from the McKearn panel are not good precipitating antibodies, and immunochemical analysis with these antibodies has been difficult. The rat anti-*Ia* mcAbs are also currently being tested in my laboratory, and at least one of these reagents will be useful for precipitating radiolabeled rat *Ia* molecules (Figure 2). We plan to test the antigen composition of the available recombinant rats with the mcAb panel as well, to determine if any of these rats display antigen products of crossovers within either *RT-1* region.

To conclude, I have summarized some of the most recent developments in the serology and genetics of the rat major histocompatibility complex. I'm looking forward to the next annual meeting of rat immunologists to be held in Philadelphia this year. I'm very grateful to Ray Owen for not having a herd of cattle in the Kerckhoff basement back in 1946, and for introducing me to the world of rats nearly ten years ago.

## References


Aptekman, P.M. and Bogden, A.E. 1955. A spontaneous ascites tumor originating and transplantable in the Wistar rat. Cancer Res. 15:89–92.

Billingham, R.W., Hodge, B.A., and Silvers, W.K. 1962. An estimate of the number of histocompatibility loci in the rat. Proc. Natl. Acad. Sci. U.S.A. 48:138–147.

Blankenhorn, E.P., Cecka, J.M., Götze, D., and Hood, L. 1978. Partial N-terminal amino acid sequence of rat transplantation antigens. Nature 274:90–92.

Blankenhorn, E.P., Cekca, J.M., Frelinger, J., Götze, D., and Hood, L. 1980. Structure of *Ia* antigens from the rat: Mouse alloantisera demonstrate at least two distinct molecular species. Eur. J. Immunol. 10:145–150.

Bodmer, W.F. 1973. A new genetic model for allelism at histocompatibility and other complex loci: Polymorphism for control of gene expression. Transplant. Proc. 5:1471–1475.

Bogden, A.E. and Aptekman, P.M. 1960. The R-1 factor, a histocompatibility antigen in the rat. Cancer Res. 20:1372–1382.

Bodgen, A. and Aptekman, P.M. 1962. Histocompatibility antigens and hemagglutinins in the rat. Ann. N.Y. Acad. Sci. 97:43–56.

Burhoe, S.O. 1947. Blood grouped in the rat *(Rattus Norvegicus)* and their inheritance. Proc. Natl. Acad. Sci. U.S.A. 33:102–109.

Butcher, G.W. and Howard, J.C. 1977. A recombinant in the major histocompatibility complex of the rat. Nature 266:362–364.

Cecka, J.M., Blankenhorn, E.P., Götze, D., and Hood, L. 1980. Microsequence analysis of *Ia* antigens from three strains of rats. Rue. J. Immunol. 10:140–144.

Cramer, D.V., Davis, B.K., Shonnard, J.W., Štark, O., and Gill, T.J. III. 1978a. Phenotypes of the major histocompatibility complex in wild rats of different geographic origins. J. Immunol. 120:179–186.

Cramer, D.V., Shonnard, J.W., and Davis, B.K. 1978b. Population genetics of the *MHC* in natural populations of rats. Rat Newsletter 4:42–46.

Davies, D.A.L. and Alkins, B.J. 1974. What abrogates heart transplant rejections in immunological enhancement? Nature 247:294–297.

Elkins, W.L., and Palm, J. 1966. Identification of a single strong histocompatibility locus in the rat by normal spleen-cell transfer. Ann. N.Y. Acad. Sci. 129:573–580.

Elsässer-Beile, U., and Günther, E. 1979. Monoclonal antibodies against $RT\text{-}1^a$ antigens. Transpl. Proc. 11:1571–1573.

Gasser, D. 1977. Current status of rat immunogenetics. Adv. Immunol. 25:93–139.

Götze, D. 1978. The major histocompatibility complex of the rat, *RT-1*. I. Serological characterization of the MNR haplotype $(RT1^m)$ in regard to cross-reacting haplotypes $RT\text{-}1^a$, $RT\text{-}1^c$, and $RT\text{-}1^b$. Immunogenetics 7:491–506.

Günther, E. 1979. Close association between particular *I*-region-determined cell surface antigens and *Ir* gene-controlled immune responsiveness to synthetic polypeptides in wild rats. Eur. J. Immunol. 9:391–401.

Günther, E., and Rüde, E. 1975. Genetic complementation of the histocompatibility-linked *Ir* genes in the rat. J. Immunol. 115:1387–1393.

Günther, E., and Štark, O. 1977. The major histocompatibility system of the rat (*Ag-B* or *H-1* system). In The Major Histocompatibility System in Man and Animals. D. Götze, ed. New York: Springer-Verlag.

Günther, E., and Štark, O. 1979. Overview: The major histocompatibility system of the rat. Transplant. Proc. 11:1550–1554.

Howard, J.C. 1978. Rat membrane alloantigen news. Rat Newsletter 4:12–17.

Howard, J.C. 1979. Rat membrane alloantigen news. Rat Newsletter 5:12–13.

Howard, J.C., Butcher, G.W., Galfre, G., and Milstein, C. 1978. Monoclonal anti-rat *MHC (H-1)* alloantibodies. Curr. Top. Microbiol. Immunol. 81:54–60.

Howard, J.C., Butcher, G.W., Galfre, G., Milstein, C., and Milstein, C.P. 1979. Monoclonal antibodies as tools to analyze the serological and genetic complexities of major transplantation antigens. Immunol. Rev. 47:139–174.

Klein, J. 1975. Biology of the Mouse Histocompatibility-2 Complex. New York: Springer-Verlag.

Kohoutova, M., Günther, E., Štark, O., Vojčik, V. 1978. Further two recombinants at the major histocompatibility complex of the rat. Folia Biol. (Praha) 24:406–407.

Kunz, H.W., Cramer, D.V., Gill, T.J. III, Coffman, K.P., Davis, B.K., and Shonnard, J.W. 1979. Studies on the $RT\text{-}1^d$, $RT\text{-}1^f$, and $RT\text{-}1^e$ haplotypes of the major histocompatibility complex in the rat. Transplant. Proc. 11:1557–1562.

Marshak, A., Doherty, P.C., and Wilson, D.B. 1977. The control of specificity of cytotoxic T-lymphocytes by the major histocompatibility complex *(AgB)* in rats and identification of a new alloantigen system showing no *AgB* restriction. J. Exp. Med. 146:1773–1790.

McKearn, T.J., Fitch, F.W., Smilek, D.E., Sarmiento, M., and Stuart, F.P. 1979. Properties of rat anti-*MHC* antibodies produced by cloned rat-mouse hybridomas. Immunol. Rev. 47:91–115.

McMaster, W.R. and Williams, A.F. 1979. Monoclonal antibodies to *Ia* antigens from rat thymus: Cross-reactions with mouse and human and use in purification of rat *Ia* glycoproteins. Immunol. Rev. 47:117–138.

Owen, R.D. 1962. Earlier studies of blood groups in the rat. Ann. N.Y. Acad. Sci. 97:37–42.

Ozato, K., Mayer, N., and Sachs, D.H. 1980. Hybridoma cell lines secreting monoclonal antibodies to mouse *H-2* and *Ia* antigens. J. Immunol. 124:533–541.

Palm, J. 1962. Current status of blood groups in rats. Ann. N.Y. Acad. Sci. 97:57–68.

Sachs, D.H., Humphrey, G.W., and Lunney, J.K. 1977. Sharing of *Ia* antigens between species. I. Detection of *Ia* specificities shared by rats and mice. J. Exp. Med. 146:381–393.

Shinohara, N., Cullen, S.E., and Sachs, D.H. 1977. *AgB*-linked analogue of *Ia* antigens in the rat. J. Immunol. 118:2083–2087.

Shonnard, J.W., Cramer, D.V., Poloskey, P.E., Kunz, H.W., and Gill, T.J. III. 1976. Polymorphism of the major histocompatibility locus in the wild Norway rat. Immunogenetics 3:193–200.

Sieck, T., Rothstein, A.M., and Wilson, D.B. 1979. Studies of the *MHC*-linked "CT" alloantigenic systems in rats. I. Neither an SD nor an LD gene product. Immunogenetics 9:165–172.

Smilek, D.E., Boyd, H.C., Wilson, D.B., Zmijewski, C.M., Fitch, F.W., and McKearn, T.J. 1980. Monoclonal rat anti-major histocompatibility complex antibodies display specificity for rat, mouse, and human target cells. J. Exp. Med. 151:1139–1150.

Soulillou, J.-P., Carpenter, C.B., d'Apice, A.J.F., and Strom, T.B. 1976. The role of non-classical, Fc receptor associated *Ag-B* antigens *(Ia)* in rat allograft enhancement. J. Exp. Med. 143:405–41.

Sporer, R., Black, G., Rigiero, C., Manson, L., and Götze, D. 1978. The major histocompatibility complex of the rat, *RT-1*. II. Biochemical evidence for a complex genetic organization. Immunogenetics 7:507–514.

Stark, O., Günther, E., Kohoutová, M., and Vojčik, V. 1977. Genetic recombination in the major histocompatibility complex (*H-1, AgB*) of the rat. Immunogenetics 5:183–187.

Stock, W. and Günther, E. 1979. Serologic analysis of two new alloantigenic systems of the rat major histocompatibility complex. Transpl. Proc. 11:1579–1581.

Wagener, D.K., Cramer, D.V., Shonnard, J.W., and Davis, B.K. 1979. Linkage disequilibrium between two genetic loci of the major histocompatibility complex in rats. Immunogenetics 9:157–164.

Hildemann, ed. Frontiers in Immunogenetics

# The *B* and *C* Systems of Cattle Revisited

Clyde Stormont

*Serology Laboratory, Department of Reproduction, School of Veterinary Medicine, University of California, Davis, California*

## Introduction

Of all the blood group systems my colleagues and I have brought to light over the past four decades, none rivals the *B* system of cattle in sheer complexity and interest. A runner-up for the number two position is the *C* system, the second most complex system in cattle. When considered alone or collectively, here is polymorphism personified, what with the *B* system involving at least 1,000 "alleles" and the *C* system around 100. Here I put alleles in quotation marks because there has always been considerable debate whether complex blood group systems of the order of *B* and *C* of cattle, Rh and MNS of human beings, and A and B of chickens are controlled by a single series of allelic genes or by closely linked genes. There is, as reviewed herein, voluminous evidence that the blood factors which comprise the *B* and *C* phenogroups of cattle are recombinable. In fact one of the objectives of this article is to bring the reader up to date on chromosome maps of the *B* and *C* regions. However, before doing so it is well to review some of the more important developments in our knowledge of those two systems.

## The Early Studies on the *B* and *C* Systems

As reviewed elsewhere (Stormont 1978), at the time the *B* and *C* systems were first brought into focus, I and my co-workers, R.D. Owen and M.R. Irwin, were working with the so-called revised or 1942 alphabet of cattle blood factors. That 38-letter alphabet, which involved blood factors A, B, $C_1$, $C_2$, F, G, H, I, J, K, $O_1$, $O_2$, $O_3$, P.Q, R, S, $T_1$, $T_2$, $U_1$, $U_2$, V, W, $X_1$, $X_2$, $Y_1$, $Y_2$, Z, A′, D′, $E'_1$, $E'_2$, $E'_3$, I′, J′, K′, L′, and Z′, took into account subtyping relationships that have all stood the test of time, and it also freed a number of letters (E, M, N, C′, F′, and G′) for use in designating additional cattle blood factors that were bound to be discovered in future years.

That number of blood factors was, at the time, wholly unprecedented, but only because it was the first systematic attempt to make use of alloimmune or isoimmune hemolysins in the study of blood groups. The cattle tests, which employ fresh-frozen, pooled rabbit serum as the source of complement, are extremely sensitive and, in my opinion, are capable of detecting the most minute structural differences in the molecules at the surface of the membrane of cattle red cells.

The key to the analysis of the *B* system was discovery of the inclusion group BGK. When tracing that group and the other combination of factors B and G in the family studies, what we (R.D. Owen, M.R. Irwin, and I) actually saw was the segregation of blood factors B, G, I, K, $O_1$, $O_2$, $O_3$, P,Q, $T_1$, $T_2$, $Y_1$, $Y_2$, A′, D′, $E'_1$, $E'_2$, $E'_3$, I′, J′, and K′ as the integrants of an extensive series of so-called antigenic complexes, later dubbed phenogroups (Stormont 1955). Those phenogroups were of the order $BGIO_1T_2A'$, $BGKO_2Y_1A'E'_3K'$, $BGKE'_2$, $BO_1Y_2D'$, $GY_2E'_1$, $IQE'_1$, $O_1T_1E'_3K'$, $O_3D'E'_3$, $O_3J'K'$, PI′, $QD'E'_1$, $T_1E'_3$, I′, and – (the absence of all 21 blood factors). This segregation was, for the contrasting pair $BGKE'_2$ and $GY_2E'_1$, in the sire family of a registered Holstein-Friesian bull, Carnation Peerless, whose family of 19 offspring and their dams had their blood types put on record along with that of Peerless, in the early 1940's.

Concomitantly, the *C* system came into view. What we saw there was the segregation of blood factors $C_1$, $C_2$, R, W, $X_1$, $X_2$, and L′ as the integrants of a series of phenogroups of the order $C_1$, $C_1R$, $C_1WX_2$, $C_1X_1$, $C_2$, $C_2RX_1$, $RWX_2$, W, $WX_2$, $X_1$, $X_2$, $X_2L'$, and – (the absence of all seven factors), as evidenced for the contrasting pair $C_1X_1$ and $X_2L'$ in the sire family of Peerless (Table 1).

Altogether, and as ultimately published some years later (Stormont et al. 1951), we identified 80 phenogroups in the *B* system and 22 in the *C* system. The evidence for those *B* and *C* phenogroups was based on an analysis of 50 sire families representing four dairy breeds (Holstein-Friesians, Guernseys, Brown Swiss, and Jerseys), with an average of 20 offspring per family. Because of the voluminous nature of the tabular data, only the segregation ratios were shown for most of the 50 sire families, including that of Peerless (Table 1), who was simply coded as Holstein bull H8. Here again the data were wholly unprecedented when considering the fact that the Rh system of human beings involved at that time only about five blood factors, as reviewed by Wiener and Wexler (1958). Most all of those original *B* and *C* phenogroups have stood the test of time. But, as indicated elsewhere in this article, many of them were split by the addition of new factors to each of the systems. Likewise, most of the phenogroups continued to grow by the addition of one or more blood factors.

Although those early data on the *B* and *C* systems were presented on the basis of multiple allelic genes, as were those published later in that decade (Bouw 1958; Braend 1959; Neimann-Sorensen 1958; Rendel 1958), the idea of closely linked genes was never dismissed.

Table 1. Segregation of B and C Phenogroups in 19 Offspring of Carnation Peerless 629480. This Bull was Coded H8 in the 1951 Report.

| | Tag numbers | | Phenogroup formulas | |
|---|---|---|---|---|
| | Dams | Offspring | | |
| H8 | | | $BGKE'_2/GY_2E'_1$ | $C_1X_1/X_2L'$ |
| | 3882 | | $O_3J'K'/Y_1$ | $C_1/$ |
| | | 4116 | $GY_2E'_1/O_3J'K'$ | $C_1X_1/$ |
| | 3937 | | $BO_1Y_2D/E'_1$ | $RWX_2/$ |
| | | 4191 | $BGKE'_2/E'_1$ | $C_1X_1/RWX_2$ |
| | | 4485 | $GY_2E'_1/E'_1$ | $C_1X_1/RWX_2$ |
| | | 4897 | $BGKE'_2/BO_1Y_2D'$ | $X_2L'/$ |
| | 4017 | | $BO_1Y_2D'/$ | $C_1X_1/C_2R$ |
| | | 4422 | $GY_2E'_1/BO_1Y_2D'$ | $X_2L_1/C_2R$ |
| | 4265 | | $GY_2E'_1/$ | $C_1X_1/$ |
| | | 4887 | $GY_2E'_1/$ | $C_1X_1/$ |
| | | 5074 | $GY_2E'_1/$ | $X_2L'/C_1X_1$ |
| | 4573 | | $GY_2E'_1/$ | $C_1X_1/X_2L'$ |
| | | 4842 | $GY_2E'_1/$ | $X_2L'/C_1X_1$ |
| | 4354 | | $BO_1Y_2D'/GY_2E'_1$ | $C_1/$ |
| | | 4949 | $GY_2E'_1/GY_2E'_1$ | $X_2L'/C_1$ |
| | 4758 | | $GY_2E'_1/O_3J'K'$ | $C_1W/X_2$ |
| | | 4992 | $BGKE'_2/O_3J'K'$ | $C_1X_1/C_1W$ |
| | 4556 | | $GY_2E'_1/$ | $C_1X_1/$ |
| | | 5043 | $BGKE'_2/GY_2E'_1$ | $C_1X_1/$ |
| | | 5155 | $GY_2E'_1/$ | $C_1X_1/$ |
| | 4829 | | $GY_2E'_1/$ | $C_1/X_2$ |
| | | 5077 | $BGKE'_2/GY_2E'_1$ | $C_1X_1/$ |
| | 4837 | | $GY_2E'_1/$ | $C_1/$ |
| | | 5086 | $GY_2E'_1/$ | $X_2L'/C_1$ |
| | 4813 | | $BGKE'_2/GY_2E'_1$ | $X_2/$ |
| | | 5095 | $BGKE'_2/BGKE'_2$ | $C_1X_1/$ |
| | 4751 | | $BGKE'_2/GY_2E'_1$ | $C_1X_2$ |
| | | 5112 | $BGKE'_2/BGKE'_2$ | $X_2L'/C_1$ |
| | 4750 | | $GY_2E'_1/O_3J'K'$ | $C_1X_1/$ |
| | | 5017 | $GY_2E'_1/GY_2E'_1$ | $C_1X_1/$ |
| | 4590 | | $GY_2E'_1/$ | $C_1/$ |
| | | 8002 | $GY_2E'_1/$ | $X_2L'/C_1$ |
| | 4559 | | $GY_2E'_1/-$ | $C_1R/$ |
| | | 8061 | $BGKE'_2/-$ | $C_1X_1/$ |

## *Expansion of the B System*

In 1950 when I joined the faculty of the School of Veterinary Medicine of the University of California, I had the opportunity to begin again the analysis of cattle blood group systems. I had with me a small supply of some but not all of the blood typing reagents from the original University of Wisconsin sources and also a small supply of a new reagent, anti-E, which I had isolated from an antiserum developed by M.B. Buddle in New Zealand. The first job was to develop an entirely new battery of blood typing reagents from alloimmune antisera produced in our local university and state herds.

In the process, a number of new factors (NF1, NF2, NF3, . . . etc.) were detected and most of those, as might be expected, were found to be members of the *B* system (Stormont 1954, 1959, 1962). For example, there were the important new factors of the *B* system, which were initially designated NF4, NF6, and NF8, but were ultimately given international status when those designations were changed to Y′, B′, and O′, respectively. Other workers in the field of cattle blood groups have had this same experience. As a result, there are always some new factors like our NF7, belonging to the *B* system, and NF35, belonging to the *C* system, which are still awaiting international recognition but will not gain such status until antibodies specific for those factors have been developed by two or more laboratories.

As a result of adding such blood factors to the *B* system as B′, F′, G′, O′, and Y′, extending the O and E′ series of subtypes, recognizing new subtyping relationships (e.g., $B_1$-$B_2$ and $I_1$-$I_2$), and expanding the family and population studies to include such breeds as the Angus, Hereford, and Milking Shorthorn, the list of *B* phenogroups continued to grow, not only in numbers of phenogroups but also in size and complexity of the phenogroup formulas. The last list of *B* phenogroups, prepared by D.F. Weseli in this laboratory, was distributed in 1959. That list contained 252 phenogroups.

Some years ago the International Society for Animal Blood Group Research delegated a committee to prepare an up-to-date list of *B* phenogroups. That committee, insofar as I am aware, has yet to issue its report, and this is not surprising in view of the fact that there are over 20 laboratories throughout the world that are engaged in studies of cattle blood groups. Consequently it is up to each laboratory to maintain its own list of *B* phenogroups and most do so by breeds. Casual inspection of the lists maintained by breeds in the author's laboratory indicates approximately 600 *B* phenogroups. The real number when all such lists are compared is certain to be more than 1,000, but there is the problem of deciding which phenogroups are duplicates of known phenogroups and which are really new. The problem arises from the fact that no two laboratories use the same battery of *B* system reagents. Consequently the symbolism for *B* system phenogroups varies from one laboratory to another, and the same is true for the *C* system. In the author's laboratory, we make every effort to limit the number of factors shown in the phenogroup formulas to those that are the most important in the diagnosis and differentiation of the phenogroups.

Of all the cattle blood group systems, most attention is given to the *B* system for two reasons: (1) the great utility of that system in solving problems of questionable parentage arising in the breeding of registered or pedigreed cattle, and (2) the value of that system in distinguishing between breeds of cattle and tracing breed relationships. With respect to the latter, these breed differences can easily be seen by listing the ten most frequent phenogroups in each of the various breeds, as done here for eight breeds of cattle (Tables 2 and 3).

Generally speaking, the sum of the frequencies of the alleles controlling the ten most frequent *B* phenogroups in any breed is usually greater than 0.80. For example,

**Table 2.** The Ten Most Frequently Encountered *B* Phenogroups in Purebred Bulls of Each of Two Breeds of American Beef Cattle and Each of Two Breeds of American Dairy Cattle. The Phenogroups are Listed in Order of Relative Frequency.

| Angus | Hereford | Holstein | Jersey |
|---|---|---|---|
| $O_1Q'$ | — | $GY_2E'_1Q'$ | $B_1GKO_2Y_1A'B'E'_3G'K'O'Y'$ |
| $O_xE'_3O'$ | $Y_1D'I'$ | — | $T_1E'_3F'$ |
| $I_2E'_1$ | $O_xA'$ | $O_xE'_3G'$ | $O_1T_1E'_3F'K'$ |
| $B_1O_1Y_2D'$ | $I'$ | $I_2$ | $B_1I'Q'$ |
| $GY_2E'_1Q'$ | $Y_1D'$ | $O_1A'$ | $O_xE'_3F'G'O'$ |
| $I_2Y_2E'_1Y'$ | $QI'Q'$ | $O_xD'E'_3F'G'O'$ | $B_2GD'$ |
| $O_1E'_1$ | $B_2I_1Y_1$ | $B_1O_1$ | $B_1GKO_xA'B'K'O'$ |
| $I'Q'$ | $O_xE'_3F'O'$ | $O_3J'K'O'7$ | $I'Q'$ |
| $B_1O_2Y_1A'E'_3G'Q'$ | $B_1GKO_xY_2A'O'$ | $B_1O_2Y_1A'E'_3G'Q'$ | $O_3J'K'O'7$ |
| $O_xT_1Y_1A'E'_3G'$ | $QQ'$ | $B_1O_1Y_2D'$ | $O_xY_1D'$ |

**Table 3.** The Ten Most Frequently Encountered *B* Phenogroups in Purebred Bulls in Each of Four "Exotic" Breeds of Cattle Recently Introduced into the United States. The Phenogroups are Listed in Order of Relative Frequency. The Number of Bulls upon Which This Survey Was Based Is Shown Within Parentheses.

| Limousin (385) | Maine-Anjou (142) | Simmental (684) | Tarentaise (29) |
|---|---|---|---|
| $B_1O_xQE'_3F'I'O'$[a] | $B_1O_2Y_1A'E'_3G'O'$ | $Q'$ | $I_1YE'_1Y'$ |
| $B_1I_1Q$[a] | $Q'$ | $O_xO'$[a] | $B_1GKO_xQE'_2F'G'$[a] |
| $B_1O_xT_1A'B'E'_3F'Q'$[a] | $B_1GKO_xY_2A'Q'$ | $B_2GO_xA'$[a] | $O_xQA'E'_1O'$[a] |
| $O_3E'_2F'J'$ | $O_1T_1E'_3F'K'$ | $O_1I'Q'$[a] | $O_3E'_2F'J'$ |
| $I'Q'$ | $O_3A'E'_4Q'$[a] | $B_1I_1Q$[a] | $B_1GO_1$ |
| $B_2G$ | $B_2GO_1Y_2$ | $O_1T_1E'_3F'I'K'$ | $O_1Q'$ |
| $B_1O_xQA'$[a] | $I'Q'$ | $Q$ | $O_xY_2O'$[a] |
| $O_xQA'B'D'E'_3$[a] | $I_1Q'$[a] | $O_xQA'E'_1O'$[a] | $Q'$ |
| $I_1Q'$[a] | $GY_2E'_1Q'$ | $O_xA'B'$[a] | $O_xO'$ |
| $GI_2J'O'$[a] | $B_1Y_1E'_2G'$[a] | $O_xY_2A'D'E'_1$ | $B_1T_1$[a] |

[a]Phenogroups not previously encountered in the long-established breeds of American cattle (e.g., those represented in Table 2).

this is true for all the breeds listed in Table 2 except Holsteins. The sum of the frequencies of the ten most frequent *B* alleles in Holsteins is only about 0.70. That breed, the most extensively studied of all American breeds, has approximately 130 *B* alleles with frequencies less than 0.001.

Many of the phenogroups in the *B* system are ubiquitous whereas others, such as the number one phenogroup in the Limousin (Table 2), are essentially breed-specific.

## *Expansion of the C System*

Until recently the *C* system has received far less attention than *B*. For example, the only "official" blood factor I have added to that system since the time of its initial description is blood factor E, which split such phenogroups as –, $C_1$, $C_2$, $C_1X_1$, $C_1WX_2$, $C_2W$, and W into E, $C_1E$, etc., as indicated in the only published list of *C* phenogroups from this laboratory (Stormont 1962). That list contained 35 phenogroups.

Since then virtually all new developments in knowledge about the *C* system have come about as the result of efforts on the part of European investigators. In that connection, I have at hand an article by Grosclaude et al. (1980) which reports the development of reagents for four new factors, F1, F6, F10, F15, in the *C* system. In tests using reagents for those factors plus reagents for $C_1$, $C_2$, E, $R_1$, $R_2$, W, $X_1$, $X_2$, C′, L′, and C″, the latter initially known as PLB-1 (Duniec et al. 1973), Grosclaude and co-workers have identified 77*C* system phenogroups in the Charolais breed alone. On the basis of that report, it can be assumed that the list of *C* phenogroups will soon exceed 100 if it has not already done so.

## *Chromosome Maps of the B Region*

The first two anomalies in the transmission of *B* alleles were documented by the author (Stormont 1954). One involved a Holstein cow of formula $BO_1Y_2d'/BO_16$ (later changed to $BO_1B'$) which produced a female calf of formula $BO_1/PY_2$ in mating to a bull of formula $PY_2/E'_1$. This was interpreted as a mutation which deleted either $Y_2D'$ from the $BO_1Y_2D'$ allele or $B'$ from the $BO_1B'$ allele. In any event, what we saw here was the reemergence, so to speak, of an old phenogroup which stands high on the list of Holstein *B* phenogroups (Table 2).

The second anomaly, which occurred in the same herd of cattle and at almost the same time, involved a cow of formula $GY_2E'_1/O_3J'K'O'7$ which produced a male calf of formula $GY_2{}^{\pm}E'_3/Py_2$ in mating to a bull of formula $BO_2Y_1A'E'_3$ (later written as $B_10_2Y_1A'E'_3G'Q')/PY_2$. As verified by absorption tests, the new phenogroup $GY_2E'_3$ was completely negative with all of our $E'_1$ and $E'_2$ reagents but did show weak reactivity with our $E'_3$ reagents. Although the parental phenogroup undoubtedly possessed factor $Q'$ in addition to G, $Y_2$, and $E'_1$, unfortunately anti-$Q'$ was not developed until almost a decade later and, in the interim, the new phenogroup became lost, but not until it was traced to second-generation offspring.

In the next eight years, as reviewed elsewhere (Stormont 1964), eight additional anomalies in the transmission of *B* alleles were recorded by workers in various laboratories. Also, Bouw et al. (1964) recorded four additional cases, thereby bringing the total number to 14. As I pointed out in my 1965 review, the general consensus among the workers who observed these anomalies—some of which, as the first two, involved a loss of one or more blood factors, others a gain of one or more blood factors, and still others both a gain and a loss of blood factors—is that most of them have come about as the result of crossing over within the confines of the complex *B* locus. However, in the absence of outside markers, there is no direct proof that this is the case.

Green (1966), working with data provided by the author, published the first two tentative maps of the *B* region which I show here in their mirror image forms in order to conform with the sequence of determinants in maps developed later (e.g., that of Bouw and Fiorentini published in 1970): G′-Y-B-O-B′ and Q-OK′-J′O′.

In the interim, while all this was going on, certain of the cattle breed registries in Europe decided to make it a requirement that any animals to enter the herd books must have their blood types officially recorded. This program began to provide an enormous amount of family data for those laboratories that performed the blood typing tests.

Thus, on the basis of a comparison of the blood groups of 30,000 Dutch cattle with those of their parents, Bouw and Fiorentini (1970) stated that they observed 57 cases in which a modification in the inheritance of *B* phenogroups had occurred. However, they recorded only 19 of those 57 cases which they considered useful in constructing what I shall refer to as the first Dutch map. That map showed 21 determinants in the following sequence: $Y_1$-Q-D′-$E'_1$-$Y_2$-$E'_3F'$-G-BGKB-P′-$O_1$-J′-$O_xO'$-$I_2$-$O_3A'$-I′.

In presenting this sequence, they diagrammed how each of the 19 cases could be accommodated on such a map by postulating a single crossover event. Bouw and Fiorentini regarded each of the 21 genetic determinants as single genes.

Stormont (1972) pointed out, on the basis of population data alone, that the Bouw and Fiorentini map of the *B* region might be satisfactory for such breeds as the Hereford, where recombination in animals of phenogroup formula $Y_1D'I'/-$ could readily generate such phenogroups as $Y_1D'$,I',$Y_1$, and D'I', all of which occur in that breed, but unsatisfactory for breeds such as the Jersey where the highly frequent inclusion group BGK of phenogroup $B_1GKO_2Y_1A'B'E'_3K'O'Y'$ is often alternative to $O_1T_1$ and $T_1$ in the phenogroups $O_1T_1E'_3F'K'$ and $T_1E'_3F'$ (Table 2), but never seems to ride with $O_1T_1$ or $T_1$. Thus population data clearly indicated that the positioning of the coding elements for BGK and $O_1$ in the Dutch map would eventually have to be changed.

A second or revised Dutch map of the *B* region was published by Ruiterkamp et al. (1977). Their map was based on 146 cases of irregular transmission observed in a sample of approximately 100,000 Dutch cattle tested over the years 1960–1974, and presumably included the 57 cases mentioned by Bouw and Fiorentini (1970), whose data were collected over the period 1960–1967.

The second Dutch map shows 15 determinants aligned in the following linear sequence: Q-$Y_2$-D'-G″-F'-$E'_1$-Q'-$I_2$-OK'-J'O'7-$I_1$-I' and, in addition, shows numerous determinants above and below the main sequence but connected to it by means of arrow diagrams. The arrows indicate that the determinants for BGK, B, G, $O_1$, $O_x$, $E'_4$, etc. must map at any of several points in the linear sequence but just where is not too clear from perusal of their article. For example, only one of the 123 recombinants, which were said to be useful in constructing the map, was shown.

In effect, the second Dutch map of the *B* region deleted $Y_1$, $E'_3$, G, BGK, B, P', $O_1$, and $O_3$ from the linear sequence of the first Dutch map, added G″, Q', K', 7, and $I_1$ to that sequence, and suspended a number of determinants above and below the main sequence. Ruiterkamp et al. (1977) compared what they described as two main gene clusters, one radiating from $E'_4$ and the other from $O_x$, with the *H-2K* and *H-2D* regions in chromosome 17 of the mouse. They saw certain similarities between the *B* system of cattle and the *H-2* system of mice. According to them, crossing over or recombination within the genes of the two main clusters was reduced about 5-fold, assuming equal chance for crossing over between all determinants. In the absence of any tabular data on the actual recombinants involved in the study, we are obliged to go along with what they did or did not say.

The most recent map of the *B* region is that developed by Grosclaude et al. (1979). It is based on 40 cases of irregular inheritance of *B* phenogroups observed in about 55,000 sire-dam-offspring comparisons in seven breeds of French cattle. In addition, 200 families from the Normande breed were typed in order to increase the amount of data for estimating the recombination rate between terminal markers. Some information about the position of several determinants was deduced from population data. The French map shows 22 determinants listed in the following linear sequence: Q-YY'-D'-$G_2$-$E'_3$G″-G'-B-$P'_1$-$E'_2$-Q'-$G_3$T-($O_2$,$O_3$K')-$I_1$($J'_1$,O')-I″-I'.

The determinants for some 22 additional factors (e.g., $BG_2K$, $G_1$, $I_2$, $O_1$, $P_1$, $E_1'E_3'$, etc.) are displayed in that map above and below the linear sequence, in variable positions indicated by means of arrows. In this manner $BG_2K$ is shown above $I_2$, which is placed above $E_3',O'$, which map somewhere between Q′ and $O_3K'$ and possibly very near T on the main circuit. A third position for $E_3'$ is indicated between YY′ on the left and B on the right, whereas $E_1'$ is indicated in a position between G′ and Q′. B′ is indicated in a position somewhere between $J_1'O'$ on the left to I′ on the right. Below the main circuit Y is shown again but this time somewhere between Q and D′. Similarly, $G_1$ is indicated between $G_2$ and B. $J_2'$ is shown between T and $O_3K'$, whereas A′ is shown between $I_1$ and I″. These are the main features of the French map which, in my opinion, will accommodate virtually all published cases of irregularities in the inheritance of *B* phenogroups on the assumption that each involved a single crossover. However, Grosclaude et al. discussed two cases that would have to involve a double exchange on the assumption that they were brought about by crossing over. But that, of course, is not a necessary assumption.

In a study of the inheritance of *B* phenogroups in the offspring of Normande bulls of formulas $I_1QD'E_1'G''/O_2I'J'K'O'$ and $I_1O_3QA'E_1'K'Q'I'/O_2I'J'K'O'$ in matings to cows that lacked the pertinent blood factors $I_1$, Q, and I″, Grosclaude et al. recorded 6 recombinants in 447 test cases involving the terminal markers Q and I′, which yields a recombination rate in centimorgans of 1.34. They also observed five recombinants in 1,266 cases involving Q and $I_1$ and three recombinants in 451 cases involving Q and I″, which yield centimorgan rates of 0.40 and 0.67, respectively.

They regarded 1.34 centimorgans as an overestimate of the rate of recombination for the terminal pair and suggested that this figure should be halved. I would challenge the validity of that conclusion for several reasons, at least one of which is inherent in the data they presented. For example, they also observed six recombinants in 2,115 test cases involving K′ and I′. This yields a recombinant rate of 0.28 centimorgans which, when considering the confidence limits listed in their report, can hardly be regarded as significantly different from the other rates. Indeed, the distance between $I_1$ and I′ may fall in the same range when adequate data are available to measure it. One thing seems clear from the overall data on B chromosome maps and that is the codon for I′ must be considerably to the right of all others.

Grosclaude et al. pointed out that certain pairs or groups of factors were not observed to occur together in the same phenogroup as, for example, Q and Y or YY′, $G_2$ and G″, $BG_2K$ and T, and A′ and J′. They stated that such oppositional relationships are better interpreted as an effect of close linkage between the determinants of these pairs of factors or groups of factors. This implies that they are of the opinion that no two determinants map at the same point. It also implies that eventually all possible combinations of the 40 or so blood factors will be found, and that is a large number of combinations. But they failed to discuss the fact that most of the recombinants yielded established phenogroups rather than new combinations of blood factors. For example, 16 of the 25 recombinants they observed in the Normande breed yielded phenogroups that were already on record in that breed. It is difficult to reconcile such observations with their suggestion that the B chromosomal region might house as many as 100 cistrons.

### *Chromosome Maps of the C Region*

In material involving a comparison of blood groups in 16,000 Dutch cattle with those of their parents, Bouw et al. (1974) observed 43 irregularities in the inheritance of *C* phenogroups. However, they mentioned that only 27 of those cases were useful in constructing a map of the *C* region. and they listed only six cases that were used to derive the following linear sequence of determinants: L′-(R,W)-C-E-X-C′, in which symbolism R represents $R_1$ and $R_2$, C represents $C_1$ and $C_2$, and X represents $X_1$ and $X_2$. Because there were no recombinants involving the respective members of these subtype series, they stated that the controlling genes can be placed on the same spot or close to each other in the map. Likewise, there were no recombinants involving R and W, so it was assumed that the genes that control those factors must map near to one another, as indicated by the use of parentheses.

Apparently none of the *C* system recombinants observed by Bouw and his co-workers yielded previously unrecognized *C* phenogroups.

In material involving 55,000 sire-dam-offspring comparisons, Guérin et al. (1980) recorded 20 cases involving irregular inheritance of *C* phenogroups in French cattle. Sixteen of the 20 recombinants were observed in Charolaise cattle and apparently five of those recombinants resulted in *C* phenogroups not previously seen in that breed. Two were observed in Normande cattle and two in the Limousine breed. The two in Normande cattle resulted in *C* phenogroups not previously seen in that breed.

Their map shows the following linear sequence:

$$
\begin{array}{l}
L'\text{-}R_2W)\text{-}C_1\text{-}E\text{-}X_2 \\
\qquad\qquad\;\; C_2 \\
\qquad\qquad\;\; C_1'' \\
\qquad\qquad\;\; C_2''
\end{array}
$$

with the determinants for $X_1$, C′, and F10 mapping at or near $X_2$, as indicated by the use of arrow diagrams. The position of the determinants for F6 and F15 was indicated by arrows in the area bounded by E on the left and X on the right.

Using L′ and C′ as terminal markers and confining the analysis to informative matings involving Charolaise sire families, Guérin et al. estimated that the operational length of the DNA coding for the *C* system blood factors is approximately 0.4 centimorgans.

## Discussion

Auditore and Stormont (1978) showed that, within the phenogroup $GY_2E_1'Q'$, anti-G effectively blocks absorption of anti-$E_1'$ and anti-$Y_2$, and the latter antibodies effectively block one another. In addition, we showed that anti-$E_1'$ is blocked by anti-Q′ but that there is no effective blocking of anti-G by anti-$Y_2$, anti-G by anti-Q′, and so on. We therefore proposed that it is not necessary to postulate more than a single molecule per phenogroup and, accordingly, no more than one gene per phenogroup. This, of course, is in line with the idea (Stormont et al. 1951; Bouw 1958; Braend 1959; Neimann-Sorenson 1958; Rendel 1958) that the *B* phenogroups can be accounted for on the basis of a single series of allelic genes.

Grosclaude et al. (1979) tell us that our interpretation of the results of the blocking experiments could be wrong, which we will admit. Moreover, they scold us, as it were, for neglecting to take into account available information about recombination within the *B* system. They contend that observations about recombination do not fit, in the present state of knowledge, with the hypothesis of control of the *B* system factors by a single gene locus. They also tell us that what is known at present regarding the number of alleles normally present at one locus, even a long one, does not fit at all with the hypothesis of only one locus controlling the huge variability of the *B* system. In support of their contentions, Grosclaude et al. suggest that a map length of 0.7 centimorgans is indicative of a sequence of at least several tens of loci and could correspond to a region embracing some 100 cistrons.

The article by Auditore and Stormont (1978) had nothing to do with recombination. If, however, we left the impression that we do not believe the factors of phenogroups such as $GY_2E_1'Q'$ are recombinable, I hasten to correct such an impression.

So it appears, once again, that I am being invited to defend the idea of multiple alleles, and I shall begin doing so by pointing out, as recently reviewed by Kolata (1980), that the genes of animals and animal viruses, unlike the genes of bacteria, come in pieces that are spread out along DNA. In between each of these pieces are long stretches of DNA whose functions are as yet poorly understood. First, and RNA copy is made of the entire length of the DNA containing the gene. Next, the copies of the extra DNA are snipped out of the long piece of RNA, and the remaining pieces are sealed together to form the messenger RNA, which then moves to the cytoplasm.

As pointed out by Kolata, there is so much extra DNA, called intervening sequences, that the initial RNA copy of the gene is actually five to ten times longer than the messenger RNA.

Two pieces of DNA can break and rejoin at virtually any point within these intervening sequences, thereby making recombination as easy within a gene as between genes. I have no difficulty at all in conceiving a *B* gene with as many as 20 or more pieces which can occur in hundreds of allelic forms. What we have in the form of the cattle blood typing test is one of the most sensitive tests ever developed to measure the full extent of allelic differentiation and to detect recombinants involving the pieces of those alleles. With such a model, who then is to say that a single locus cannot support more than a few dozen alleles? The same argument applies to the *C* locus and all other blood group loci that are not conserved from the standpoint of evolution.

And then there is the notion (Ruiterkamp et al. 1977) that control of the *B* system is vested in a series of gene clusters. One of the most thoroughly analyzed genetic systems is that involving the so-called arom gene cluster of *Neurospora crassa* (as reviewed by Giles 1978). Until about 1970, the arom gene cluster was believed by almost all workers in *Neurospora* genetics to involve a minimum of five genes which encode five enzymes catalyzing reactions 2 through 6 in the polyaromatic biosynthetic pathway. Moreover, mutants were obtained that lacked individual activities for each of the five enzymes and those mutants mapped in discrete, nonoverlapping segments of the arom region.

As pointed out by Giles in his 1978 review, biochemical studies over the years 1967–1977 have conclusively established that the basic subunit of the arom aggregate is actually a single pentafunctional polypeptide chain. This indicates that the arom gene cluster, and others like it, is actually a single gene, and Giles cites a 1977 report by Gaertner and Cole in which they now refer to a gene cluster as a "cluster gene."

Grosclaude et al. (1979) seem to be unaware that rates of recombination comparable with those they report for pairs of terminal or near-terminal markers in the *B* system have also been reported for genetic traits encoded by a single series of allelic genes. For example, no one so far as I know has ever proposed that closely linked genes code for the electrophoretic variants of the enzyme 6PGD that occur in a variety of species including human beings. In a study of electrophoretic forms of 6PGD in a population of Japanese quail, Ohno et al. (1969) recorded 11 recombinants in 1,011 progeny from 26 mating pairs. This yields a rate of 1.1 units on the centimorgan scale.

This and other cases involving high rates of intragenic recombination are reviewed in Ohno's (1970) monograph. In that context, he discusses the principle that "polymorphism generates more polymorphism" and illustrates how new alleles can be readily generated by recombination and how a single locus can support many alleles even in the confines of a very small breeding population.

And now I am reminded of one of the four explanations advanced by Stormont et al. (1951) in discussing the *B* and *C* systems. We suggested that a gene may be subject to precise modification through mutation at any of a number of different points. One limited area on a *B* allele, for example, may be concerned with the specificity detected serologically in the ultimate gene product as G, another with the specificity called I, and so on, which was really a daring thing to suggest at that time. Had we gone one step further and suggested that the various points within such a gene may be recombinable and that many of the *B* alleles could be generated in that manner, we would have arrived at a point in history which is now being verified on many different fronts.

So much for genetic maps of the *B* and *C* regions. Elsewhere I intend to stir up the subject of linear subtyping relationships. It is necessary to do so because it is evident from the report of Grosclaude et al. (1979), as well as some earlier reports on cattle blood groups, that the serological criterion for deciding whether two or more blood factors are related as linear subtypes is being overlooked. For example, the notion that Y′ is a linear subtype of $Y_1$ and $Y_2$ (Grosclaude et al. 1979) is without serological foundation, as will be pointed out elsewhere.

## References

Auditore, J.J., and Stormont, C. 1978. The cell surface distribution of alloantigens of the bovine erythrocyte. Immunogenetics 6:457.

Bouw, J. 1958. Blood Group Studies in Dutch Cattle Breeds. Wageningen: H. Veenman and Zonen.

Bouw, J., and Fiorentini, A. 1970. Structure of loci controlling complex blood group systems in cattle. In Proceedings XIth European Conference on Animal Blood Groups and Biochemical Polymorphism, Warsaw, 1968. The Hague: Dr. W. Junk N.V.

Bouw, J., G.E. Nasrat, and C. Buys. 1964. The inheritance of blood groups in the blood group system *B* of cattle. Genetica 35:47.

Bouw, J., Buys, C., and Schreuder, I. 1974. Further studies on the genetic control of the blood group system *C* of cattle. Anim. Blood Groups Biochem. Genet. 5:105.

Braend, M. 1959. Blood Groups of Cattle in Norway. Skandinavisk Bladforlag.

Duniec, M., Stawarz, K., Buys, C., and Bouw, J. 1973. A closed system within blood group locus *C* of cattle. Anim. Blood Groups Biochem. Genet. 4:185.

Giles, N. 1978. The organization, function and evolution of gene clusters in eucaryotes. Am. Naturalist 112:641.

Green, P. 1966. Towards a tentative map of the genetic determinants of the *B* blood group system of cattle. Immunogenet. Lett. 4:188.

Grosclaude, F., Guerin, G., and Houlier, G. 1979. The genetic map of the *B* system of cattle blood groups as observed in French breeds. Anim. Blood Groups Biochem. Genet. 10:199.

Grosclaude, F., Alaux, M.T. Houlier, G., and Guerin, G. 1980. The *C* system of cattle blood groups. I. Additional factors in the system. Anim. Blood Groups Biochem. Genet., in press.

Guerin, G., Grosclaude, F., and Houlier, G. 1980. The *C* system of cattle blood groups. II. Partial genetic map of the system. Anim. Blood Groups Biochem. Genet., in press.

Kolata, G.B. 1980. Genes in pieces. Science 207:392.

Neimann-Sorensen, A. 1958. Blood Groups of Cattle. Copenhagen: A/S Carl Fr. Mortensen.

Ohno, S. 1970. Evolution by Gene Duplication. New York: Springer-Verlag.

Ohno, S., Steinus, C., Christian, L., and Schipmann, G. 1969. De novo mutationlike events at the 6PGD locus of the Japanese quail, and the principle of polymorphism breeding more polymorphism. Biochem. Genet. 3:417.

Rendel, J. 1958. Studies of cattle blood groups. IV. The frequency of blood group genes in Swedish cattle breeds, with special reference to breed structure. Acta Agric. Scand. 8:192.

Ruiterkamp, W.A., Spek, C.M., and Bouw, J. 1977. Gene clusters in the blood group system *B* of cattle. Anim. Blood Groups Biochem. Genet. 8:231.

Stormont, C. 1954. On the genetics and serology of the *B* system of bovine blood groups. Proceedings IXth International Congress of Genetics (Bellagio 1953). Caryologia (Supplement) 6 (Part II): 1205.

Stormont, C. 1955. Linked genes, pseudoalleles and blood groups. Am. Naturalist 89:105.

Stormont, C. 1959. On the application of blood groups in animal breeding. Proceedings Xth International Congress of Genetics (Montreal 1958). Genet. Today 1:206.

Stormont, C. 1962. Current status of blood groups in cattle. Ann. N.Y. Acad. Sci. 97:251.

Stormont, C. 1964. Mammalian immunogenetics. Proceedings XIth International Congress of Genetics (The Hague 1963) 3:715.

Stormont, C. 1972. The language of phenogroups. Haematol. 6:73; In Current Topics in Immunohematology and Immunogenetics. Alexander S. Wiener Festschrift, ed. Budapest: Akadamiai Kiado.

Stormont, C. 1978. The early history of cattle blood groups. Immunogenetics 6:1.

Stormont, C., Owen, R.D., and Irwin, M.R. 1951. The *B* and *C* systems of bovine blood groups. Genetics 36:134.

Wiener, A.S., and Wexler, I.B. 1958. Heredity of the Blood Groups. New York: Grune and Stratton.

Hildemann, ed. Frontiers in Immunogenetics

# Where Are Rhesus Monkeys on the Immunogenetics Tree?

W.H. Stone, J.L. VandeBerg, and M. Curie-Cohen

*Laboratory of Genetics and Wisconsin Regional Primate Research Center, University of Wisconsin, Madison, Wisconsin*

## Introduction

It was with great pleasure that we accepted the invitation to participate in this symposium honoring Dr. Ray D. Owen, not only because of our personal admiration for Ray Owen, but also because of the significant role he played in launching the immunogenetic studies of rhesus monkeys.

In 1962, Owen and Anderson identified five blood group factors in rhesus monkeys; they used multispecific sera produced by heteroimmunization of rabbits with rhesus erythrocytes (red blood cells—RBC). The antibodies in these sera behaved as incomplete agglutinins and thus required the addition of goat antirabbit γ-globulin (Coombs reagent) to complete the reactions. Family studies were not possible, but the frequencies of these factors in a population of 447 monkeys suggested that two factors were controlled by independent loci. Two other factors appeared to be alleles of a third independent locus, whereas the fifth factor was associated (perhaps cross-reactive or in a haplotype) with one of the first two. Although three independent blood group systems were described then, no further genetic studies were done, and the antisera are no longer available. These studies were initiated to monitor the repopulation of RBC following bone marrow transplantation in irradiated recipients. Unfortunately, this goal was never adequately realized, partly because the Coombs test is not suitable for separating mixed populations of RBC and partly because the antisera were multispecific. However, Ray Owen will be gratified to know that this study was finally performed in our laboratory some ten years later in collaboration with Dr. Hans Balner (Primate Center, The Netherlands). Using our monospecific alloimmune blood typing reagents we were able to follow the proportion of the two RBC types in radiation chimeras as the recipients' cells gradually replaced those of the donors (unpublished).

It is interesting that Owen and Anderson (1962) attempted to produce antirhesus lysins in chickens, but they abandoned this approach because they observed that several samples of RBC that were negative in the hemolytic test with a given antiserum were nevertheless capable of absorbing out all of the antibodies from that antiserum. Workers in the field of histocompatibility are painfully aware of a similar phenomenon which they refer to as CYNAP (cytotoxicity negative, absorption positive), but we doubt if they are aware that Owen and Anderson had earlier observed its analogue, "LYNAP" (lysis negative, absorption positive), in the rhesus monkeys.

The early 1960's are historically significant in rhesus immunogenetics; not only did Owen and Anderson publish their paper in 1962, but just two years earlier, seven regional primate research centers were established by the NIH. Prior to this, genetic studies of nonhuman primates were practically impossible since pedigreed animals in breeding colonies were not available. Since that time, however, the genetics of nonhuman primates has attracted a growing interest, particularly in behavior and population studies. It is already clear that immunogenetic polymorphisms are key parameters in these and in other studies of nonhuman primates (Stone 1975, 1980).

At the Wisconsin Regional Primate Research Center (WRPRC), a large number of rhesus monkeys has been available for our immunogenetic research. From a foundation colony of about 1,000 feral monkeys obtained primarily from India, over 2,400 monkeys have been born at Wisconsin since 1955. Currently, WRPRC maintains about 1,000 monkeys (639 ♀♀ and 399 ♂♂) in the breeding colony. We also have available two troops that have been set up for the purpose of studying reproductive behavior. One troop contains 60 monkeys (8 mature males, 21 mature females, and 31 juveniles); the other contains 50 monkeys (2 mature males, 19 mature females, and 29 juveniles). In addition, we have been able to study a population of 302 rhesus born at the primate laboratory operated by the U.W. Psychology Department. Both parents of almost all these captive-born monkeys are known with certainty. There are many large sire families in our primate colonies; the largest single family in our center includes a male, 76 children, 67 grandchildren, and 8 great-grandchildren, and several other pedigrees extend over five generations. This large number of pedigreed rhesus has enabled us to confirm the mode of inheritance for most of our immunogenetic markers.

We have developed a computer data base system to collect and to analyze data on the rhesus population at our center. Currently, the data for each monkey include pedigree and phenotype information from 32 blood group factors representing 13 loci, and 4 electrophoretic polymorphisms. Our computer system also maintains inventory records. Analysis programs have been developed to solve disputed paternity cases, to screen for inconsistent pedigree and inheritance patterns, to search for maternal-fetal incompatibilities, and to generate pedigrees. Finally, this system will allow tests for linkage to be implemented routinely. This computer system greatly increases the accuracy and utility of our data and facilitates further collection of phenotype and pedigree information. We believe that it will serve as a prototype for record systems of other nonhuman primate colonies.

Our objective in this paper is to describe the major polymorphisms found in rhesus blood (the blood groups, electrophoretic polymorphisms and the major histocompatibility system) and to illustrate how we have used them in our laboratory to study a variety of biological questions.

## Blood Groups

Our laboratory has applied the classical immunogenetic approach—an approach to which Ray Owen has contributed significantly—to study the rhesus blood groups (Stone 1967). Initially, we immunized monkeys with blood from their offspring. Since rhesus monkeys do not possess allospecific, naturally occurring antibodies—a fact also reported by Owen and Anderson (1962)—intravenous alloimmunizations could be made without fear of transfusion reactions. The resulting immune sera were absorbed until they behaved as monospecific reagents. Our operational criterion for serological monospecificity was that each reactive blood sample had to be capable of absorbing out the antibodies against every other reactive sample. In other words, the presumed monospecific reagent could not be fractionated further by absorption with any sample of reactive blood cells. Although this criterion depends heavily on the source and the number of samples tested, it has proved very efficient as an adjunct to genetic tests for monospecificity. In general, the factors detected by monospecific reagents behaved as simple codominant Mendelian traits (as do practically all polymorphic immunogenetic traits). As each new blood group factor was discovered, it was tested for its relationship with every other factor. Suggestive evidence for association was sometimes obtained from 2 × 2 contingency tests. However, these tests often yield spurious results since associations may be due to many factors, such as nonrandom mating as a result of the population structure in rhesus monkey colonies (Duggleby et al. 1972). By having pedigreed monkeys, we have been able to study each pair of factors in families to determine if they were controlled by independent, closely linked, or allelic genes.

Because monkeys are extremely expensive to raise and to maintain, they are generally shared by several investigators. As a result, it is not always possible to obtain repeated blood samples from particular monkeys. To obviate this problem, we have stored frozen blood samples from more than 3,000 of our monkeys. In addition, we have developed a microtiter agglutination procedure that permits typing of extremely small quantities of blood cells (0.125% suspension) and greatly increases the dilution at which the blood typing reagents can be used (Sullivan et al. 1976). More recently we have discovered that the addition of Ficoll 400 (a synthetic, high-molecular weight polymer of sucrose and epichlorohydrin which greatly reduced the zeta potential) obviates the need for Coombs reagent to detect incomplete antibodies (unpublished). This technical advance eliminates the need for repeatedly washing and resuspending the cells, and it significantly increases the dilution at which some blood typing reagents can be used.

Table 1 summarizes the blood group systems described by our laboratory. We have developed 32 operationally monospecific reagents (agglutinins), 23 of which define 13 genetically independent blood group systems (loci). The other nine re-

**Table 1.** The Blood Group Systems of Rhesus Monkeys Detected by the Wisconsin Laboratory.

| Systems | No. of reagents | Detectable alleles | Phenotypes Number | Phenotypes Kinds | Genotypes Number | Genotypes Kinds |
|---|---|---|---|---|---|---|
| G | 6[a] | $G^1, G^2, G^3, G^4$ | 9 | $G_1$, $G_1G_3$, $G_1G_4$<br>$G_2$, $G_2G_3$, $G_2G_4$<br>$G_3$, $G_3G_4$<br>$G_4$ | 10 | $G^1/G^1, G^1/G^2, G^1/G^3, G^1/G^4$<br>$G^2/G^2, G^2/G^3, G^2/G^4$<br>$G^3/G^3, G^3/G^4$<br>$G^4/G^4$ |
| H | 2 | $H^1, H^2$ | 3 | $H_1$, $H_1H_2$, $H_2$ | 3 | $H^1/H^1, H^1/H^2, H^2/H^2$ |
| I | 2 | $I^1, I^2$ | 4 | $I_1$, $I_1I_2$<br>$I_2$, i | 6 | $I^1/I^1, I^1i, I^1/I^2$<br>$I^2/I^2, I^2/i, i/i$ |
| M | 3 | $M^1, M^2, M^3$ | 7 | $M_1$, $M_1M_2$, $M_1M_3$<br>$M_2$, $M_2M_3$<br>$M_3$, m | 10 | $M^1/M^1, M^1/m, M^1/M^2,$<br>$M^1/M^3, M^2/M^2, M^2/m,$<br>$M^2/M^3, M^3/M^3, M^3/m, m/m$ |
| N | 2 | $N^1, N^2$ | 4 | $N_1$, $N_1N_2$<br>$N_2$, n | 6 | $N^1/N^1, N^1/n, N^1/N^2$<br>$N^2/N^2, N^2/n, n/n$ |
| J, K, L, O<br>P, Q, R, S | 1 ea. | $J^1, 3K^1, L^1, O^1$<br>$P^1, Q^1, R^1, S^1$ | 2 ea. | $J_1$, j<br>$K_1$, k<br>etc. | 3 ea. | $J^1/J^1, J^1/j, j/j$<br>$K^1/K^1, K^1/k, k/k$<br>etc. |
| Unknown | 9 | reagents 31-39 | | — | — | — |

[a]Two of these reagents help distinguish among the different genotypes.

agents have not yet been studied sufficiently to determine whether or not they define new systems. Two systems (*G* and *H*) are "closed" with no recessive null alleles; thus the genotype can be inferred directly from the phenotype. All of the other systems contain a null allele, so pedigree data are usually required to determine accurately the genotype of a monkey from phenotypic data. Other blood group factors have been reported in rhesus by Moor-Jankowski and Socha (1978). Although we have not extensively compared their reagents with ours, it appears that most of them are multispecific. Very little genetic data concerning their factors are available, so no additional blood group loci have been identified using their reagents.

Table 2 illustrates the inheritance of several blood group systems in a rhesus sire family. The monkey numbered 342 is the father of AA51 and AA09, listed below their respective mothers. Since G2 and G3 are subtypes of G1, they behave as recessive to G1; thus the genotype of 096 cannot be determined for the *G* system; however, AA09 must be $G^1/G^2$, having inherited $G^2$ from his father and $G^1$ from his mother. Similarly, AA51 and AA09 must both have genotype $I^2/i$. Since AA09 has the null phenotype of the *M* system, the sire, 342, must be $M^3/m$. Careful analysis of these data can further elucidate the genotypes.

## Biochemical Polymorphisms

New technics for electrophoresis and isoelectric focusing, coupled with novel staining methods for localizing enzymes and other proteins after electrophoresis, have permitted great advances in the genetics of protein polymorphisms over the past 25 years. Only in the past decade, though, have these technics been extensively employed in studies of rhesus. In particular, the proteins in the serum and erythrocytes of rhesus have revealed a large array of genetic variability. Somatic cell hybridization technics have been used recently to localize 32 genes on 13 of the 21 rhesus chromosomes (Pearson et al. 1979).

A polymorphic locus can be defined as one for which the most common allele in a particular population has a frequency of less than 0.99 (Harris and Hopkinson 1972). Twenty-two such loci have been discovered among the serum or erythrocyte

**Table 2.** Genotypes of a Sire, His Mates, and Their Offspring.

| Animal | Abbreviated blood type | | | | |
|---|---|---|---|---|---|
| | G | H | I | L | M |
| ♂ 342 | $G^2/G^2$ | $H^1/H^2$ | $i/i$ | $l/l$ | $M^3/?$ |
| ♀ 068 | $G^2/G^4$ | $H^1/H^1$ | $I^2/?$ | $L^1/?$ | $M^3/?$ |
| AA51 | $G^2/G^2$ | $H^1/H^2$ | $I^2/?$ | $L^1/?$ | $M^3/?$ |
| ♀ 096 | $G^1/?$ | $H^1/H^1$ | $I^1/I^2$ | $l/l$ | $m/m$ |
| AA09 | $G^1/?$ | $H^1/H^1$ | $I^2/?$ | $l/l$ | $m/m$ |
| ♀ 035 | $G^2/G^4$ | $H^1/H^1$ | $I^1/?$ | $L^1/?$ | $m/m$ |
| W93 | $G^2/G^2$ | $H^1/H^1$ | $i/i$ | $l/l$ | $M^3/?$ |

proteins of rhesus (Table 3). This number has been derived from studies of rhesus from widely disparate localities; no single population of rhesus would be expected to exhibit all of these polymorphisms. At least 24 additional loci are thought to be monomorphic; i.e., they have exhibited no genetic variation in electrophoretic studies (Table 4).

It seems certain that many new polymorphisms will be discovered for the following reasons: First, some markers listed as monomorphic have been studied only in populations from a single geographic area; second, staining technics are now available for additional loci not yet surveyed in rhesus, and new staining technics for more enzymes are rapidly becoming available; third, the application of protein separation technics that have higher resolving power may enable new polymorphisms to be discovered. Indeed, when Donald Shreffler was a graduate student in Ray Owen's laboratory, he was unable to detect hemoglobin polymorphism in rhesus by electrophoresis (Owen and Anderson 1962); not until the advent of isoelectric focusing was an α-chain variant discovered (Basch 1972).

Biochemical polymorphisms have been used extensively to study the genetic composition of wild populations. In one study, blood was collected from 31 rhesus from Thailand, 32 from West Pakistan, 60 from China, and 82 from India. The proportion of the 29 loci that were polymorphic in the four populations ranged from 21% to 38%, close to the range typically observed in most animal species (Nozawa et al. 1977). Mean heterozygosity per individual ranged from 6% to 10%, again within the typical range of 5–15%. Hence rhesus are similar to most other animal species in the extent of their genetic variability.

A wealth of phenotypic data is available for many of the rhesus polymorphisms. The phenotypic frequencies are suggestive of autosomal codominant inheritance, which is expected by analogy with other mammalian species for which pedigree data have been accumulated. In our studies of rhesus monkeys, autosomal codominant inheritance for 6PGD, GPI, CA-C, and Tf has been unequivocally demonstrated (VandeBerg and Stone 1978a, 1978b, and unpublished). Genetic studies are important because intraspecific variation for a particular marker is occasionally caused by nongenetic factors. More than one isozyme geneticist has observed an apparent polymorphism, seemingly in Hardy-Weinberg equilibrium, only to discover that the three phenotypes were an artifact of stepwise degradation process.

Of all the genetic markers now used in rhesus, transferrin (Tf) is among the most valuable. Although Tf is polymorphic in many species, it rarely exhibits as many allelic forms with as high a level of heterozygosity as in rhesus. We have observed 11 allelic forms of Tf *(A, B, C, D', D, E, F'', F, G, H', H)* in feral rhesus imported from India, and two additional allelic forms *(D'', F')* have been described elsewhere (Beuttner-Janusch et al. 1974). The most common allele (*C*) had a gene frequency of 0.48 in our feral animals; three other alleles had frequencies greater than 0.05; and six more had frequencies greater than 0.01. Two hundred thirty-one of the 329 feral animals (70%) were heterozygous for Tf; the most common genotype *(C/C)* was shared by 23% of the population. Sixty-six genotypes are theoretically possible in our colony, and we have observed 46 of them. Thus the Tf system is very powerful for identifying individual monkeys.

**Table 3.** Polymorphic Enzymes and Proteins in Rhesus Detected by Electrophoretic Technics.

| Protein or polypeptide | Abbreviation | Blood component | Putative no. of alleles | References |
|---|---|---|---|---|
| 1. Acid phosphatase | ACP | RBC | 2 | Nozawa et al. 1977 |
| 2. Adenosine deaminase | ADA | RBC | 3 | Nozawa et al. 1977 |
| 3. α-Antitrypsin, protease inhibitor | Pi | serum | 2 | Omoto et al. 1970; Nozawa et al., 1977 |
| 4. Carbonic anhydrase B | CA-B | RBC | 3 | Tashian et al. 1971 |
| 5. Carbonic anhydrase C | CA-C | RBC | 2[a] | Nozawa et al. 1977 |
| 6. Complement component 3 | C3 | serum | 3 | Alper et al. 1971 |
| 7. Complement component 6 | C6 | serum | 3 | Hall and Alper 1977 |
| 8. NADH-diaphorase | DIA-A | RBC | 4 | Los and Meera Khan 1977 |
| 9. NADPH-diaphorase | DIA-B | RBC | 2 | Meera Khan and Balner 1972 |
| 10. Group-specific component | Gc | serum | 2 | Alper et al. 1971 |
| 11. Glucose-phosphate isomerase | GPI | RBC | 5[b] | Nozawa et al. 1977 |
| 12. Hemoglobin-α chain | Hb-α | RBC | 2 | Basch 1972 |
| 13. Isocitrate dehydrogenase | ICD | RBC | 3 | Ishimoto et al. 1974, Nozawa et al. 1977 |
| 14. Lactate dehydrogenase-A polypeptide | LDH-A | RBC | 2 | Nozawa et al. 1977 |
| 15. Malate dehydrogenase 1 | MDH-1 | RBC | 2 | Nozawa et al. 1977 |
| 16. Peptidase C | PEP-C | RBC | 2 | Meera Khan and Balner, 1972 |
| 17. Phosphoglucomutase 1 | PGM-1 | RBC | 3 | Nozawa et al. 1977 |
| 18. Phosphoglucomutase 2 | PGM-2 | RBC | 2 | Nozawa et al. 1977 |
| 19. Phosphogluconate dehydrogenase | 6PGD | RBC | 2[a] | Meera Khan and Balner 1972 |
| 20. Properdin factor B | Bf | serum | 6 | Ziegler et al. 1975 |
| 21. Thyroxin binding prealbumin | TBPA | serum | 2 | Weiss et al. 1971, Nozawa et al. 1977 |
| 22. Transferrin | Tf | serum | 13[c] | see Buettner-Janusch et al. 1974 |

[a]These alleles have been confirmed by extensive pedigree data (VandeBerg and Stone 1978a and unpublished).

[b]Two of these alleles have been confirmed by extensive pedigree data (VandeBerg and Stone 1978b).

[c]Ten of these alleles have been confirmed by extensive pedigree data (VandeBerg et al. 1980).

**Table 4.** Monomorphic Enzymes and Proteins in Rhesus.

| Protein or polypeptide | | Abbreviation | Blood component | References |
|---|---|---|---|---|
| 1. | Adenylate kinase 1 | AK-1 | RBC | Meera Kahn and Balner 1972 |
| 2. | Albumin | ALB | serum | Berg and Balner 1972 |
| 3. | Alkaline phosphatase | ALP | serum | Nozawa et al. 1977 |
| 4. | Amylase | AMY | serum | Nozawa et al. 1977 |
| 5. | Catalase | CAT | RBC | Kulkarni 1970 |
| 6. | Ceruloplasmin | Cp | serum | Nozawa et al. 1977 |
| 7. | Cholinesterase | ChEs | serum | Nozawa et al. 1977 |
| 8. | Esterase $A_1$ | $ESA_1$ | RBC | Nozawa et al. 1977 |
| 9. | Glucose-6-phosphate dehydrogenase | G6PD | RBC | Meera Khan and Balner 1972 |
| 10. | Glutamate oxaloacetate transaminase-cytoplasmic | GOT-1 | RBC | Meera Khan and Balner 1972 |
| 11. | Glyceraldehyde-3-phosphate dehydrogenase | GAPDH | RBC | Buettner-Janusch and Sockol 1977 |
| 12. | Glyoxalase I | GLO-I | RBC | VandeBerg et al., unpublished |
| 13. | Haptoglobin | Hp | serum | see Jolly and Barnicot 1966 |
| 14. | Hemoglobin-$\beta$ chain | Hb-$\beta$ | RBC | see Nute 1974 |
| 15. | Inorganic pyrophosphatase | PP | RBC | VandeBerg et al., unpublished |
| 16. | Lactate dehydrogenase-B polypeptide | LDH-B | RBC | Nozawa et al. 1977 |
| 17. | $\alpha_1$-Macroglobulin | $\alpha_2$ | serum | Nozawa et al. 1977 |
| 18. | Nucleoside phosphorylase | NP | RBC | Buettner-Janusch and Sockol 1977 |
| 19. | Peptidase A | PEP-A | RBC | Meera Khan and Balner 1972 |
| 20. | Peptidase B | PEP-B | RBC | Meera Khan and Balner 1972 |
| 21. | Phosphoglycerate kinase A | PGK-A | RBC | Meera Khan and Balner 1972 |
| 22. | Pyruvate kinase | PK | RBC | VandeBerg et al., unpublished |
| 23. | Superoxide dismutase 1 | SOD-1 | RBC | Meera Khan and Balner 1972 |
| 24. | Uridine monophosphate kinase | UMPK | RBC | VandeBerg et al., unpublished |

In one of the zoo troops previously mentioned, the proportion of homozygotes for Tf has almost doubled in less than two generations even though the gene frequencies have not changed. Furthermore, homozygotes for rare alleles have appeared. This illustrates the consequences of inbreeding in a closed population.

Equally provocative in our studies of rhesus transferrins is an aberrant segregation ratio in heterozygotes for the *C* and *D′* alleles (VandeBerg et al. 1980). The *C* allele was transmitted to 72 offspring, whereas the *D′* allele was transmitted to only 41 ($P < 0.01$). Aberrant ratios were observed in both sexes and could not be attributed to maternal-fetal incompatibilities. Segregation ratios for all other heterozygous genotypes did not differ significantly from 1:1. More detailed studies of this phenomenon are in progress.

## Allotypes

Rapacz (1978) has defined a low-density lipoprotein (LDL) polymorphism in rhesus monkeys. He has produced five alloimmune antisera (anti-Lmp1, 2, 3, 4, and 11) against lipoprotein fractions obtained by ultracentrifugation (density < 0.085 g/ml). All five typing sera behaved as monospecific reagents in double diffusion gel precipitation tests. Preliminary genetic studies of these allotypes indicate that they are controlled by autosomal codominant genes, but it is not known whether they are allelic or closely linked. Significantly, serum from an Lmp1 monkey never reacts with anti-Lmp11 unless the monkey is heterozygous ($Lmp^1/Lmp^{11}$), in which case the Lmp1 and Lmp11 specificities are carried on different molecules. In contrast, the serum from Lmp2, Lmp3, or Lmp4 monkeys also reacts with anti-Lmp11, and each of these specificities is carried on the same molecule along with Lmp11. This implies that each of the Lmp haplotypes can code for a unique specificity as well as for another one shared by many haplotypes in the series. Compatible with this notion is that anti-Lmp11 cross-reacts with all human and swine sera tested, whereas anti-Lmp1, 2, 3, and 4 do not. This remarkable immunogenetic model has been demonstrated for the LDL polymorphism of swine (Rapacz 1978), which may well be the paradigm for the LDL polymorphisms in humans and in other species.

At least two other lipoprotein polymorphisms have been detected by immunological technics in rhesus sera (Berg and Balner 1972). The Lp(a) lipoprotein is especially interesting because it has been suggested as a risk factor for coronary heart disease (Berg et al. 1974). About 57% of rhesus were classified as "reactors" in tests with antiserum against human Lp(a) antigen. Berg and his colleagues suggested that the presence of this antigen may be governed by an autosomal dominant gene, but others suggested that Lp(a) is a quantitative trait determined polygenically (Harvie and Schultz 1980; Albers et al. 1974). The other polymorphic lipoprotein antigen, Lt(a), was present in about 80% of rhesus screened with antihuman Lt(a) antiserum, but the reactions were difficult to score and genetic data were limited.

Our laboratory has attempted to define allotypes in rhesus monkeys using alloimmune precipitating sera. We have defined one system, A1, controlled by a dominant autosomal gene (unpublished). Preliminary immunoelectrophoretic analysis suggests that the A1 determinant is carried by a macroglobulin molecule. An immunoglobulin (IgG) allotype has been described in rhesus by Kruisbeek et al. (1974). We also have preliminary evidence for at least two new IgG allotypes (unpublished). Neither system is related to the human group specific component (Gc), which is also polymorphic in rhesus (Table 3).

## The Use of Immunogenetic Markers for Determination of Parentage

Using all of our 13 blood group systems and four electrophoretic polymorphisms (6GPD, GPI, CA-C, and Tf), we can detect over $1 \times 10^9$ different phenotypes representing about $1 \times 10^{11}$ possible genotypes. Obviously, these markers provide a very powerful tool for identification and parentage determination (Sullivan et al 1977, 1978).

An illustration of the use of blood typing in assigning parentage is shown in Table 5. This case involved a study of mating behavior in which a female was placed with a group of four males. On the basis of observed mating behavior, the dominant male was initially recorded as the father of the offspring. However, our blood typing revealed that this infant must have come from a father who had the alleles $I^1$ and $N^2$ and either of the alleles $G^1$ or $G^4$. The dominant male had none of these alleles; among the four possible fathers, only one had $I^1$, $N^2$, and $G^4$ and therefore must have been the father.

Using all 17 of our immunogenetic loci, we can exclude a randomly chosen male as the father with a theoretical probability of over 90%. Our actual success rate, however, is slightly lower. The parentage of 52 of 161 monkeys born at the WRPRC in 1978 were disputed; 44 of 145 monkeys were disputed in 1979 (Table 6). This large number is not to be construed as the result of poor husbandry at our primate center. Almost all of the monkeys whose parentage was unknown belonged to groups housed together in three-generation "nuclear families." We were able to assign a single male to 43 of the 52 and 35 of the 44 cases for a combined success rate of 81%.

**Table 5.** Example of Disputed Parentage Case in Rhesus Monkeys Solved by Blood Typing.

| Animal | (I.D.) | Abbreviated blood type | | | | |
|---|---|---|---|---|---|---|
| Offspring | | $G^1/G^4$ | $I^1/I^1$ | $k/k$ | $L^1/-$ | $N^2/n$ |
| Mother | | $G^1/G^4$ | $i/i$ | $k/k$ | $L^1/-$ | $n/n$ |
| Listed father | Fa | $G^2/G^2$ | $i/i$ | $k/k$ | $L^1/-$ | $n/n$ |
| Alternative fathers: | 1 | $G^2/G^4$ | $i^1/-$ | $k/k$ | $l/l$ | $N^2/-$ |
| | 2 | $G^4/G^4$ | $i/i$ | $k/k$ | $L^1/l$ | $N^2/n$ |
| | 3 | $G^1/G^2$ | $i/i$ | $k/k$ | $L^1/l$ | $N^2/n$ |

*(Source: Adapted from Stone (1980) with permission.)*

**Table 6.** Disputed Parentage Cases.

| Colony | Years | Number born | Disputed | Solved (%) |
|---|---|---|---|---|
| WRPRC | 1978 | 161 | 52 | 43 (0.83) |
| WRPRC | 1979 | 145 | 44 | 35 (0.80) |
| Zoo | 1973–79 | 155 | 155 | 77 (0.50) |

In our colony of monkeys at the Madison zoo, we have been able to resolve only 77 (50%) of the 155 paternity cases. These are two troops of monkeys that have remained isolated and under observation since 1972. The relatively low success rate in these troops is due to the large number and close familial relationships between the breeding males. In one zoo troop, we also compared the actual parentage determined by the immunogenetic parameters with the observed mating behavior. Although the dominant male was observed in about 80% of all matings, he actually fathered less than 50% of the infants born into the troop. The moral of the story is, "Monkey see, monkey not necessarily do!" Preliminary data also suggest avoidance of mother-son matings, independent of age and rank restrictions. Both of these sociogenetic behaviors will effect the amount of inbreeding occurring within the troop. We have observed also a distinct age effect in mating; each year, dominant males contribute less to both the number of observed matings and the number of offspring. (We are indebted to Ms. Debbie Yoshahara for her cooperation in these studies.)

## The Major Histocompatibility Complex of Rhesus (RhLA)

Remarkable progress has been made in defining the MHC of rhesus monkeys by Balner and his co-workers (see Balner 1980 for extensive references). The present status of the rhesus MHC can best be illustrated by the genetic map shown in Figure 1. Although the exact position of these genes is uncertain, this map represents the best estimate at this time.

The close similarity of this gene family to that of humans, mice, and other mammalian species is immediately obvious. At the left end of the map, we find the *Bf* locus, which codes for a factor (B) that is involved with complement function and the sequence of events leading to eventual lysis of a cell by the alternate complement pathway. The *Ir* locus (previously called "GL") controls the humoral antibody response to synthetic linear copolymers of glutamic acid and lysine (or alanine) and conjugates with the hapten dinitrophenol. Just to the right of *Ir* is the *D/DR* region. The *D* locus is analogous to the *D* locus of humans and the *LAD* loci of mice, which are involved in the mixed lymphocyte culture (MLC) reactions. The *DR* region of rhesus encodes for eight antigens that are analogous to the *Ia* antigens of mice and B-cell antigens of humans. As in humans, there are also *Ia*-like antigens (*Ia'*, *Ia"*) which are not controlled by the *DR* locus; the *Ia'* gene maps within the

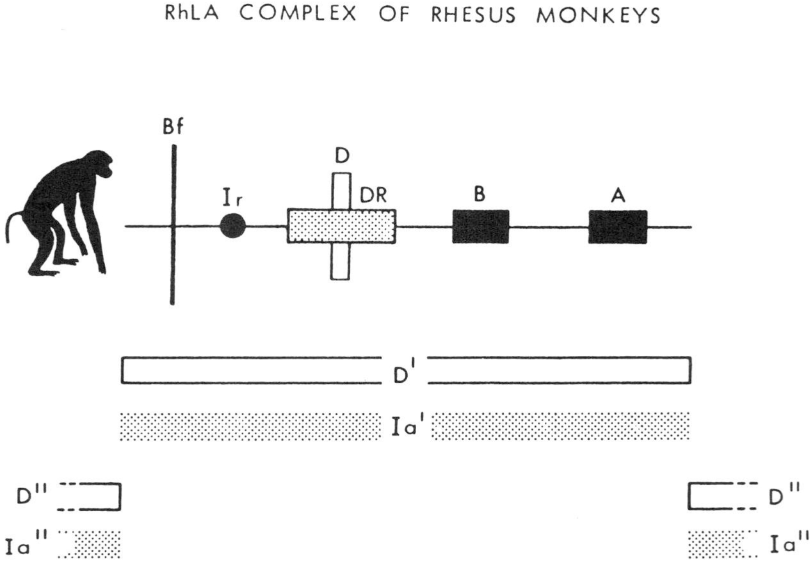


**Figure 1.** A model for the RhLA of rhesus monkeys. (Adapted from Balner (1980) with permission.)

*RhLa* region, whereas the *Ia''* gene does not. Similarly, there are D-like antigens (D′) that map within the region, and some (D″) that do not. It is not known if the D or *DR* antigens of rhesus are identical or merely strongly associated. Finally, the *A* and *B* loci encode for 13 and 14 serologically defined antigens, respectively. These loci, along with the Tf locus, are the most polymorphic systems known in rhesus.

## Why Don't Rhesus Monkeys Get Hemolytic Disease?

Curiously, the Rh factor responsible for hemolytic disease of the newborn in humans is not detectable as an alloantigenic factor on RBC of rhesus monkeys. Moreover, hemolytic disease of the rhesus monkey has never been clearly demonstrated. Our studies (Sullivan et al. 1976; Stone et al. 1980; Stong et al. unpublished) have shown that transplacental alloimmunization occurs frequently (in about 20% of all pregnancies) but hemolytic disease does not result. Neither have we been able to induce any symptoms of hemolytic disease by hyperimmunizing pregnant females with the blood of their mates or by passively immunizing newborn monkeys with high-titered incompatible antiserum; newborn monkeys whose cells are heavily coated with antibodies escape the disease.

By following the survival of $^{51}$Cr-labeled erythrocytes that were injected into rhesus recipients, we have shown that rhesus possess two mechanisms that eliminate allogeneic erythrocytes: sequestration followed by phagocytosis by reticuloendothelial cells, primarily in the liver and spleen; and intravascular hemolysis involving the activation of complement. In general, however, rhesus erythrocytes coated with alloantibodies usually survive as well as uncoated cells in the rhesus circulation. Robin Stong in our laboratory has developed an *in vitro* model for erythrocyte sequestration using monocytes isolated from rhesus monkey peripheral blood. Apparently rhesus monocytes possess trypsin-sensitive Fc receptors. Moreover, the *in vitro* results parallel the *in vivo* results; that is, antibody-coated RBC that are rapidly cleared from the circulation *in vivo* are also readily phagocytized *in vitro* and those that are not cleared *in vivo* are not phagocytized *in vitro*. Recently we discovered some hyperimmune monkeys that rapidly sequester transfused incom-

**Figure 2.** The "phylogency" of rhesus immunogenetics.

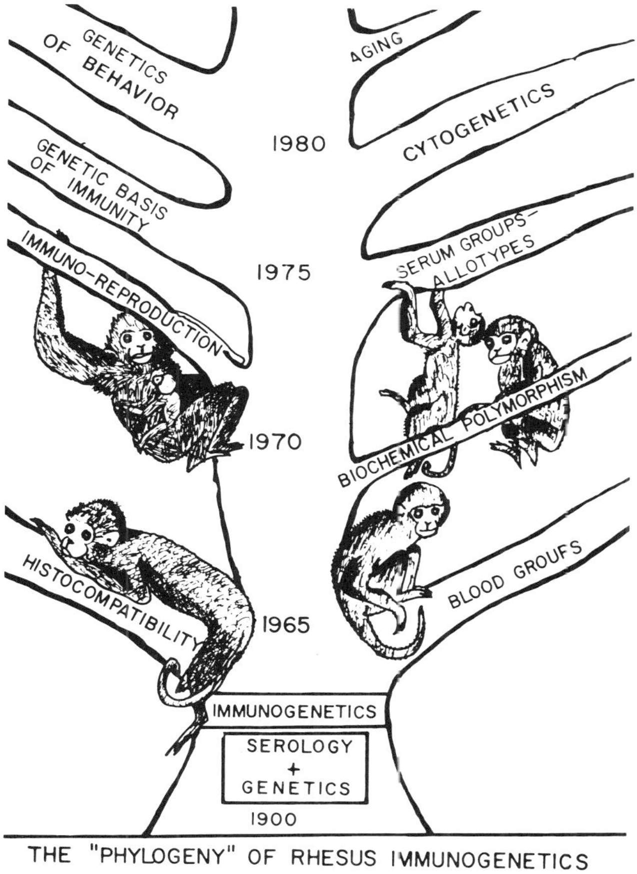

patible cells. As might be expected, RBC coated with these antibodies *in vitro* and then injected into a third nonimmune recipient were also rapidly cleared. These results suggest that the vast majority of rhesus monkeys produce a class of alloimmune antibodies against RBC that do not opsonize cells. It may be that these antibodies belong to an IgG subclass that cannot interact with the Fc receptors on phagocytic cells. In humans, $IgG_2$ and $IgG_4$ do not bind to the Fc receptors on monocytes, and $IgG_4$ does not fix complement at the C1 step. Antibody specificity and the corresponding antigen density on the rhesus RBC may also play a role. We are currently investigating these hypotheses.

## Summary and Conclusions

More than 40 polymorphic loci have been identified in rhesus. The 17 loci routinely typed in our laboratory can define more than a trillion different phenotypes in this species. Obviously, if all 40 loci were typed, the total genetic variability would be astronomical.

In 1962 Owen and Anderson stated, "A great deal of further diversity remains to be identified within this species and awaits only the investment of effort in this direction." It would appear that this prediction has been more than amply fulfilled and that—as shown in Figure 2—the rhesus monkey is firmly perched on the immunogenetic tree. Finally, we might add that this is what happens when Ray Owen "monkeys" around!

ACKNOWLEDGMENTS

We wish to thank Mr. Charles Blystad, Ms. Kathy Benforado, Mr. Kent McLaughlin, and Ms. Lesleigh Luttrell for excellent technical assistance and our graduate student, Robin Stong, for permission to cite her thesis work on hemolytic disease of the newborn. We also thank Mr. Charles Kahn for his expert computer services and Dr. Mary Ruth McMahan for drawing to our attention several key references in Table 3. Of course, we are grateful to all who have contributed to the immunogenetic profile of the rhesus monkey.

This paper is number XVI in a series entitled "Immunogenetic Studies of Rhesus Monkeys." The work described from our laboratory was supported in part by NIH Grants HD 07385, RR-00167, HD 11200, and RR01216.

This work represents paper No. 2441, Laboratory of Genetics, and No. 20-003, Wisconsin Regional Primate Research Center.

## References

Albers, J.J., Wahl, P., and Hazzard, W.R. 1974. Quantitative genetic studies of the human plasma Lp(a) lipoprotein. Biochem. Genet. 11:475–486.

Alper, C.A., Robin, N.I., and Refetoff, S. 1971. Genetic polymorphism in rhesus C3 and Gc globulin. J. Immunol. 107:96–98.

Balner, H. 1980. The DR system of rhesus monkeys; a brief review of serology, genetics and relevance to transplantation. Transplant. Proc. 12, in press.

Basch, R.S. 1972. Hemoglobin polymorphism in the rhesus macaque. Nature New Biol. 238:238–240.

Berg, K. and Balner, H. 1972. Serum protein polymorphisms in rhesus monkeys. Medical Primatology Proceeding of 3rd Conference on Experimental Medicine and Surgery in Primates. Lyon, 1972, Part 1. Basel: Karger, pp. 327–335.

Berg, K., Dahlen, G., and Frick, M.H. 1974. Lp(a) lipoprotein and pre-$B_1$-lipoprotein in patients with coronary heart disease. Clin. Genet. 6:230–235.

Buettner-Janusch, J., Mason, G.A., Dame, L., Buettner-Janusch, V., and Sade, D.S. 1974. Genetic studies of serum transferrins of free-ranging rhesus macaques of Cayo Santiago, *Macaca mulatta* (Zimmerman, 1780). Am. J. Phys. Anthrop. 41:217–232.

Buettner-Janusch, J. and Sockol, M. 1977. Genetic studies of free-ranging macaques of Cayo Santiago. 1. Description of the population and some non-polymorphic red cell enzymes. Am. J. Phys. Anthropol. 47:371–374.

Duggleby, C.R., Duggleby, W.F., and Stone, W.H. 1972. Immunogenetic studies of rhesus monkeys. III. Statistical analysis of relationships between antigenic (blood group) factors of rhesus monkeys. Transplant. Proc. 4:113–117.

Hall, J.E. and Alper, C.A. 1977. Genetic polymorphism of the sixth component of complement (C6) in the rhesus monkey. J. Immunol. 119:253–255.

Harris, H. and Hopkinson, D.A. 1972. Average heterozygosity per locus in man: An estimate based on the incidence enzyme polymorphisms. Ann. Hum. Genet. 36:9–20.

Harvie, N.R. and Schultz, J.S. 1970. Studies of Lp-lipoprotein as a quantitative genetic trait. Proc. Nat. Acad. Sci. U.S.A. 66:99–103.

Ishimoto, G., Kuwata, M., and Shotake, T. 1974. Polymorphism of red cell NADP dependent isocitrate dehydrogenase in macaque monkeys. J. Anthrop. Soc. Nippon 82:52–58.

Jolly, C.J. and Barnicot, N.A. 1966. Serum and red-cell protein variations of the Celebes black ape. Folio Primatol. 4:206–220.

Kruisbeek, A.M., Radl, J., and Swart, A.C.W. 1974. Allotypic markers of rhesus monkey immunoglobulin. G. Eur. J. Immunol. 4:448–450.

Kulkarni, A.R. 1970. A survey of genetic variants in six erythrocyte proteins in *Macaca mulatta* and *Macaca nemestrina*. Ph.D. Thesis, University of Wisconsin—Madison.

Los, W.R.T. and Meera Khan, P. 1977. Red cell NADH-diaphorase polymorphism in *Macaca mulatta*. J. Hum. Evol. 6:227–230.

Meera Khan, P. and Balner, H. 1972. Polymorphic enzymes in rhesus monkeys and chimpanzees. In Medical Primatology. Proceedings of the 3rd Conference on Experimental Medicine and Surgery in Primates. Lyon, 1972, Part 1, Basel: Karger, pp. 363–371.

Moor-Jankowski, J. and Socha, W.W. 1978. Blood groups of macaques: A comparative study. J. Med. Primatol. 7:136–145.

Nozawa, J. Shotake, T., Ohkura, Y., and Tanabe, Y. 1977. Genetic variations within and between species of Asian macaques. Japan. J. Genet. 52:15–30.

Nute, P.E. 1974. Multiple hemoglobin a-chain loci in monkeys, apes, and man. Ann. N.Y. Acad. Sci. 241:39–60.

Omoto, K., Harada, S., Tanaka, T., Nigi, H., and Prychodko, W. 1970. Distribution of the electrophoretic varients of serum alpha$_1$-antitrypsin in six species of macaques. Primates 11:215–228.

Owen, R.D. and Anderson, D.R. 1962. Blood groups in rhesus monkeys. Ann. N.Y. Acad. Sci. 97:4–8.

Pearson, P.L., Roderick, T.H., Davisson, M.T., Garver, J.J., Warburton, D., Lalley, P.A., and O'Brien, S.J. 1979. Report of the committee on comparative mapping. Cytogenet. Cell Genet. 25:82–95.

Rapacz, J. 1978. Lipoprotein immunogenetics and atherosclerosis. Am. J. Med. Genet. 1:377–405.

Stone, W.H. 1967. Immunogenetics of type-specific antigens in animals. In Advances in Immunogenetics. T.J. Greenwalt, ed. Philadelphia: J.P. Lippincott, pp. 173–215.

Stone, W.H. 1975. Immunogenetic studies of rhesus. In The Rhesus Monkey. G.H. Bourne, ed. New York: Academic Press, pp. 304–336.

Stone, W.H. 1980. How might immunogenetics relate to cardiovascular disease in nonhuman primates? In The Use of Nonhuman Primates in Cardiovascular Disease. S.S. Kalter, ed. Austin: University of Texas Press, pp. 387–425.

Stone, W.H., Stong, R., Blazkovec, A., Blystad, C., and Houser, W.D. 1980. Animal models of erythrocyte destruction (Why aren't the erythrocytes of the newborn rhesus monkey destroyed by maternal antibodies?) In Immunobiology of the Erythrocyte. The 11th American Red Cross Sci. New York: A.R. Liss, Inc., in press.

Sullivan, P.T., Blystad, C., and Stone, W.H. 1976. Immunogenetic studies of rhesus monkeys. VII. A simple hemagglutination technique for blood typing. J. Immunol. Methodol. 14:31–36.

Sullivan, P.T., Blystad, C., and Stone, W.H. 1977. Immunogenetic studies on the rhesus monkey *(Macaca mulatta)*. XI. Use of blood groups in problems of parentage. Lab. Ann. Sci. 27:348–351.

Sullivan, P.T., Blystad, C., and Stone, W.H. 1978. Immunogenetic studies of rhesus monkeys. X. The O, P. Q, R and S blood group systems. Immunogenetics. 7:125–130.

Sullivan, P.T., Duggleby, C., Blystad, C., and Stone, W.H. 1976. Immunogenetic studies of rhesus monkeys. V. Transplacental immunization in *Macaca mulatta* as a result of maternal-fetal blood group incompatibility. Immunogenetics. 3:473–479.

Tashian, R.W., Goodman, M., Headings, V.E., Desimone, J., and Ward, J.H. 1971. Genetic variation and evolution in the red cell carbonic anhydrase isozymes of macaque monkeys. Biochem. Genet. 5:183–200.

VandeBerg, J.L., Benforado, K., and Stone, W.H. 1980. Transferrin polymorphism in rhesus monkeys. Isozyme Bull. 13:107.

VandeBerg, J.L., and Stone, W.H. 1978a. Biochemical genetics of macaques. I. 6-Phosphogluconate dehydrogenase polymorphism in *Macaca mulatta* and *Macaca speciosa*. Biochem. Genet. 16:373–377.

VandeBerg, J.L., and Stone, W.H. 1978b. Biochemical genetics of macaques. II. Glucose-phosphase isomerase polymorphism in rhesus monkeys. Biochem. Genet. 16:691–694.

Weiss, M.L., Goodman, M., Prychodko, W., and Tanaka, T. 1971. Species and geographic distribution patterns of the macaque prealbumin polymorphism. Primates 12:75–80.

Ziegler, J.B., Alper, C.B., and Balner, H. 1975. Properdin factor B and histocompatibility loci linked in rhesus monkeys. Nature 254:609–610.

# SECTION II:

# Genetics of Immune Responsiveness

Hildemann, ed. Frontiers in Immunogenetics

# The Arrangement, Rearrangement, and Diversification of Antibody Genes

Henry Huang, Stephen Crews, and Leroy Hood

*Division of Biology, California Institute of Technology, Pasadena, California*

## Introduction

The immunoglobulin genes require DNA rearrangements for their proper expression. These gene rearrangements operate upon the genetic elements that code for the immunoglobulin variable region (*V* Genes) as well as upon the constant region genes (*C* genes).

That immunoglobulin genes undergo rearrangements during differentiation was first proposed by Dreyer and Bennett (1965). Results from subsequent genetic, serological, and protein structural studies were all consistent with their proposal. The results may be summarized as follows (Figure 1; Hood et al. 1975). Immunoglobulins are coded for by three multigene families on separate autosomes. The κ and λ families code for the immunoglobulin L-chain, and the H family codes for the H-chain. Each family consists of a cluster of *V* genes separate from one or a few *C* genes. During B-cell development a *V* gene is joined to a *C* gene to create a functional gene.

The advent of recombinant DNA technology made it possible to examine the immunoglobulin genes directly. Besides confirming the prevailing picture of immunoglobulin genes, these molecular studies revealed hitherto unsuspected features of this fascinating system. We will first describe the two different kinds of DNA rearrangements operating upon antibody genes and then discuss how DNA rearrangements as well as other mechanisms contribute to generate a potentially enormous immunoglobulin repertoire. The existence of many genetic elements, which together code for a single polypeptide, requires a clear definition of the terminology. We define a "segment" to mean a protein sequence, and define a "gene segment" to mean the DNA that encodes the segment. We retain the terms "*V* gene" and

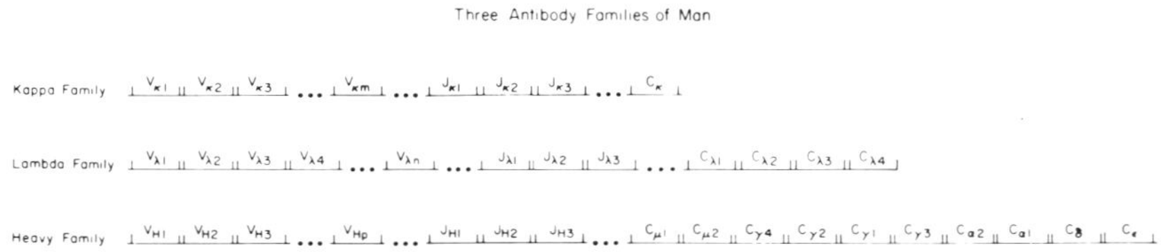


**Figure 1.** The antibody multigene families.

"*C* gene" to mean those genetic elements that encode the antibody *V* region and *C* region, respectively. Thus the $V_\lambda$ gene is composed of $L_\lambda$, $V_\lambda$, and $J_\lambda$ gene segments, which encode for the $L_\lambda$, $V_\lambda$, and $J_\lambda$ segments, respectively. The $V_\lambda$ and $J_\lambda$ segments together make up the *V* region of the mature λ polypeptide chain. The $C_\lambda$ gene encodes the λ constant region.

## V-J Joining

Tonegawa and his colleagues (Brack and Tonegawa 1977; Brack et al. 1978; Bernard et al. 1978) first showed that $V_\lambda$ and $C_\lambda$ genes are separate in the germline and are joined during B-cell differentiation (Figure 2). In the germline the $V_\lambda$ and $C_\lambda$ genes are separated by a stretch of DNA of unknown size. The $L_\lambda$ gene segment codes for a leader peptide sequence, similar to the leader peptides of most secretory proteins, which is used to extrude the nascent polypeptide through the endoplasmic reticulum membrane and into the cisternae (Blöbel and Dobberstein 1975). It is removed from the mature polypeptide (Milstein et al. 1972). The $L_\lambda$ gene segment

**Figure 2.** Top: Germline arrangement of λ genes. Bottom: λ genes in a differentiated plasma cell.

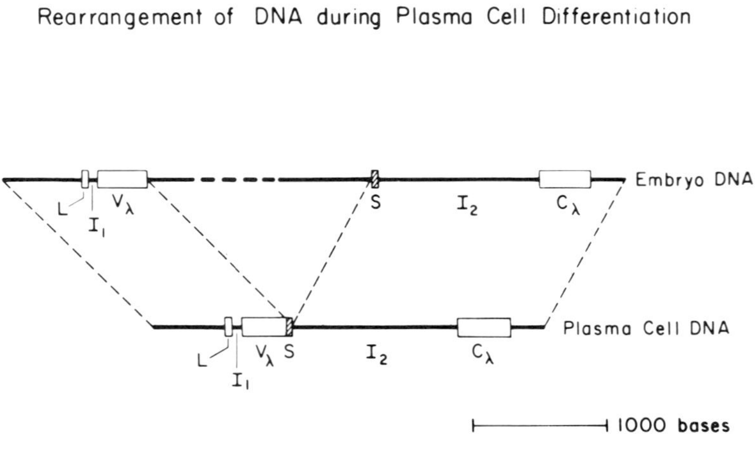

is separated from the $V_\lambda$ gene segment by a small stretch of intervening sequence. The $V_\lambda$ gene segment codes for most of the λ chain *V* region, including the first and second hypervariable regions. The third hypervariable region is coded for by the 3′ end of the $V_\lambda$ segment, and by a separate $J_\lambda$ (joining) gene segment which is located 5′ to the $C_\lambda$ gene. During B-cell differentiation, V-J joining fuses, through a site-specific recombination event, the 3′ end of the $V_\lambda$ gene segment to the 5′ end of the $J_\lambda$ gene segment to form a contiguous coding sequence. The intervening DNA is believed to be looped out and deleted during the V-J joining event. There are conserved palindromic sequences 3′ to the *V* gene segment and 5′ to the *J* gene segment (Bernard et al. 1978; Sakano et al. 1979) which are likely to be recognition sites used in the apposition and fusion of the *V* and *J* gene segments (Figure 3). The joined structure, termed the *V* gene, can then be transcribed. The primary transcript is processed to remove the intervening sequences between $L_\lambda$ and $V_\lambda$ gene segments and between the $J_\lambda$ gene segment and the $C_\lambda$ gene to give the mature mRNA which contains an uninterrupted polypeptide coding sequence. An identical type of V-J joining event occurs in the κ family (Seidman et al. 1979; Sakano et al. 1979). We will see later that the *H* family has an extra level of complexity with regard to DNA rearrangements.

## $C_H$ Switch

During B-cell differentiation, the first immunoglobulin made belongs to the IgM class (Raff 1976; Cooper et al. 1976). Subsequently, the cell may switch to make immunoglobulin of a different class (e.g., IgG or IgA). The same *V* regions of both

**Figure 3.** A site-specific model for V-J joining. *p* denotes conserved palindromic sequences.

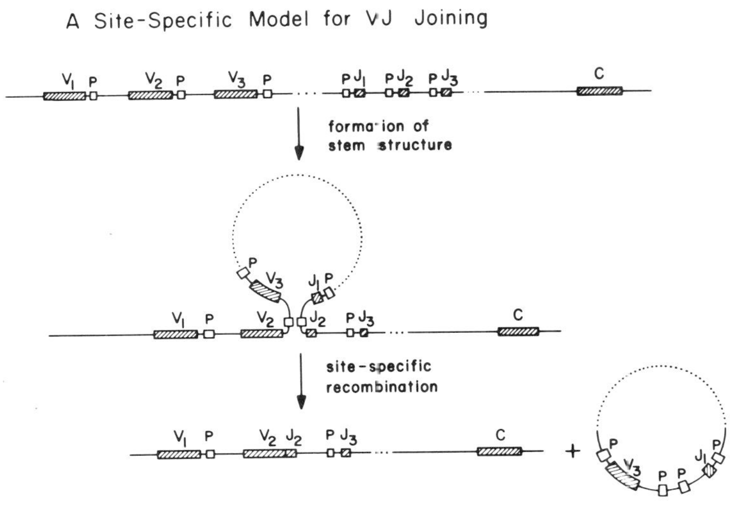

H and L-chains are retained during the class or $C_H$ switch (Pernis et al. 1976). Davis et al. (1980) compared the functional α chain gene of the M603 (IgA-producing) myeloma with its germline counterparts. As expected, the germline M603 $V_H$ gene segment and the $C_\alpha$ gene are represented in the mature gene (Figure 4), but in addition there is a stretch of DNA which is located 5′ to the $C_\mu$ gene in the germline, and which includes the $J_H$ gene segment. A mechanistic explanation of the tripartite α gene is that the $V_H$ gene segment initially was joined to a $J_h$ gene segment located 5′ to the $C_\mu$ gene (Figure 5). At this stage the cell would synthesize IgM molecules. Subsequently, a $C_H$ switch brought in the $C_\alpha$ gene, which displaced the $C_\mu$ gene. (The intervening DNA is believed to be deleted in this process (Honjo and Kataoka 1978; Cory and Adams 1980; Coleclough et al. 1980; Rabbitts et al. 1980; Yaoita and Honjo 1980a,b).) This results in the tripartite nature of the α gene, and the cell now synthesizes IgA molecules. Since all known $J_H$ gene segments are located 5′ to the $C_\mu$ gene (Early et al. 1980; Sakano et al. 1980), this suggests that all B-cells must at least transiently synthesize IgM molecules but can then synthesize molecules of other classes upon $C_H$ switching.

There are therefore two kinds of DNA rearrangements found in immunoglobulin families. One joins $V$ and $J$ gene segments to give functional immunoglobulin $V$ genes. The second operates only upon the H-chain family, and it allows the sequential combination of any antigen-binding activity coded by a $V_H$ gene with a number of different effector functions coded by the various $C_H$ genes.

## Sources of Immunoglobulin Diversity

There are three major sources of immunoglobulin diversity. First, there are multiple germline genes. Second, owing to the separate nature of immunoglobulin genes, the individual gene segments may be joined in a combinatorial fashion, thus gen-

**Figure 4.** The M603 heavy chain gene and its germline counterparts.

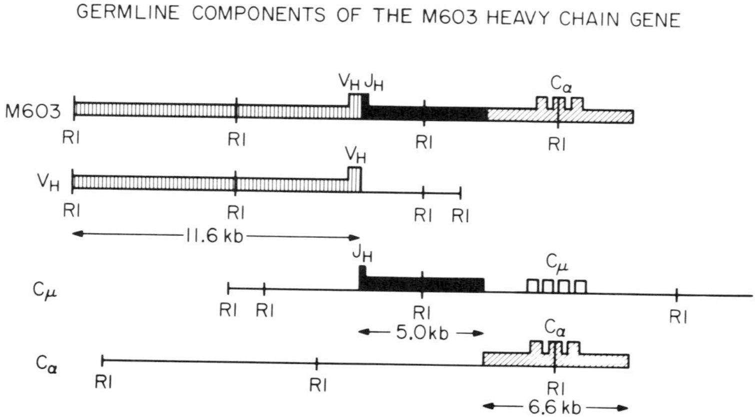

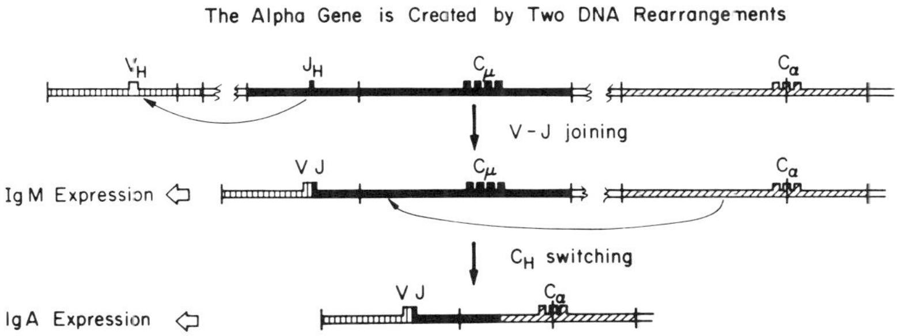


**Figure 5.** The tripartite structure of the M603 heavy chain gene is created by two DNA rearrangements.

erating many possible coding sequences and therefore many possible antigen-binding sites. For example, if each of three *V* gene segments can join to three *J* gene segments, nine *V-J* combinations result. Third, the joining event is nonprecise and creates junctional diversity (Figure 6). For example, the terminal CCC codon of the $V_\kappa$ gene segment may join to the initial TGG codon of the $J_\kappa$ gene segment to create a hybrid codon CGG which codes for arginine. Similarly, joining may occur at other sites, thus giving the different protein sequences shown in Figure 6. Note that deletion or insertion of a codon may also occur. The only constraint in this nonprecise joining is that frame shifts will not be expressed as functional polypeptides.

## Diversity of κ Chains

Amino acid sequence studies have shown that κ-chains may be divided into groups, each group being defined as sequences that differ by three or fewer residues over the amino-terminal 23 residues (Potter 1978; Weigert et al. 1978). The members of one group can be clearly distinguished from members of a different group. Altogether some 30–50 $V_\kappa$ groups are known (Hood et al. 1974; Weigert and Riblet 1976). Studies at the DNA level showed that each group is coded by up to ten germline genes (Rabbitts 1977; Lenhard-Schuller et al. 1978; Seidman et al. 1978; Valbuena et al. 1978). Thus there may be 300–500 $V_\kappa$ gene segments. It is also known that there are four $J_\kappa$ gene segments. Therefore one source of κ-chain diversity is in having multiple *V* and *J* germline gene segments.

Each of the 300–500 $V_\kappa$ gene segments may join with any of the four $J_\kappa$ gene segments. Thus combinatorial joining makes possible some 1,200–2,000 $V_\kappa$ region sequences.

In Figure 6 we showed how nonprecise joining may increase κ-chain diversity. When κ protein sequences are examined, every one of the possibilities shown in Figure 6 is observed (Weigert et al. 1980). Thus junctional diversity generated by nonprecise recombinatorial events appears to be an important somatic mechanism

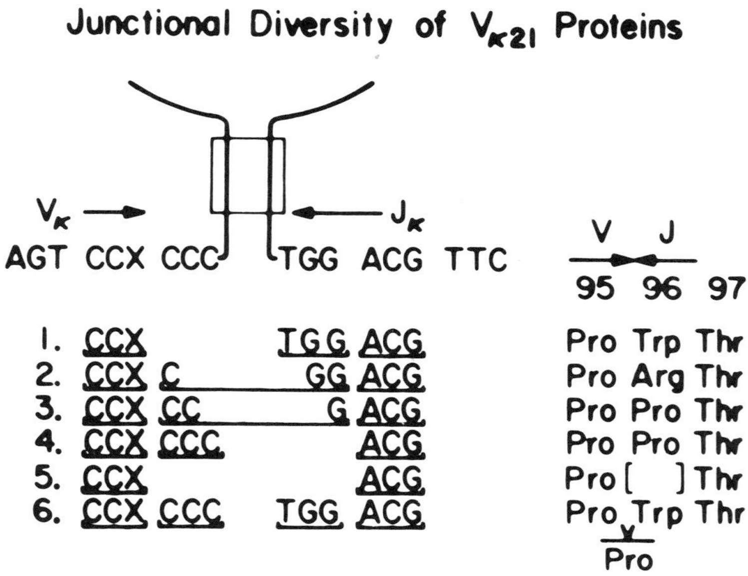


**Figure 6.** Generation of junctional diversity by nonprecise joining. Pro = proline, Trp = tryptophan, Thr = threonine, Arg ≥ arginine, X = any base.

for generating diversity. This is a functionally significant increase in diversity, since the site of joining codes for residues inside the antigen-binding cleft and diversity at this position will influence antigen binding (R. Poljak, personal communication).

In summary, the diversity of κ-chains originates from three types of diversification mechanisms: germline genes, combinatorial V-J joining, and somatic junctional diversification.

## H-Chain Diversity

The sources of H-chain diversity are similar to that found for κ-chains, but with an extra level of complexity. There are at least 20 $V_H$ groups (Barstad et al. 1978). Again, we and others using Southern hybridization have found up to 10 $V_H$ gene segments for each group (Figure 7; Kemp et al. 1979), so there may be 200 or more $V_H$ gene segments. There are four known $J_H$ gene segments, all situated 5′ to the $C_\mu$ gene (Early et al. 1980; Sakano et al. 1980). Thus, one source of H-chain diversity is multiple germline gene segments.

Unlike the $V_L$ gene which consists of fused $V_l$ and $J_L$ gene segments, the $V_H$ gene results from a fusion of $V_H$, $D$ (diversity), and $J_H$ gene segments. The existence of the $D$ gene segment was predicted from protein sequence data (Figure 8; Schilling et al. 1980). $V_H$ region protein sequences can be divided into three segments: $V_H$, $D$, and $J_H$. When the $V_H$ segments are arranged by $V_H$ groups, it is clear that $V_H$,

$D$, and $J_H$ may be independently sorted into different combinations. For example, the $V_H$ segment of M104E is distinct from the $V_H$ segment of H8, yet they have the same $J_H$ segment; while M104E and Hdex4 have identical $V_H$ segments, the $J_H$ segments are different. The $D$ segments show the greatest diversity, both in sequence replacements and in size, which can be two (or less) to 14 residues long (Figure 8; Schilling et al. 1980; Early et al. 1980; Sakano et al. 1980).

Direct evidence for $D$ gene segments was provided by DNA sequence studies comparing a complete M603 myeloma $V_H$ gene with its germline counterparts, the $V_H$ and $J_H$ gene segments (Early et al. 1980). It was found that a region of the M603 $V_H$ gene cannot be contributed by either the $V_H$ or the $J_H$ gene segments (Figure 9). Thus this $D$ gene segment must come from elsewhere. There are two

**Figure 7.** Southern hybridization of S107 $V_H$ gene probe to EcoR1 digested BALB/c liver DNA (left) and to Charon 4A clones (right), which contain $V$ genes which hybridize to the S107 probe.

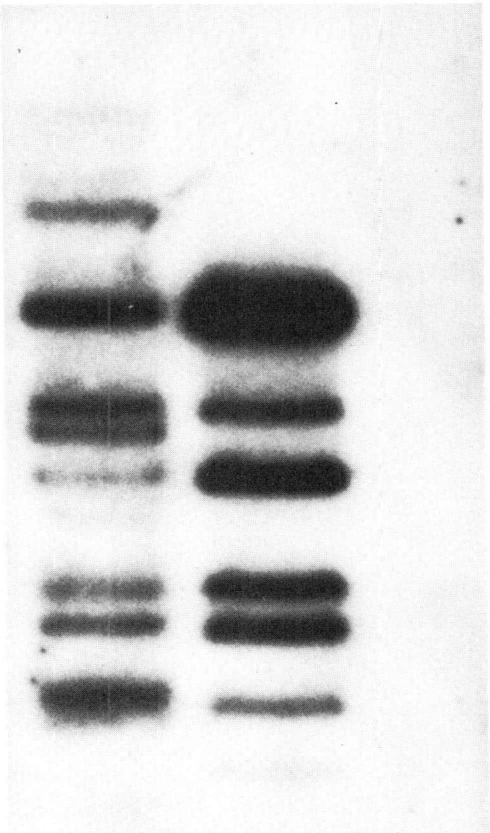

| Protein | Specificity | V segment | D segment | J segment |
|---|---|---|---|---|
| M104E, Hdex16 | 1,3 Dextran | SSSTAYMQLNSLTSEDSAVYYCARD | YD | WYFDVWGAGTTVTVSS |
| Hdex8 | " | ---G--------------------- | -- | ---------------- |
| J558 | " | ------------------------- | RY | ---------------- |
| Hdex9 | " | --N--F------------------- | RY | ---------------- |
| Hdex10 | " | ------------------------- | VN | ---------------- |
| Hdex6 | " | ------------------------- | SH | ---------------- |
| Hdex3 | " | ------------------------- | R- | ---------------- |
| Hdex17 | " | ------------------------- | SY | ---------------- |
| Hdex7 | " | ------------------------- | A- | ---------------- |
| Hdex12 | " | ------------------------- | GN | ---------------- |
| Hdex2 | " | ------------------------- | NY | ---------------- |
| Hdex1 | " | ------------------------- | NY | H----V---------- |
| Hdex5 | " | ------------------------- | SN | Y---Y--Q---L---- |
| Hdex4 | " | ------------------------- | K- | Y---Y--Q---L---- |
| Hdex15 | " | ------------------------- | SS | Y---Y--Q---L---- |
| Hdex18 | " | ------------------------- | RY | Y---Y--Q---L---- |
| Hdex11 | " | ------------------------- | -- | F---Y--Q---L---- |
| Hdex13 | " | ------------------------- | GN | YR-AY--Q--L--- |
| Hdex14 | " | ------------------------- | RY | YAM-Y--Q--S----- |
| T15,S63,S107,Y5236 | Phosphorylcholine | -Q-IL-L-M-A-RA--T-I------ | YYGSSY | --------------- |
| H8 | " | -Q-IL-L-M-A-RA--T-I------ | ---N-- | ---------------- |
| W3207 | " | -Q-IL-F-M-A-RA--T-I-----N | --KYDL | --V---------- |
| M603 | " | -Q-IL-L-M-A-RA--T-I-----N | ----T | ------------- |
| M167 | " | -Q-VL-L-M-A-RA--T-T---T-- | ADYGDSYF | G------------ |
| M511 | " | -Q-IL-L-M-A-RA--T-I------ | GDYG-SY | --------------- |
| A4 | 2,1 Levan | -K-SV-L-M-N-RA--TGI---TTG | [ ] | [ ]-AY--Q--L--- |
| E109 | " | -K-SVFL-M-N-RA--TGIH--TTG | [ ] | [ ]-AY--Q--L--- |
| U61 | " | -K-SV-L-M-N-RA--TGI---TTG | [ ] | [ ]-AY--Q--L-P- |
| A47N | " | -K-SV-L-M-N-RA--T-I---STG | [ ] | [ ]-AY--Q--L--- |
| M315 | DNP | -ENQFFLK-D-V-[ ]T-T----G- | NDH | L---Y--Q---L--- |
| M21 | Unknown | PKN-LFL-MT--R---T-M-----H | GNYPW | YAM-Y--Q--S----- |
| M173 | Unknown | AKN-L-L-MSKVR---T-L-----S | PY | YAM-Y--Q--S----- |
| T601 | Galactan | AKN-L-L-MSKVR---T-L-----G | GYY | G--------------- |
| X44 | " | AKN-L-L-MSKVR---T-L-----L | H-- | G-AAY--Q--L----A |
| X24 | " | AKN-L-L-MSKVR---T-L-----G | --- | G---Y--Q---L---- |
| J539 | " | AKNSL-L-MSKVR---T-L-----L | H-- | G-NAY--Q--L----A |

**Figure 8.** A compilation of $V_H$ region protein sequences.

possibilities for the origin of the *D* gene segment. First, it may be created by some enzymatic activity when the $V_H$ and $J_H$ gene segments are joined. Second, it constitutes a bona fide germline gene segment. We favor the latter possibility. The strongest evidence for a germline origin of *D* is that identical *D*-coded sequences have been found in four independently isolated myelomas (T15, S107, S63, Y5236; see Figure 8). This makes it unlikely that *D* is due to enzymatic activities. This is

**Figure 9.** Comparison of M603 $V_H$ gene and the corresponding germline $V_H$ and $J_H$ gene segments.

DNA SEQUENCES OF MYELOMA AND GERMLINE $V_H$ AND $J_H$ GENE SEQUENCES

| | 96 | 97 | 98 | 99 | 100a | 100b | 100c | 100d | 100e | 100f | 100g | 100h | 101 | 102 | 103 |
|---|---|---|---|---|---|---|---|---|---|---|---|---|---|---|---|
| Amino-acid sequence | C | A | R | D/N | -/Y | -/Y | -/G | -/S | -/T | -/W | -/Y | -/F | -/D | -/V | -/W |
| Germline $V_{HPC}$ | TGT | GCA | AGA | GAT | GCA | CAC | AGT | GAG | AGG | ACG | TCA | TTG | TGA* | GCC | CAG |
| M603 $V_H J_H$ | TGT | GCA | AGA | AAT | TAC | TAC | GGT | AGT | ACC | TGG | TAC | TTC | GAT | GTC | TGG |
| Germline $J_{HPC}$ | ACA | GAG | GCA | GAA | CAG | AGA | CTG | TGC | TAC | TGG | TAC | TTC | GAT | GTC | TGG |

$V_H$ (96–99) | $D_H$ (100a–100d) | $J_H$ (100e–103)

because in the absence of a proliferation of enzymes the same enzyme must perform seemingly conflicting tasks. It must show fidelity in creating the same *D* gene segment in four separate instances, yet must be able to generate the extremely diverse sequence and length heterogeneity generally found in the *D* gene segment.

Our model of *V-D-J* joining is shown in Figure 10 (Early et al. 1980). The $V_H$ gene segment is joined to the *D* gene segment which in turn is joined to a $J_H$ gene segment located 5′ to the $C_\mu$ gene.

It is readily apparent that the use of a third gene segment will greatly increase the diversity arising from combinatorial joining. Thus, for example, with 200 $V_H$, five *D*, and four $J_H$ gene segments, 4,000 different *VDJ* combinations are possible.

The existence of two junctional bounderies in the $V_H$ genes doubles the potential junctional diversity when compared to the single junctional boundary in $V_L$ genes. An example of junctional diversity is shown in Figure 11. Insertions, deletions, and hybrid codons are found exactly at the borders between $V_H$ and *D* and between *D* and $J_H$ gene segments in the three myeloma mRNA sequences shown (Early et al. 1980). An interesting observation is that *D*-$J_H$ junctional insertion or deletion can involve more than one codon (Early et al. 1980; Sakano et al. 1980). Although this has not been seen at the $V_L$-$J_L$ junction, it cannot yet be excluded as an additional possibility for diversification.

An additional source of diversity may occur because of the presence of two junctional boundaries (Hood and Early 1980). Joining that causes a frame shift in the *D* at one boundary may be compensated for at the other boundary by an appropriate joining that restores the reading frame. Thus a given *D* gene segment may be used in any of all three reading frames, provided that no termination codons are embedded in it.

Since the *D* gene segment codes for sequences lying in the antigen-binding cleft (R. Poljak, personal communication), germline diversity of *D* and junctional diversity at the *D* boundaries will contribute to diversity of antigen-binding sites.

In summary, the diversity of $V_H$ genes originate from three types of mechanisms. First, there are multiple germline $V_H$ and $J_H$ (and probably *D*) gene segments.

**Figure 10.** A model for the joining of $V_H$, *D*, and $J_H$ gene segments. Flanking arrows denote conserved palindromic sequences.

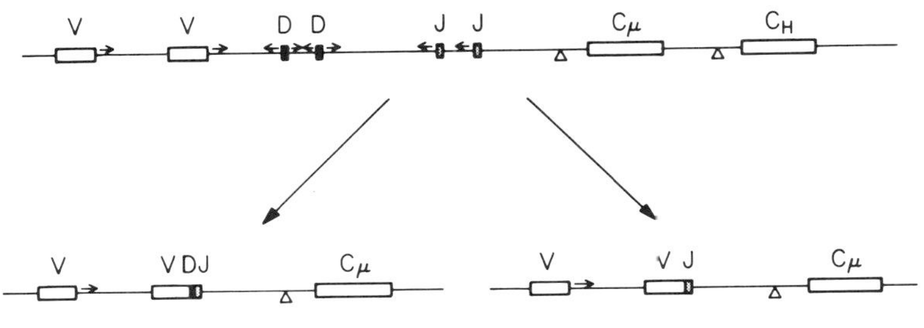

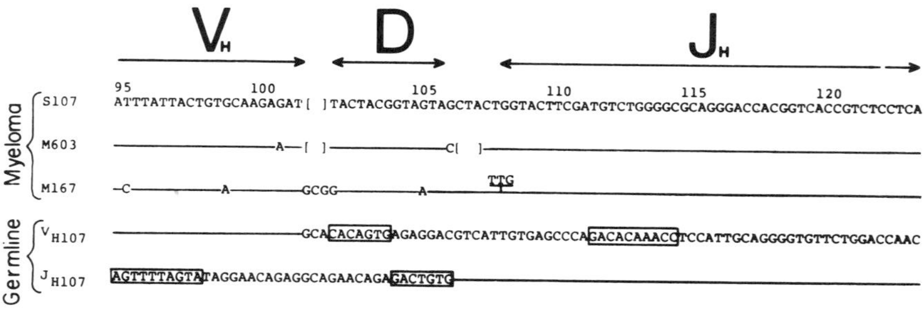

**Figure 11.** Junctional diversity at the $V_H$-$D$ and $D$-$J_H$ junctional boundaries. Three myeloma mRNA sequences are compared.

Second, there is the combinatorial joining of $V_H$ to $D$ to $J_H$ gene segments. Third, there is extensive junctional diversity at the $V_H$-$D$ and the $D$-$J_H$ junctions.

We have seen that the split genes of immunoglobulins make possible the coding of an enormous protein diversity by a relatively few gene segments. One wonders if the strategies of split genes, combinatorial mechanisms, and junctional diversity are also used in other biological systems (Hood et al. 1977).

ACKNOWLEDGMENTS
This research was supported by NSF Grant PCM 76-81546 and USPHS Grant AI 09072. S.C. is supported by NIH training Grant GM 07616. All experiments involving recombinant organisms were conducted in accordance with the NIH Guidelines on Recombinant DNA.

## References

Barstad, P., Hubert, J., Hunkapiller, M., Goetze, A., Schilling, J., Black, B., Eaton, B., Richards, J., Weigert, M., and Hood, L. 1978. Immunoglobulins with hapten-binding activity: Structure-function correlations and genetic implications. Eur. J. Immunol. 8:497–503.

Bernard, O., Hozumi, N., Tonegawa, S. 1978. Sequences of mouse immunoglobulin light chain genes before and after somatic changes. Cell 15:1133–1144.

Blöbel, G. and Dobberstein, B. 1975. Transfer of proteins across membranes. I. Presence of proteolytically processed and unprocessed nascent immunoglobulin light chains on membrane-bound ribosomes of murine myeloma. J. Cell Biol. 67:835–851.

Brack C., Hirama, M., Lenhard-Schuller, R., and Tonegawa, S. 1978. A complete immunoglobulin gene is created by somatic recombination. Cell 15:1–14.

Brack, C. and Tonegawa, S. 1977. Variable and constant parts of the immunoglobulin light chain gene of a mouse myeloma cell are 1250 nontranslated bases apart. Proc. Nat. Acad. Sci. U.S.A. 74:5652–5656.

Coleclough, C., Cooper, C., and Perry, R.P. 1980. Rearrangement of immunoglobulin heavy chain genes during B-lymphocyte development as revealed by studies of mouse plasmacytoma cells. Proc. Natl. Acad. Sci. U.S.A. 77:1422–1426.

Cooper, M.D., Kearney, J.F., Lydyard, P.M., Grossi, C.E., and Lawton, A.R. 1976. Studies of generation of B-cell diversity in mouse, man and chicken. Cold Spring Harbor Symp. Quant. Biol. 41:139–145.

Cory, S. and Adams, J.M. 1980. Deletions are associated with somatic rearrangements of immunoglobulin heavy chain genes. Cell 19:37–51.

Davis, M.M., Calame, K., Early, P.W., Livant, D.L., Joho, R., Weissman, I.L., and Hood, L. 1980. An immunoglobulin heavy-chain gene is formed by at least two recombinational events. Nature 283:733–739.

Dreyer, W.J. and Bennett, J.C. 1965. The molecular basis of antibody formation: A paradox. Proc. Natl. Acad. Sci. U.S.A. 54:864–868.

Early, P., Huang, H., Davis, M., Calame, K., and Hood, L. 1980. An immunoglobulin heavy chain variable region gene is generated from three segments of DNA: $V_H$, $D$ and $J_H$. Cell 19:981–992.

Honjo, T. and Kataoka, T. 1978. Organization of immunoglobulin heavy chain genes and allelic deletion model. Proc. Natl. Acad. Sci. U.S.A. 75:2140–2144.

Hood, L., Barstad, P., Loh, E., and Nottenburg, C. 1974. Antibody diversity: An assessment. In The Immune System. Genes, Receptors, Signals. E.E. Sercarz, A.R. Williamson, and C.F. Fox, eds. New York: Academic Press, pp. 119–139.

Hood, L., Campbell, J.Y., and Elgin, S.C.R. 1975. The organization, expression, and evolution of antibody genes and other multigene families. Ann. Rev. Genet. 9:305–353.

Hood, L. and Early, P. 1980. Organization and rearrangements of heavy chain variable region genes. In Immunoglobulin Genes and B-Cell Differentiation. J.R. Battisto and K.L. Knight, eds. New York: Elsevier North Holland pp. 7–15.

Hood, L., Huang, H.V., and Dreyer, W.J. 1977. The area-code hypothesis: The immune system provides clues to understanding the genetic and molecular basis of cell recognition during development. J. Supramol. Struct. 7:531–559.

Kemp, D.J., Cory, S., and Adams, J.M. 1979. Cloned pairs of variable region genes for immunoglobulin heavy chains isolated from a clone library of the entire mouse genome. Proc. Natl. Acad. Sci. U.S.A. 76:4627–4631.

Lenhard-Schuller, R., Hohn, B., Brack, C., Hirama, M., and Tonegawa, S. 1978. DNA clones containing mouse immunoglobulin κ-chain genes isolated by *in vitro* packaging into phage λ coats. Proc. Natl. Acad. Sci. U.S.A. 75:4709–4713.

Milstein, C., Brownlee, G.G., Harrison, T.M., and Mathews, M.B. 1972. A possible precursor of immunoglobulin light chains. Nature New Biol. 239:117–120.

Pernis, B., Forni, L., and Luzzati, A.L. 1976. Synthesis of multiple immunoglobulin classes by single lymphocytes. Cold Spring Harbor Symp. Quant. Biol. 41:175–183.

Potter, M. 1978. Antigen-binding myeloma proteins of mice. Adv. Immunol. 25:141–212.

Rabbitts, T.H. 1977. A molecular hybridization approach for the determination of the immunoglobulin V-gene pool size. Immunol. Rev. 36:29–50.

Rabbitts, T.H., Forster, A., Dunnick, W., and Bentley, D.L. 1980. The role of gene deletion in the immunoglobulin heavy chain switch. Nature 283:351–356.

Raff, M.C. 1976. Development and modulation of B-lymphocytes: Studies on newly formed B-cells and their putative precursors in the hemopoietic tissues of mice. Cold Spring Harbor Symp. Quant. Biol. 41:159–162.

Sakano, H., Hüppi, K., Heinrich, G., and Tonegawa, S. 1979. Sequences at the somatic recombination sites of immunoglobulin light chain genes. Nature 280:288–294.

Sakano, H., Maki, R., Kurosawa, Y., Roeder, W., and Tonegawa, S. 1980. The two types of somatic recombination necessary for generation of complete immunoglobulin heavy chain genes. Nature 286:676–683.

Schilling, J., Clevinger, B., Davie, J.M., and Hood, L. 1980. Amino acid sequence of homogeneous antibodies to dextran and DNA rearrangements in heavy chain *V* region gene segments. Nature 283:35–40.

Seidman, J.G., Leder, A., Edgell, M.H., Polsky, F., Tilghman, S.M., Tiemeier, D., and Leder, P. 1978. Multiple related immunoglobulin variable-region genes identified by cloning and sequence analysis. Proc. Natl. Acad. Sci. U.S.A. 75:3881–3885.

Seidman, J.G., Max, E.E., and Leder, P. 1979. A κ-immunoglobulin gene is formed by site-specific recombination without further somatic mutation. Nature 280:370–375.

Valbuena, O., Marcu, K.B., Weigert, M., and Perry, R.P. 1978. Multiplicity of germline genes specifying a group of related mouse κ-chains with implications for the generation of immunoglobulin diversity. Nature 276:780–784.

Weigert, M., Gatmaitan, L., Loh, E., Schilling, J., and Hood, L. 1978. Rearrangement of genetic information may produce immunoglobulin diversity. Nature 276:785–790.

Weigert, M., Perry, R., Kelley, D., Hunkapiller, T., Schilling, J., and Hood, L. 1980. The joining of *V* and *J* gene segments creates antibody diversity. Nature 283:497–499.

Weigert, M. and Riblet, R. 1976. Genetic control of antibody variable regions. Cold Spring Harbor Symp. Quant. Biol. 41:837–846.

Yaoita, Y. and Honjo, T. 1980a. Deletion of immunoglobulin heavy chain genes accompanies the class switch rearrangement. Biomed. Res., 1:164–175.

Yaoita, Y. and Honjo, T. 1980b. Deletion of immunoglobin heavy chain genes from expressed allelic chromosome. Nature 286:850–853.

Hildemann, ed. Frontiers in Immunogenetics

# Regulation of Memory B-Cell Development and Expression

Leonore A. Herzenberg, Takeshi Tokuhisa, F. Timothy Gadus, Samuel J. Black[1], and Leonard A. Herzenberg

*Department of Genetics, Stanford University School of Medicine, Stanford, California*

## Introduction

Contributing this chapter has a special significance for me in that it provides an opportunity to acknowledge formally Ray Owen's influence in shaping my career. Since I've never had any official academic connection with Ray, few people know even that our paths have crossed. Nonetheless, I first learned about antigens, antibodies, and the power of immunogenetic methods as an auditor in his course and, because of his encouragement, I published some years later my first paper in immunology (Herzenberg and Gonzales 1962).

This came about as follows: While working as a half-time technician in my husband's laboratory shortly after we came to Stanford University, I collected a series of observations demonstrating maternal immunization to paternal antigens in the mouse. I considered these studies an amusing side project; however, when I described them to Ray, he took the work quite seriously and suggested that I publish what I had found. I demurred, pointing out that I didn't have a bachelor's degree and didn't see myself as a publishing scientist. Ray then countered by saying (rightly) that degrees as such were irrelevant and that if I was going to do research I should be prepared to put it into a journal of record. "Otherwise," he said, "you're just wasting your time."

Duly chastened, but also very pleased that Ray thought these studies were publishable, I wrote up what I had done. That paper, published nearly 20 years ago, constituted the first link in a chain of studies that eventually led (through allotype suppression) to the work I shall describe here on the regulation of memory B-cell

[1]Current address: International Laboratory for Research on Animal Diseases, P. O. Box 30709, Nairobi, Kenya.

development and expression. Thus it is perhaps understandable that I consider Ray "my professor" and am pleased at the opportunity to thank him for launching me on a life's activity that I have thoroughly enjoyed.

I am also pleased to be able to record here what may have been one of Ray's earliest forays into the education and encouragement of women in science, an area in which he has distinguished himself recently at Caltech. Ray will always be better known and appreciated for his own scientific achievements; but his quiet, behind-the-scenes activity in helping young people realize their potential has multiplied his effectiveness many times over, much to the benefit of us all.

Turning now to scientific matters: My co-authors join me for the remainder of this chapter, in which we first summarize our work describing the antigen-dependent differentiation of memory B-cells and the mechanisms that control the development of high-affinity memory populations and then move to a description of a newly recognized regulatory mechanism that, we have shown (Herzenberg et al. 1980a), can be induced to selectively suppress the expression of individual IgG memory B-cell clones according to the isotype, allotype, and combining-site commitment (specificity and affinity) of the clone. This "hapten-specific" mechanism, which can suppress production of all the lowest affinity antibody in a heterogeneous response, may also be active (as indicated later) in immune response *(Ir)* gene control and immunologic tolerance.

## Regulation of Memory B-Cell Development

B-cell memory development can be characterized as an antigen-stimulated increase in precursors of antibody-forming cells (afc) for a given antigen and, especially with time and repeated antigenic stimulation, a selective expansion of high affinity precursors (Burnet 1957; Siskind and Benacerraf 1969). These two events, namely memory generation and affinity maturation, have generally been considered to be different manifestations of the same ongoing selection-expansion process; however, our recent studies (Herzenberg et al. 1980b; Black et al. 1980) demonstrate that they occur at different stages during memory development and can be regulated independently. In addition, these studies suggest that the presence or absence of surface IgD receptors may play a crucial role in determining the potential for affinity maturation in memory populations.

Memory B-cells were shown some time ago to carry surface IgG immunoglobulins that indicate the isotype and allotype commitment of these cells with respect to the antibodies their progeny afc will produce Okumura et al. 1976; Mason 1976). These memory B-cells also sometimes carry surface IgD immunoglobulins expressed on the "virgin" B-populations from which the memory cells were drawn (Mason 1976). Both $IgD^+$ and $IgD^-$ B-cells from primed donors give rise to adoptive IgG memory responses.

The $IgD^+$ memory cells are precursors of $IgD^-$ memory cells; however, $IgD^+$ memory populations can persist indefinitely in primed donors, either as a major or minor portion of the total memory cell pool. The relative proportions of $IgD^+$ and

$IgD^-$ memory cells in a given animal are determined by the strength of the priming stimulus and the availability of T-cell help to support differentiation from $IgD^+$ to $IgD^-$ (Herzenberg et al. 1980b).

$IgD^+$ memory cells taken from donors primed under a variety of conditions always give rise to predominantly low-affinity adoptive responses while their progeny $IgD^-$ memory cells in the same donors uniformly give rise to higher-affinity responses characteristic of secondary responses to strong antigenic stimuli (Herzenberg et al. 1980b). These data, which support and extend conclusions from our earlier studies (Black et al. 1978, Okumura et al. 1976b), indicate that affinity maturation initiates with the emergence of the $IgD^-$ memory population and proceeds mainly, if not exclusively, within this population thereafter. Thus the transition from early ($IgD^+$) to mature ($IgD^-$) memory is required for the development of high affinity response.

The affinity differential between early and mature memory populations does not appear to be due to selective differentiation of higher affinity $IgD^+$ memory cells into the $IgD^-$ memory pool. The selective forces responsible for affinity maturation therefore appear to operate mainly in mature memory cell populations that have already lost IgD receptors; or, stated conversely, little or no selection toward high affinity memory appears to occur among memory cells that retain IgD receptors (Herzenberg et al. 1980b).

In discussing these findings, we have suggested that the IgD receptors themselves are responsible for maintaining early memory populations at a lower average affinity than $IgD^-$ populations in the same animal. The IgD receptors, we argue, serve to increase the antigen-binding capacity of lower affinity memory cells. Accordingly, these cells can survive, expand, and differentiate (to $IgD^-$) at antigen concentrations that select against expansion of low-affinity memory cells no longer carrying IgD receptors. When antigen is limiting, $IgD^-$ memory populations will be selectively expanded to higher average affinities, whereas coexisting $IgD^+$ populations will retain their initial affinity profile.

This hypothesis suggests that mechanisms regulating expression and loss of IgD receptors are central to the adaptability of the immune system in its response to invading pathogens. Two related roles can be envisioned for the IgD receptors in this regard. First, they extend the lower boundary of the affinity range of early memory cell populations induced by a given antigenic stimulus and therefore broaden the diversity of responses obtainable from these populations. Second, they support the persistence of low-affinity memory populations under conditions where antigen becomes limiting and eventually disappears. These persisting populations then serve as a diversely reactive reservoir from which mature memory populations can be drawn. This can yield higher affinities either for the original antigen or, more importantly, for related antigens that the animal may subsequently encounter. Thus the existence of IgD receptors on early memory cells maintains the full range of responsiveness despite ongoing selective expansion of (mature) memory populations to produce antibodies with high combining affinities for individual antigens. The flexibility inherent in such an organizational system, we believe, could be expected to account for the evolutionary development of IgD receptors and the regulatory capabilities that support operation of the system.

Our data (Herzenberg et al. 1980b) also bears on the roles played by helper T-cells during memory development. Earlier studies have shown that affinity maturation is regulated by the availability of helper T-cells. Gershon and Paul (1971) demonstrated a marked reduction in the capacity for development of high-affinity responses in T-depleted animals reconstituted with limiting T-cell doses. We have shown an apparently similar impairment in affinity maturation in the Igh-1b* memory population in mice depleted (by allotype suppressor T-cells) of the helper T-cells required specifically to help 1b* allotype B-cells (Okumura et al. 1976b). We have also shown that the failure in affinity maturation in allotype-suppressed mice is due to the selective inability of the suppressed environment to support a normal transition from an $IgD^+$ population to a predominantly $IgD^-$ population (Herzenberg et al. 1980b). These studies, coupled with the demonstration that carrier-specific helper T-cells are required for tbe expansion of $IgD^-$ memory populations (Black et al. 1980), provide a partial understanding of the mechanisms through which T-cells regulate memory B-cell development and thus regulate the quality as well as the quantity of antibody responses.

## Regulation of Memory B-Cell Expression: the Hapten-Specific Regulatory System

Affinity maturation in memory B-cell populations, however, does not necessarily assure the production of high affinity antibody. As we have recently shown (Herzenberg et al. 1980a), a partial suppression of antihapten responses can be routinely generated. The production of high affinity IgG antibody is specifically suppressed while memory expansion and maturation is allowed to proceed normally. This suppression often persists through multiple hapten-carrier stimulations; however, it can also be reversed or its induction prevented by appropriate protocol modifications.

The effector mechanism responsible for this suppression is hapten-specific and is closely intertwined with the mechanisms responsible for allotype and idiotype suppression, and for the control of individual IgG isotype and allotype representation in IgG responses. In addition, carrier-specific suppression and perhaps genetic non-responsiveness appears to be mediated through the hapten-specific system. Thus we see this system, which has gone unrecognized as such until now, as perhaps the central regulatory mechanism in the humoral response.

This view is consistent with the properties of the theoretical regulatory cell interaction circuits we have recently described. The core regulatory circuit in this

*Our previous allotype notation is replaced here by a new notation system recently agreed upon by investigators in the field (Green 1979). Igh-1a and Igh-1b (previously called Ig-1a and Ig-1b) are allotypes of $IgG_{2a}$ isotype immunoglobulins; Igh-4a and Igh-4b are $IgG_1$ allotypes; and Igh-5a and Igh-5b are IgD allotypes. For simplicity, these allotypes will subsequently be referred to as 1a, 1b, etc., in the text.

model, for example, displays both idiotype and allotype/isotype specificity and can thus provide both hapten-specific and Ig-specific regulation. Furthermore, auxiliary regulatory circuits sensitive to antigen and other environmental stimuli may initially induce the core circuit into either a suppression or help mode. A shift from one configuration to the other, when changes occur in the environment, provides a potentially rational explanation for some of the more puzzling properties of hapten-specific regulation. Although the induction of hapten-specific suppression by exposure of carrier-primed mice was not predicted by the circuits as drawn, and although our studies on hapten-specific suppression were not initiated as a test for this model, they have yielded data which fulfill several of its key theoretical predictions.

**Figure 1.** Carrier-priming prevents hapten-carrier stimulation of antihapten antibody responses. (BALB/c × SJL)$F_1$ hybrids were used for these experiments. BALB/c and BAB/14 mice showed similar results. Data for Igh-1a ($IgG_{2a}$) allotype anti-DNP responss are shown in this figure. Protocol and assay details are described in the legend for Table 1. (●-●-●) primed with 100 μg KLH at −6 weeks; (▲-▲-▲) no prior antigenic exposure.

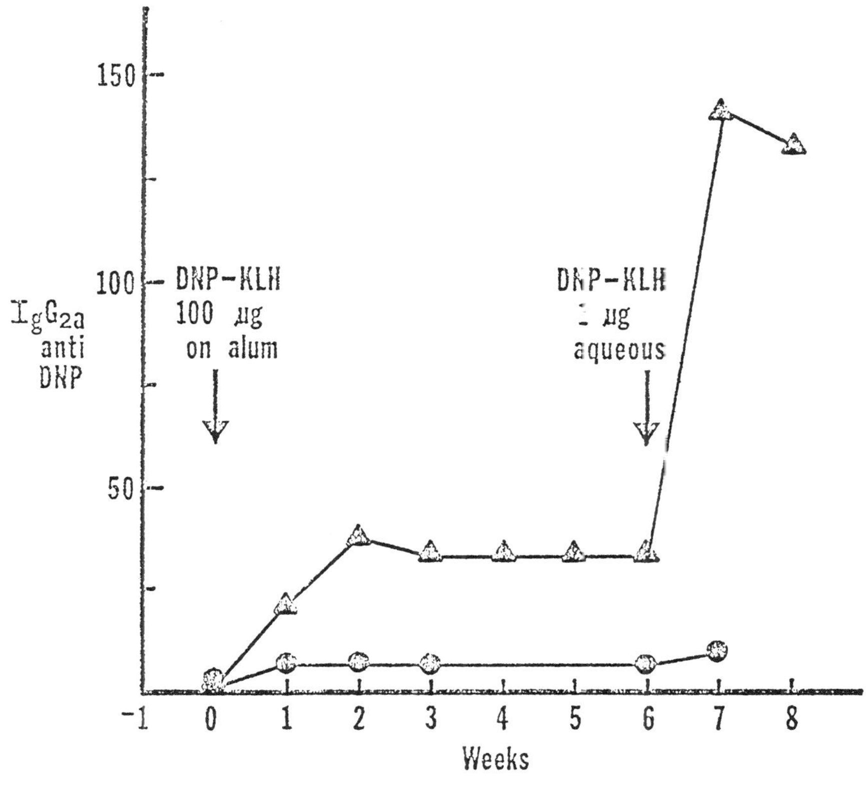

These studies introduce a novel protocol for inducing "hapten-specific" suppression of a large portion of an *in situ* IgG antihapten response, e.g., to the anti-2,4,-dinitrophenyl (DNP) hapten: Mice are primed first with carrier protein, such as keyhole limpet hemocyanin (KLH) and then exposed to hapten conjugated to the carrier protein (i.e., DNP-KLH). This carrier/hapten-carrier immunization sequence, which might be expected to augment antihapten responses, surprisingly results in a persistent and specific suppression of high affinity anti-DNP antibody production without interfering with the production of anticarrier antibody or the development of anti-DNP memory (see Figures 1 and 2, and Tables 1 and 2).

The induction of suppression for the anti-DNP response requires exposure to a carrier protein and subsequent exposure to hapten on that carrier. Once this sequence is complete, antibody responses to DNP on the same or a different carrier are suppressed, although responses to both carriers are normal. Exposure to a carrier followed by exposure to hapten on a different carrier, however, does not produce suppression, i.e., hapten must be presented on the same carrier used for priming (see Figure 3). Although the actual suppression is specific for production of antibodies reactive with the hapten, the mechanism responsible for induction of suppression has a clearly defined carrier-specific component.

**Figure 2.**

PRODUCTION OF ANTI-HAPTEN ANTIBODY IS SUPPRESSED IN CARRIER-PRIMED MICE STIMULATED WITH HAPTEN-CARRIER CONJUGATE

| Antigenic Exposures* (time in weeks) | | | $IgG_{2a}$ Antibody Responses† |
|---|---|---|---|
| -6 | 0 | 6 | Anti-DNP Mean $K_a$ (x $10^6$) |
| KLH | - | - | - |
| KLH | DNP-KLH | - | <0.3 |
| KLH | DNP-KLH | DNP-KLH | <0.3 |
| - | DNP-KLH | | 5 |
| - | DNP-KLH | DNP-KLH | 100 |

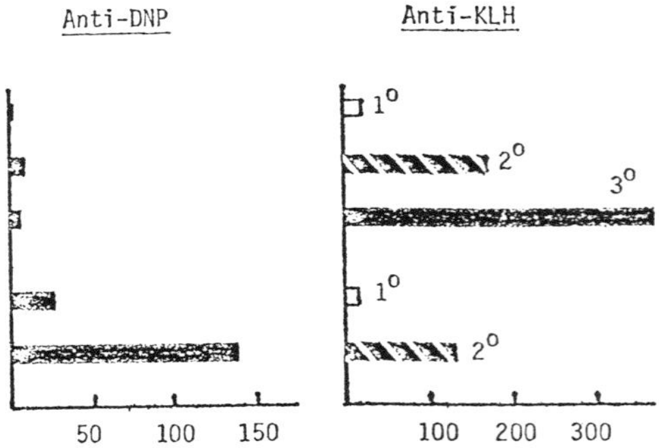


*100 μg on alum

†Response measured 1 week after last indicated stimulation; RIA units shown are relative to "standard" antiserum pools for each antigen.

**Table 1.** Carrier-Priming Reduces the Amount and Affinity of Antihapten Responses Stimulated by the Hapten-Carrier Conjugate but Does not Interfere with Anticarrier Response.

| Antigenic Stimulation | | | In situ Igh-1a antibody responses[a] | | |
|---|---|---|---|---|---|
| | | | | Anti-DNP | |
| Group | Protocol | Time (weeks) | Anti-KLH units[b] | μg/ml | Mean $K_a$ ($\times 10^6$) |
| I. | Hapten-carrier first | | | | |
| | DNP-KLH (100 μg on alum) | → 0 | | | |
| | | 2 | 15 | 35 | (5) |
| | | 6 | 15 | 30 | (8) |
| | DNP-KLH (1 μg aqueous) | → 6 | | | |
| | | 7 | 130 | 140 | (100 |
| | | 8 | 120 | 120 | (500) |
| II. | Carrier first | | | | |
| | KLH (100 μg on alum) | → −6 | | | |
| | | −4 | 20 | <1 | (<0.3) |
| | DNP-KLH (100 μg on alum) | → 0 | | | |
| | | 2 | 170 | 5 | (<0.3) |
| | | 6 | n.d. | 5 | (<0.3) |
| | DNP-KLH (1 μg aqueous) | → 6 | | | |
| | | 7 | 370 | 9 | (0.5) |
| III. | Hapten-carrier first | | | | |
| | DNP-KLH (100 μg aqueous) | → 0 | | | |
| | | 2 | 4 | 3 | (<0.3) |
| IV. | Carrier first | | | | |
| | KLH (100 μg on alum) | → −6 | | | |
| | DNP-KLH (100 μg aqueous) | → 0 | | | |
| | | 2 | 140 | 5 | (<0.3) |

[a]Response measured at indicated times. Igh-1b responses were similar.

[b]Relative to a standard adoptive secondary response serum.

## "Carrier-Specific" Suppression May Be Mediated by the Hapten-Specific Mechanism

The induction of suppression by exposure to carrier proteins, commonly called carrier-specific suppression, is generally believed to result from the induction of suppressor T-cell populations that interfere with delivery of carrier-specific help and thus suppress IgG antibody production. All of the available evidence from studies of this type of suppression, however, are consistent with the actual mechanism being the carrier-specific induction of hapten-specific suppression rather than the interference with carrier-specific help. That is, these studies have shown that exposure to carrier-proteins induces populations of T-cells specifically reactive with the carrier proteins and capable of suppressing antibody responses to determinants

**Table 2.** Hapten-Carrier Stimulation of Antihapten Memory B-Cells is Normal in Carrier-Primed Mice.

| Memory B-cell donors | | | Adoptive IgG anti-DNP response | |
|---|---|---|---|---|
| | Form of antigenic stimulation | | | |
| Group | KLH | DNP-KLH | Units | Mean $K_a$ ($\times 10^6$) |
| I | [a] | Alum | 73 | 10 |
| II | Alum | Alum | 73 | 8 |
| III | [a] | Aqueous | 18 | 0.7 |
| IV | Alum | Aqueous | 50 | 8 |

[a]No KLH injection.

*Note*: Donors (BALB/c $\times$ SJL) were sacrificed from groups listed in Table 1 three weeks after the first indicated stimulation with DNP-KLH. Splenic B-cells were prepared by cytotoxic depletion of T-cells using monoclonal anti-Thy-1.2 (30-H12, J. Ledbetter, Stanford University). Cells obtained from $10^7$ spleen cells were cotransferred with $2 \times 10^6$ nylon-passed syngeneic T-cells from KLH-primed donors (100 $\mu$g on alum plus $10^9$ *B. pertussis* at least 6 weeks before transfer). Recipients (650 R irradiated BALB/c) were stimulated with 1 $\mu$g aqueous DNP-KLH (i.v.) at time of transfer and bled one week later for assay. Assay details are described in the legend for Table 1. Igh-1b ($IgG_{2a}$) response data are shown here. Igh-1a ($IgG_{2a}$) and $IgG_1$ response data were similar. Responses in mice receiving nylon T (no donor B) were 3 units of very low affinity antibody. The proportion of $IgD^+$ memory (also an index of memory population maturity[3] was similar in Groups I, II, and IV, and higher in Group III, indicating less maturation (to $IgD^-$) in mice primed with aqueous antigen. Anti-KLH memory was similar in Groups I, II, and IV, and lower in Group III.

**Figure 3.** Homologous hapten-carrier conjugate induces hapten-specific suppression in carrier-primed mice. Each indicated antigenic stimulation was given as 10 $\mu$g of antigen on alum, i.p. Responses were measured 1 week after last indicated stimulation; RIA units shown are relative to "standard" antiserum pools for each antigen. Mean $K_a$ (in parentheses in figure) was determined from RIA binding. Assay details are described in the legend for Table 1.

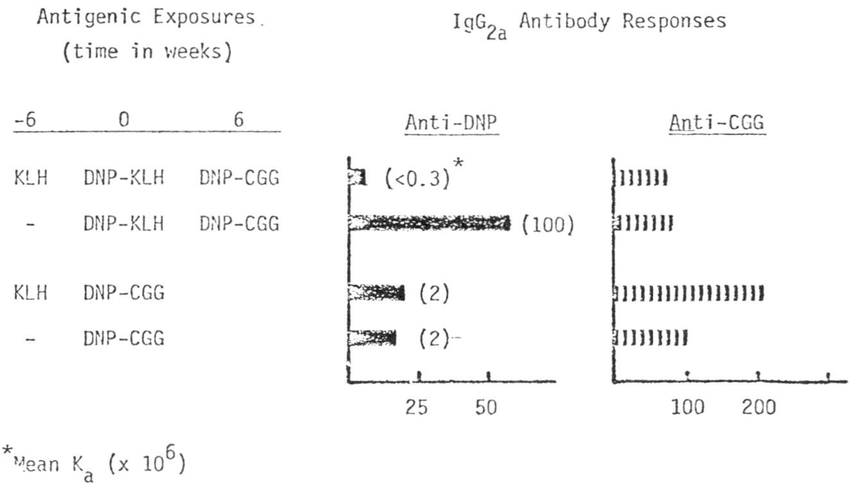

on these carrier proteins. However, this suppression has been measured in hapten-carrier systems in which the antihapten response is taken as a measure of suppression; thus it is entirely possible that the carrier-specific suppressor cells induced interact with the hapten-carrier conjugates in the test system and consequently induce a specific suppression of the antihapten antibody response without in any way interfering with carrier-specific help for such responses.

To test this possibility, we therefore conducted a series of experiments in which we followed similar *in situ* protocols used in the early carrier-specific suppression studies, except that we tested both the antihapten and anticarrier antibody responses. Depletion of carrier-specific help should affect both responses equally, whereas induction of hapten-specific suppression should affect only the antihapten response. The results of these studies indicated that hapten-specific suppression is induced. This was then confirmed by showing that subsequent exposure to hapten on an unrelated carrier stimulated responses to the new carrier but failed to stimulate even a primary level IgG anti-hapten response (T. Tokunisa, F. T. Gadus and L. A. Herzenberg, in preparation). At present there is no direct evidence to indicate that carrier-specific suppression depletes carrier-specific help. However, suppression in this system can be accounted for by the carrier-specific induction of cells that induce hapten-specific suppression when exposed to hapten-carrier conjugates.

## Other Immunoregulatory Defects May Be Mediated by Hapten-specific Suppression

These findings raise the question whether the hapten-specific suppression mechanism serves as a common channel through which diverse regulatory systems such as immunologic tolerance and *Ir* gene control ultimately control antibody production. In essence this argument states that although the initial mechanisms operating in these systems may differ considerably, they ultimately lead to the generation of signals that induce a suppression with characteristics similar to the suppression induced by the carrier/hapten-carrier exposure sequence. That is, regardless of the underlying causes, the non-responsive condition will be mediated by a common mechanism which, once induced to suppress antibodies to a given set of haptenic determinants, will suppress responses to those determinants under most stimulatory conditions.

Since this hypothesis is currently under examination, the following discussion is intended mainly to illustrate how and why we believe the various regulatory systems make use of the hapten-specific mechanism and to provide a basis for consideration of the types of experimental protocols that test the validity of our arguments. Therefore we discuss several published findings with respect to their potential consistency with our arguments without attempting to consider alternative explanations in detail. This method of presentation would clearly be unsatisfactory if we were attempting to prove our point through these examples; however, it serves our purposes here in raising the question of whether the hapten-specific mechanism provides a means for integrating signals from diverse regulatory systems.

We have, of course, demonstrated only that hapten-specific suppression can be induced for antibody responses to the artificial DNP hapten. The broad heterogeneity of such responses, however, suggests that similar suppression should be inducible for antibody produced to any haptenic determinant on an immunizing molecule whether or not that determinant constitutes an integral part of the molecular structure. Thus we see all antibody production as potentially controllable by hapten-specific suppression units (circuits?) that regulate production of unique antibody molecules according to the combining site specificity and heavy chain structure of those molecules.

The induction of suppression for a given set of antibody molecules, our data suggest, requires exposure to the hapten recognized by these molecules under conditions where the animal is predisposed towards suppression induction. These conditions may be defined by pre-immunization with the carrier on which the determinant is presented (as in the carrier/hapten-carrier suppression induction protocol), or may be intrinsic to the regulatory system operant in the animal (as in allotype suppression). Apparently, they need share only one attribute: a sufficiently strong impetus to suppression induction must outweigh the forces favoring antibody responses, such as those in already on-going responses.

## Regulatory Circuits: A Model for How a Hapten-Specific Regulation Could Integrate Signals from Diverse Regulatory Systems

We tend to view the suppression mechanism itself as having properties similar to the core regulatory circuit in the theoretical model we have proposed (Herzenberg et al., 1980). That is, it consists of a set of cell interactions with two relatively stable states. One permits dominance of the Ig-specific helper T-cell population required to help B-cells producing the relevant antibody, and the other permits dominance of a hapten-specific suppressor T-cell population that depletes this helper T-cell population. The initial stabilization of this circuit into a help or suppression mode can be determined by a relatively small excess in the amount of helper versus suppressor activity generated by signals from "auxiliary" circuits that sense environmental conditions. Once the circuit has stabilized, however, a substantially greater differential is required to shift it to the opposite configuration.

These properties, whether or not derived from cell circuit interactions such as we have proposed, are consistent with the characteristics of hapten-specific suppression vis-a-vis its ease of induction *de novo* and its relative but not absolute stability following repeated antigenic stimulation. Thus this model offers a convenient way of concretely viewing the cell interactions responsible for the properties of the hapten-specific mechanism. Bear in mind that the actual cell interactions responsible for those properties may be quite different.

The auxiliary circuits on the model as drawn are clearly inadequate to explain the induction of hapten-specific suppression by any of the mechanisms under discussion since these circuits were intentionally simplified by excluding information relating to such regulatory systems. The principle of auxiliary circuits that sense environmental stimuli and translate these stimuli into signals that determine the configuration to which the core circuit is induced (or maintained), however, has much to recommend it for the arguments we make here. Since this configuration depends on whether helper or suppressor cells are initially generated in excess, auxiliary inputs can take two general forms (i.e., they can influence suppressor development or they can influence help), with multiple inputs of each type being possible for any given circuit. Thus, in effect, the core circuit can be seen as an integrating device that accumulates signals from a variety of regulatory systems and finally transmits a single decision to help or suppress the production of the antibody it regulates.

In essence, this view allows regulatory mechanisms to be divided according to their relationship to the antigenic molecule. A central "hapten-specific" mechanism with interactions based on the combining site specificity of the regulated antibody can be postulated for haptenic determinants on the antigen. We can also define a series of auxiliary mechanisms that regulate according to the ways antigenic molecules are recognized and presented to the hapten-specific mechanism. Thus, in the carrier/hapten-carrier sequence, the carrier-induced populations of cells that predispose an animal to induction of suppression may be part of an auxiliary carrier-specific mechanism interacting with the hapten-specific mechanism (probably through a hapten-carrier "bridge"). This would result in the dominance of hapten-specific suppressor cells and thus in the suppression of anti-hapten production.

The mechanisms responsible for immunologic tolerance and *Ir* gene control can similarly be treated within this conceptual framework as having a carrier-specific induction component and a hapten-specific effector component. Suppression of responses would occur to all haptenic determinants on the antigen rather than just to additional haptens presented on the carrier at a later time. This requires only that the carrier-priming events which lead to induction of suppression occur sufficiently rapidly or efficiently. The integral haptenic determinants on the antigen must be treated as if they were new determinants on a carrier to which the animal has already been primed.

## Hapten-Specific Regulation in Immunologic Tolerance?

Data from studies of tolerance induction to external antigens are consistent with this view, since tolerance mechanisms in general appear very similar to the mechanisms responsible for "carrier-specific" suppression. This we suggest is actually the carrier-specific induction of hapten-specific suppression. The ability of animals exposed neonatally (tolerized) to human gamma globulin (HGG) to suppress responses to HGG and to DNP-HGG (Benjamin, 1975; Waters et al. 1979) for example, could be explained by the induction of an HGG-specific cell population that then induces hapten-specific suppression for haptens on the HGG moelcule.

If this were true, however, once suppression for anti-DNP responses has been induced by exposure to DNP-HGG, the animal should remain non-responsive to DNP even when the hapten is presented on an unrelated carrier.

This prediction is at odds with the prevailing view that carrier-specific suppression is responsible for immunologic tolerance (Basten et al. 1978). It is currently being tested directly in collaboration with Dr. Cory Waters, University of Alberta, Canada. A complicated series of more or less forgotten adoptive transfer experiments already challenges the strict carrier-specificity of the tolerance mechanism. In these experiments, Basten and co-workers (Basten et al. 1975) showed that T-cells from mice tolerant to human gamma globul in (HGG) supress adoptive secondary anti-DNP responses to DNP-HGG but not to DNP-KLH, *unless* the DNP-KLH and DNP-HGG are presented together, at which time the response to DNP on KLH also fails. These findings, as Basten pointed out implicate hapten-specificity as well as carrier-specificity in the suppressive mechanism.

The successful suppression of adoptive secondary anti-DNP responses by HGG-tolerant splenic populations suggests that these populations may be more efficient for inducing hapten-specific suppression than the carrier-primed populations we used in our adoptive transfer studies. Thus, if our supposition that similar mechanisms operate in induction of carrier/hapten-carrier suppression and tolerance is correct, tolerant animals may provide a better source of cells for obtaining hapten-specific suppression in adoptive transfer assays.

## Hapten-Specific Regulation in *Ir* Gene Control?

These arguments, stated for immunologic tolerance, can also be applied with little modification to mechanisms responsible for the non-responsiveness observed for antigens under *Ir* gene control. For example, hapten-specific suppression could clearly account for the tendency of non-responder animals to show impaired IgG but relatively normal IgM responses to the relevant antigens (McDevitt 1968). Similarly, the reliance on hapten-specific suppression to control antibody production is consistent with evidence showing that mechanisms akin to idiotype suppression control responses in non-responder animals (Germain et al. 1979).

The responses obtained to DNP conjugated to antigens under *Ir* gene control also support this argument. Non-responder animals to the GT antigen, for example, produce severely restricted anti-DNP responses to GT anti-DNP even though these animals produce highly heterogeneous responses to DNP on other carriers (Green et al. 1969). Such restricted responses, we would expect, are representative of the small, low-affinity responses we obtain in responses under hapten-specific suppression. Thus these findings suggest that if the non-responder animals are subsequently re-exposed to DNP on a neutral carrier, they would fail to produce an anti-DNP response commensurate with that expected following multiple stimulation with the hapten. If so, then hapten-specific suppression would appear to be the effector mechanism for *Ir*-gene controlled non-responsiveness.

Existent evidence is consistent with the idea that the induction of suppression in

*Ir* gene-controlled responses may result from disproportionate carrier-priming. In other words, non-responsive animals may rapidly become carrier-primed to *Ir* gene controlled antigens and then be induced to hapten-specific suppression rather than help for determinants on these antigens. This could explain why non-responder animals produce poor responses to an antigen when it serves as its own carrier, but produce strong IgG responses when it is complexed with a protein, e.g., methylated-BSA, which can serve as a normal (non-genetically controlled) carrier for the (genetically controlled) antigen (Kapp et al. 1974a). The demonstration that initial exposure to the antigen in its native state prevents subsequent antibody production to the antigen complexed to methylated BSA is also easily interpretable within this framework (Kapp et al. 1974b).

These findings would therefore predict that hapten-specific suppression for responses to DNP will be induced by exposure to DNP conjugated to an antigen under *Ir* gene control. Experiments to test this hypothesis are in progress; but again, supporting data can currently be drawn from the literature. Animals primed with DNP on a non-controlled carrier and thus producing a normal primary response to DNP appear to terminate their total IgG anti-DNP production when exposed to DNP conjugated to a carrier under *Ir* gene control (Paul et al. 1970). If the reduction in anti-DNP response reported in this study results from the induction of hapten-specific suppression, then these results would suggest that antigens under particular *Ir* gene control are more effective than other antigens in reversing ongoing immune responses. We have shown that the carrier/hapten-carrier sequence induces suppression only for the $IgG_{2a}$ anti-DNP response in animals already responding to DNP on an unrelated carrier.

Evidence from several other types of regulatory systems suggests that they too can be explained by a version of the carrier/hapten-carrier suppression induction sequence. For example, antigenic competition (Humphrey and White 1970) appears to derive from the physical association of two antigens injected closely enough together so the first serves as carrier for the second. The multigenic control of $IgG_{2a}$ responses to sheep cell antigens (Seman et al. 1978) demonstrates many of the properties of the mechanism described here.

## Closing Comments

In sum, we have proposed a broad sweeping revision of the current views on how immunoregulatory systems operate. We have presented suggestive evidence indicating that the hapten-specific regulatory system provides a common channel through which these systems contribute to response control, and have added the idea that the carrier/hapten-carrier sequence provides the means through which suppression is generated in these systems. More important, however, we have described how these hypotheses can be directly tested. In all systems except possibly antigenic competition, our proposals make one simple prediction: if non-responsiveness is generated for a given antigen and the animal is then exposed to DNP conjugated to that antigen, hapten-specific suppression will be generated for the anti-DNP response and the animal will subsequently fail to respond to DNP presented on an unrelated carrier. Responses to other haptenic determinants on this carrier, however, will be normal and the animal will develop normal populations of anti-DNP memory B-cells revealable by adoptive transfer assays of T-depleted speen cells, appropriately supplemented.

The demonstration that a number of regulatory systems utilize carrier/hapten-carrier-type mechanisms would perhaps surprise us all; but it would also make it easier to explain why the immune system has evolved a complex mechanism that substantially impairs responses to new haptenic determinants on a previously encountered carrier. Essentially, the negative value of being unable to respond to such determinants could be seen as the price paid for having developed a versatile system that can selectively regulate individual isotypes and idiotypes and can integrate signals from the variety of specialized mechanisms co-existing in a single animal.

The well-known tendency for cytotoxic responses to increase when antibody responses are decreased (Cohn 1975), however, introduces a possible positive value to the development of hapten-specific suppression for new determinants on a carrier. If we were to assume that the core circuit provides help for antibody responses in its "help" configuration and help for cytotoxic responses in its "suppression" configuration, then the carrier/hapten-carrier exposure sequence can be seen as a mechanism for generating cytotoxic responses to variant organisms. In addition, if we were to assume that animals can become "carrier-primed" for self determinants early in life but be prevented (perhaps by clonal deletion) from using such help to generate cytotoxic responses to self antigens, then the system would be ideally suited to dealing with viral infections. In other words, it would be initialized to generate cytotoxic responses to new (viral) determinants on the (self) carrier to which it has been primed. This argument is somewhat fanciful and clearly has many problems to be resolved before an adequate hypothesis could be advanced; nevertheless, we mention it here because it offers yet another way in which the hapten-specific mechanism could play a role in integrating various signals so the overall response meets the needs defined by the nature of the antigenic challenge.

ACKNOWLEDGMENTS
The organizers of this program deserve many thanks for bringing us all together to celebrate Ray's birthday. The authors also wish to thank Mr. Milton Wise for the excellent illustrations we have included herein and Ms. Jean Anderson for assistance in preparation of this manuscript.

## References

Basten, A., Miller, J.F.A.P., and Johnson, P. 1975. T-cell-dependent suppression of an anti-hapten antibody response. Transplant. Rev. 26:130.

Basten, A., Miller, J.F.A.P., Loblay, R., Johnson, P., Gamble, J., China, E., Pritchard-Briscoe, H., Callard. R., and McKenzie, I.F.C. 1978. T-cell-dependent suppression of antibody production. I. Characteristics of suppressor T-cells following tolerance induction. Eur. J. Immunol. 8:360.

Benjamin, D.C. 1975. Evidence for specific suppression in the maintenance of immunological tolerance. J. Exp. Med. 141:635.

Black, S.J., van de Loo, W., Loken, M.R., and Herzenberg, L.A. 1978. Expression of IgD by murine lymphocytes. Loss of surface IgD indicates maturation of memory B-cells. J. Exp. Med. 147:984–996.

Black, S.J., Tokuhisa, T., Herzenberg, L.A., and Herzenberg, L.A. 1980. Memory B-cells at successive stages of differentiation: Expression of surface IgD and capacity for self renewal. Eur. J. Immunol. 10:846–851.

Burnet, F.M. 1957. A modification of Herne's theory of antibody production using the concept of clonal selection. Austral. J. Sci. 20:67.

Cohn, M. 1975. The logic of cell interactions in determining immune responsiveness. In Molecular Approaches to Immunology, vol. 9. E.E. Smith and D.W. Ribbons, eds. New York: Academic Press.

Eardley, D.D. and Gershon, R.K. 1975. Feedback induction of suppressor T-cell activity. J. Exp. Med. 142:524.

Germain, R.H., Ju, S.T., Kipps, T.J., Benacerraf, B., and Dorf, M.E. 1979. Shared idiotypic determinants on antibodies and T-cell derived suppressor factor specific for random terpolymer L-glutamic acid$^{60}$-L-alanine$^{30}$-L-tyrosine$^{10}$. J. Exp. Med. 149:613.

Gershon, R.K. and Paul, W.E. 1971. Effect of thymus derived lymphocytes on the amount and affinity of anti-hapten antibody. J. Immunol. 106:872.

Green, M.C. 1979. Fenetic nomenclature for the immunoglobulin loci of the mouse. Immunogenetics 8:89.

Green, I., Benacerraf, B., and Stone, S.M. 1969. The effect of the amount of microbacterial adjuvants on the immune responses of strain 2, strain 13, and Hartley strain guinea pigs to DNP-PLL and DNP-GL. J. Immunol. 103:403.

Herzenberg, L.A. and Gonzales, G. 1962. Appearance of *H-2* agglutins in outcrossed female mice. Proc. Natl. Acad. Sci. U.S.A. 48:570–573.

Herzenberg, L.A., Tokuhisa, T., and Herzenberg, L.A. 1980. Carrier-priming leads to hapten-specific suppression. Nature 285:664.

Herzenberg, L.A., Black, S.J., Tokuhisa, T., and Herzenberg, L.A. 1980. Memory B-cells at successive stages of differentiation: Affinity maturation and role of IgD receptors. J. Exp. Med. 151:1071–1087.

Herzenberg, L.A., Black, S.J., and Herzenberg, L.A. 1980. Regulatory circuits and antibody responses. Eur. J. Immunol. 10:1–11.

Humphrey, J.H. and White, R.G. 1970. Immunology for Students of Medicine (third edition). Oxford, England: Blackwell Scientific Publications, p. 143.

Kapp, J.A., Pierce, C.W., and Benacerraf, B. 1974a. Genetic control of immune responses *in vitro*. III. Tolerogenic properties of the terpolymer L-glutamic acid$^{60}$-L-alanine$^{30}$-L-tyrosine$^{10}$ (GAT) for spleen cells from non-responder($H\text{-}2^s$ and $H\text{-}2^q$) mice. J. Exp. Med. 140:172–198.

Kapp, J.A., Pierce, C.W., Schlossman, S., and Benacerraf, B. 1974b. Genetic control of immune responses *in vitro*. V. Stimulation of suppressor T-cells in non-responder mice by the terpolymer L-glutamic acid$^{60}$–L-alanine$^{30}$-L-tyrosine$^{10}$ (GAT). J. Exp. Med. 140:648–659.

Mason, D.W. 1976. The class of surface immunoglobulin on cells carrying IgM memory in rat thoratic duct lymph: The size of the subpopulation mediating IgG memory. J. Exp. Med. 143:1122.

McDevitt, H.O. 1968. Genetic control of the antibody response. III. Qualitative and quantitative characterization of the antibody response to (T,G)-A-L in CBA and C57 mice. J. Immunol. 100:485.

Okumura, K., Julius, M.H., Tsu, T., Herzenberg, L.A., and Herzenberg, L.A. 1976a. Demonstration that IgG memory is carried by IgG bearing cells. Eur. J. Immunol. 6:467–472.

Okumura, K., Metzler, C.M., Tsu, T.T., Herzenberg, L.A., and Herzenberg, L.A. 1976b. Two stages of B-cell memory development with different T-cell requirements. J. Exp. Med. 144:345.

Paul, W.E., Katz, D.H., Goidl, E.A., and Benacerraf, B. 1970. Carrier function in antihapten immune responses. II. Specific properties of carrier cells capable of enhancing antihapten antibody responses. J. Exp. Med. 132:283.

Scott, D.W. 1974. Are suppressor cells responsible for tolerance to a soluble antigen? In Immunological Tolerance. D.H. Katz and B. Benacerraf, eds. New York: Academic Press, p. 503.

Seman, M., Chevalier, F., and Stanislawski, M. 1978. Evidence for independent genetic regulation of the expression of different antibody classes in anti-sheep red blood cell responses. Eur. J. Immunol. 8:262.

Siskind, G.W. and Benacerraf, B. 1969. Cell selection by antigen in the immune response. Adv. Immunol. 10:1.

Tada, T. 1974. The mode and sites of action of suppressor T-cells in the antigen-induced differentiation of B-cells. In Immunological Tolerance. D.H. Katz and B. Benacerraf, eds. New York: Academic Press, p. 471.

Tada, T., and Takemori, T. 1974. Selective roles of thymus-derived lymphocytes in the antibody response. I. Differential suppressive effect of carrier-primed T-cells on hapten-specific IgM and IgG antibody responses. J. Exp. Med. 140:239.

Waters, C.A., Pilarski, L.M., Wegmann, T.G., and Diener, E. 1979. Tolerance-induction during ontogeny. I. Presence of active suppression in mice rendered tolerant to human $\gamma$-globulin *in utero* correlates with the breakdown of the tolerant state. J. Exp. Med. 149:1135.

Hildemann, ed. Frontiers in Immunogenetics

# Genetic Factors Influencing the Immunogenicity of Thy-1 Cell Surface Antigens

Tommy C. Douglas,[1] Phil Lake,[2]
Helena Skarvall,[3] and Patti Dawson[1]

[1]*Medical Genetics Center, University of Texas Health Science Center, P.O. Box 20334, Astrodome Station, Houston, Texas;* [2]*Imperial Cancer Research Fund, Tumour Immunology Unit, Dept. of Zoology, University College London, Gower Street, London WC1, United Kingdom;* [3]*Basel Institute for Immunology, Grenzacherstrasse 487, CH-4058 Basel, Switzerland*

## The Thy-1 Alloantigen System

Upon being accepted as a graduate student in the Division of Biology at Caltech, I was assigned to Ray Owen's laboratory although I (T.C.D.) had expressed a primary interest in neurochemistry. I found Ray's lab very congenial and eventually spent a considerable amount of time trying to think of a thesis topic which would somehow relate immunogenetics to the nervous system. In a review by Boyse and Old (1969), I found that the Thy-1 antigens of the mouse (then called theta; Reif and Allen 1964; Snell 1971) were expressed at very high levels in two organs: thymus and brain. In addition to having an unusual tissue distribution, these cell surface antigens are genetically polymorphic and display striking patterns of expression during ontogeny (Reif and Allen 1966a; Raff 1971; Schachner and Hämmerling 1974). Most inbred mouse strains are homozygous for the allele *Thy-1$^b$* and express the Thy-1.2 antigenic determinant, but a small number of strains including AKR/J are homozygous for *Thy-1$^a$* and express the determinant Thy-1.1. This alloantigen system seemed to be just what I was looking for.

To produce specific anti Thy-1 reagents, we decided to use the sublines AKR/J and AKR/Cum which are closely-related but Thy-1 incompatible (Schlesinger and Hurvitz 1969; Acton et al. 1973; Krog 1976). Recipient animals were given six weekly intraperitoneal injections of approximately $1 \times 10^7$ Thy-1 incompatible cells and bled 5 to 11 days later. Elizabeth Blankenhorn, who was working in the Owen laboratory as a technician prior to beginning her graduate studies, noticed that the titers of anti Thy-1.2 sera produced in this way were consistently lower than those of the anti-Thy-1.1 sera. We solved the problem of obtaining stronger anti-Thy-1.2 reagents by using a more conventional strain combination; AKR/J mice were injected with thymus cells from the more distantly-related strain C3H/HeJ. When tested against C3H/HeJ or C3H/St (Thy-1.2) thymus cell targets[1] in a complement-dependent microcytotoxicity assay (Douglas 1972) two representative AKR/J anti-C3H antisera had titers of 1/512 and 1/1024 whereas two representative AKR/J anti-AKR/Cum sera had titers of 1/16 and 1/64. The immediate need for a stronger anti-Thy-1.2 reagent had been met, and it was not until several years later that I returned to the question of why C3H thymus cells can induce stronger anti-Thy-1.2 responses than do AKR/Cum cells. We report here on the results of some additional experiments which have been done since my departure from Ray's laboratory.

## Anti-Thy-1 Serum Antibody Responses

During my period as a postdoctoral fellow, Helena Skarvall and I found that the Danish strain AKR/ABom produces anti-Thy-1.2 responses which are similar to those of AKR/J; animals of this strain which had been hyperimmunized with C3H/HeJ thymocytes produced higher titers of anti-Thy-1.2 cytotoxic antibodies than did those which had been hyperimmunized with AKR/Cum thymocytes. To determine how early the circulating antibody levels of these two groups began to diverge, we collected individual blood samples 2 to 21 days after primary intraperitoneal injection of $1 \times 10^7$ thymocytes and 2 and 4 days after an identical secondary injection. Two-fold dilutions of these antisera were tested in the microcytotoxicity assay using AKR/Cum thymus cells as targets (Figure 1A). By days 8 and 10 of the primary response, a larger proportion of mice in the anti-C3H group had detectable levels of anti-Thy-1.2, but the average titers of the positive sera in the two groups were similar. Clear differences between the anti-C3H and anti-AKR/Cum groups first appeared in the secondary response. This difference was more marked among mice which had been injected with 10-fold fewer thymus cells (Figure 1B).

## Primary Anti-Thy-1 Plaque-Forming Cell (PFC) Responses

To follow the anti-Thy-1 cytotoxic antibody responses at the cellular level we decided to use a complement-dependent cytolytic plaque assay with thymus cells as targets (Fuji et al. 1971; Taylor and Bennett 1973).[2] Using this assay it was

[1]These data were gleaned from our original immunization records. Subsequent experiments have shown that the titers of these two types of antisera also differ markedly when determined with AKR/Cum thymus cell targets, which lack some of the "contaminating" non-Thy-1 alloantigens present on C3H cells (Acton et al. 1973; Frelinger and Murphy 1976).

[2]Only direct plaques have been studied in the present experiments. Virtually all of the PFC detected by this assay appear to be producing IgM, since more than 90% of them can be inhibited by 2-mercaptoethanol (Fuji et al. 1971), and our preliminary results indicate that more than 99% of them are inhibitable by a sheep antiserum specific for mouse IgM.

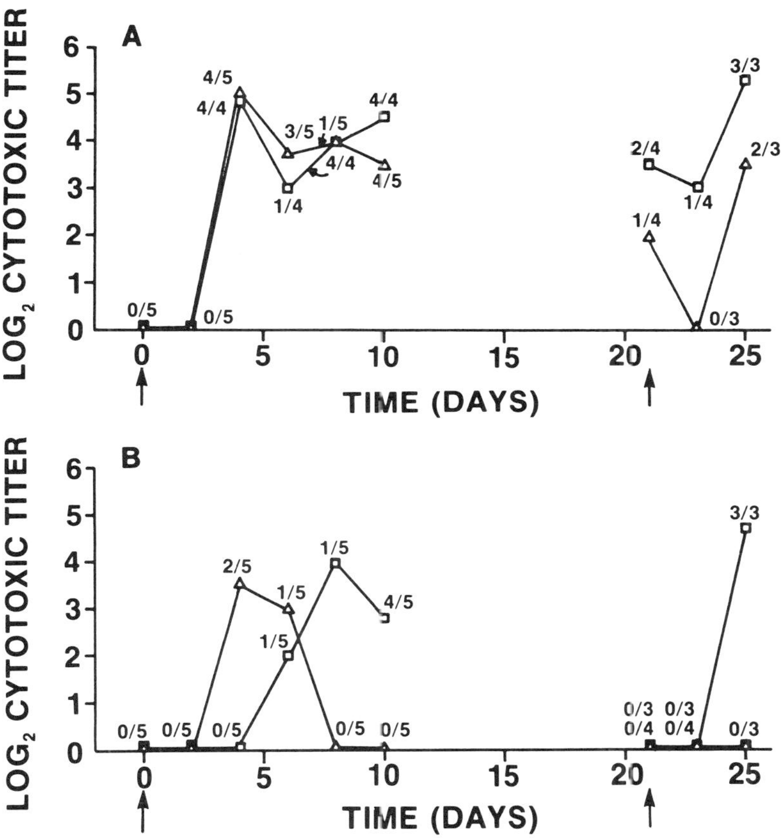


**Figure 1.** Anti-Thy-1.2 responses of AKR/ABom mice immunized with AKR/Cum or C3H/HeJ thymocytes. At the times indicated by arrows, animals were injected with $1 \times 10^7$ (upper panel) or $1 \times 10^6$ (lower panel) thymus cells from strain AKR/Cum (triangles) or C3H/HeJ (squares). Data are presented as average $\log_2$ titers of those sera which showed positive complement-dependent cytotoxicity against AKR/Cum thymus cells. The number next to each point indicates the proportion of positive sera at that time.

readily apparent that the primary anti-Thy-1.2 response of AKR/J mice to C3H thymocytes greatly exceeded that to AKR/Cum thymocytes (Table 1). The largest difference between these responses (a factor of 10) occurred on day 6 when the anti-C3H response was at its peak. AKR/ABom responders showed a similar pattern, the anti-C3H response being 40-fold higher than that against AKR/Cum on day 6. Injection of strain CBA thymocytes into AKR/J recipients resulted in a primary PFC response similar in magnitude and kinetics to that seen when C3H cells were used as immunogen (Lake and Douglas 1978).

**Table 1.** Primary PFC Responses of AKR/J or AKR/ABom Mice Immunized with Thy-1.2-Positive Thymocytes.[a]

| Day[b] | Recipient | Donor[c] AKR/Cum ♀ | C3H ♀ | p[d] |
|---|---|---|---|---|
| 3 | AKR/J ♀ | 6.4±0.5 (5)[e] | 31.8±5.0 (4) | <0.01 |
| 4 | AKR/J ♀ | 49.5±16.6 (4) | 143.5±15.4 (4) | <0.025 |
| 5 | AKR/J ♀ | 23.4±5.2 (5) | 109.0±26.9 (6) | <0.025 |
| 6 | AKR/J ♀ | 26.7±5.6 (10) | 267.0±27.2 (9) | <0.0005 |
| 7 | AKR/J ♀ | 18.6±1.8 (5) | 135.4±44.0 (5) | <0.05 |
| 9 | AKR/J ♀ | 55.2±10.8 (5) | 109.2±16.4 (5) | <0.05 |
| 11 | AKR/J ♀ | 33.0±7.2 (6) | 16.2±4.9 (5) | n.s.[f] |
| 4 | AKR/ABom ♀ | 8.0±2.9 (6) | 20.7±7.2 (6) | n.s. |
| 6 | AKR/ABom ♀ | 5.5±1.0 (6) | 218.8±49.8 (6) | <0.005 |

[a]See the footnote to Table 2 for a detailed description of the PFC assay. Data are presented as the arithmetic mean number of PFC per $6 \times 10^6$ immune spleen cells ± std. error of the mean. Target cells were AKR/Cum thymocytes. Average spleen cell yield was $7.2 \pm 0.2 \times 10^7$ (N = 65).

[b]Days elapsed between antigen injection and PFC assay.

[c]Each immunizing inoculum consisted of $4 \times 10^7$ donor thymocytes injected via the lateral tail vein.

[d]In each case the response to C3H thymocytes is compared with that to AKR/Cum thymocytes determined on the same number of days following antigen injection. Spleen cells from each mouse were tested in triplicate, the arithmetic mean number of PFC per dish being treated as a single point. Probability values are based on a one-tailed t-test as modified by Cochran for the case in which $\sigma 1 \neq \sigma 2$ (Snedecor and Cochran 1967).

[e]The number of recipient animals per group is given in parentheses.

[f]n.s. = anti-C3H response not significantly greater than anti-AKR/Cum response.

To be certain that the PFC assay was giving a true picture of the anti-Thy-1 response it was necessary to show that this assay was both specific and linear. In a control experiment to test the specificity of the PFC assay for Thy-1, immune anti-Thy-1.2 spleen cells ($6 \times 10^6$ per assay dish) were tested for their ability to form plaques on layers of target cells from 5 different strains of mice (Table 2). Large numbers of anti-Thy-1.2 PFC were detected using target cells from the *Thy-1^b^* strains C3H/HeJ, CBA/ABom, or AKR/Cum, but very few autoantibody-producing PFC could be seen with target cells from the *Thy-1^a^* strains AKR/J or AKR/ABom. The degree of Thy-1 specificity found in this experiment is comparable with that reported elsewhere (Fuji et al. 1971; Lake 1976). To maximize the specificity of the PFC assay for Thy-1 in all experiments, AKR/ABom and AKR/J anti-Thy-1.2 responses have been evaluated with AKR/Cum target cells, and AKR/Cum anti-Thy-1.1 responses on AKR/J or AKR/ABom target cells.

To determine the linearity of the PFC assay, varying numbers of anti-Thy-1.2 immune spleen cells were plated together with the standard concentration of Thy-1.2 target cells. This kind of control is important when nucleated cells are used as targets because if too many spleen cells are added these can obscure plaques of stained thymocytes, thereby causing underestimation of the frequency of PFC (Fuji et al. 1971; Taylor and Bennett 1973). As can be seen from Figure 2, spleen cell densities of 6 × $10^6$ per plate do not present a problem; a relatively constant estimate of approximately 36 PFC per million spleen cells was obtained over a wide range of spleen cell densities.

A trivial explanation of the enhanced immunogenicity of C3H or CBA thymocytes might be that these cells simply express higher levels of Thy-1.2 determinants, but quantitative absorption experiments indicate that this is not the case. The numbers of CBA or C3H/HeJ thymocytes required to absorb the cytotoxic activity of standard anti-Thy-1.2 sera were approximately equivalent to the number of AKR/Cum thymocytes required to achieve the same result.

The explanation which we favor for the augmented immunogenicity of C3H thymocytes is that these cells express one or more non-Thy-1 alloantigenic determinants for which AKR/Cum and AKR/J are matched, but for which C3H and AKR/J differ. According to this hypothesis, these foreign antigens can augment the specific anti-Thy-1.2 response by serving as immunological "carriers" for the otherwise poorly-immunogenic Thy-1.2 determinant. This type of explanation is consistent not only with the weak immunogenicity of Thy-1.2 on AKR/Cum thymocytes, but also with the low antibody responses which are often obtained when closely-related donor and recipient strains are used for the production of antibodies against *H-2*, TL, or Ly antigens (Shen et al. 1975; Wernet and Lilly 1975; Dorf and Stimpfling 1977).

**Table 2.** Specificity of the PFC Assay for Thy-1.

| | | | Target cells | |
|---|---|---|---|---|
| **Recipient** | **Donor** | **PFC** | **Strain** | **Thy-1** |
| AKR/ABom | C3H/HeJ | 412.0±29.5 (3) | C3H/HeJ | b |
| | | 579.0±102.6 (3) | CBA/ABom | b |
| | | 516.7±11.4 (3) | AKR/Cum | b |
| | | 1.0±0.6 (3) | AKR/J | a |
| | | 6.7±1.2 (3) | AKR/ABom | a |

*Note*: A pool of immune spleen cells from 3 AKR/ABom mice which had received 3 injections of C3H/HeJ thymocytes was used in this experiment. Data are presented as the arithmetic mean number of PFC per dish ± std. error (3 dishes per group). In each case 24 × $10^6$ immune spleen cells suspended in 0.2 ml of Dulbecco's Modified Eagle Medium (DMEM:Gibco H-16) + 1% fetal calf serum (FCS) were mixed at 39-39.5°C with 80 × $10^6$ target thymus cells suspended on 0.2 ml DMEM + 1% FCS and 1.6 ml of DMEM containing 0.5% agarose. One-half ml of this mixture was spread evenly in each 60 × 15 mm tissue culture dish (Falcon 3002), which contained an underlayer of 1 ml of 1% agarose in Dulbecco's phosphate buffered saline, pH 7.4 (PBS:Dulbecco and Vogt 1954). After the cell-containing layer had solidified, 5 ml of DMEM + 1% FCS were added to each dish. The dishes were incubated for 1 hr at 37°C in 95% air, 5% $CO_2$, then washed with 4 ml PBS, drained, and treated with 1.6 ml rabbit complement at a dilution (1/10) determined in preliminary experiments. After one hour's incubation at 37°C in 95% air, 5% $CO_2$, each plate was washed twice with PBS as before and stained for 15 minutes with 2 ml of 0.16% trypan blue dissolved in 0.9% NaCl. Dishes were then washed twice more with PBS and stored at 4°C until plaques were counted (within several hours) using a 15 x stereomicroscope with diffuse white illumination.

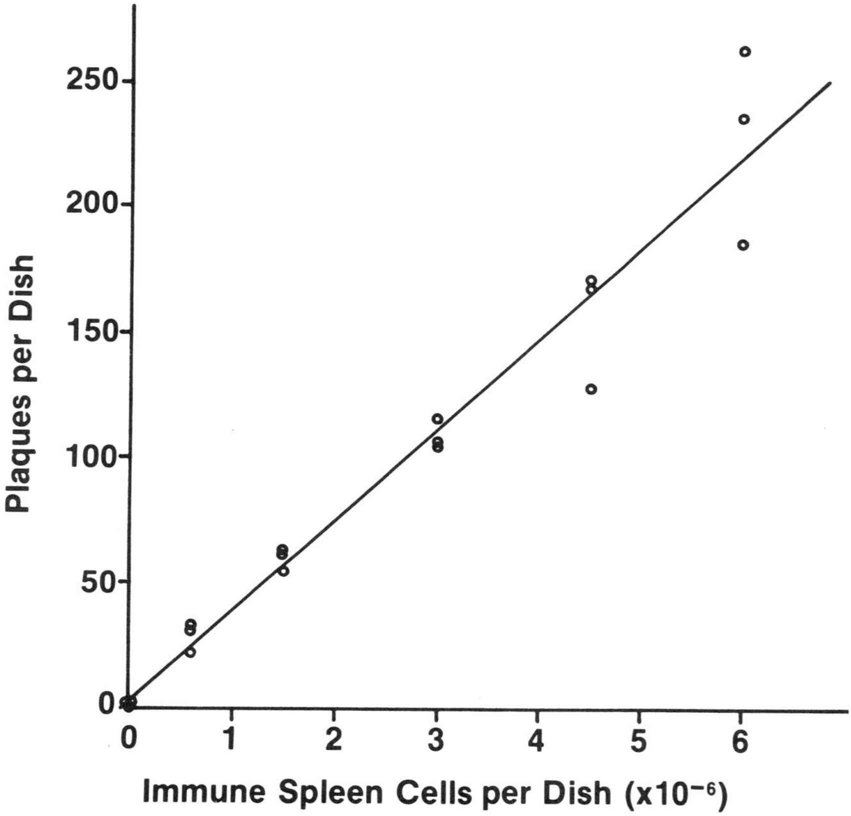


**Figure 2.** Linearity of the PFC assay. A pool of spleen cells collected from two AKR/ABom females on the fourth day following secondary immunization with C3H/HeJ thymocytes was used as a source of PFC. Replicate dishes containing a constant number of AKR/Cum target thymus cells ($20 \times 10^6$) and varying numbers of anti-C3H spleen cells ($0\text{-}6 \times 10^6$) were assayed for PFC. Each point represents the number of plaques scored in a single assay dish. The slope of the least-squares regression line is approximately 36 PFC per $1 \times 10^6$ spleen cells.

Because alloantigens are usually expressed in a dominant or codominant manner, this model predicts that the thymocytes of F1 hybrids between strains C3H and AKR/Cum should express both "carrier" and Thy-1.2 determinants. These cells should therefore induce augmented anti-Thy-1.2 responses in AKR/ABom or AKR/J recipients. The results of experiment 1 in Table 3 (lines 1–3) confirm that this is indeed the case. A similar situation also exists with respect to anti-Thy-1.1 responses. AKR/Cum mice immunized with AKR/ABom or AKR/J thymocytes produce low numbers of PFC, but augmented responses are obtained when thy-

**Table 3.** The "Carrier" Effect in Primary PFC Responses Against F1 Hybrid Thymocytes.

| Recipient | Donor | PFC | Antigen | p |
|---|---|---|---|---|
| AKR/ABom ♀ | AKR/Cum ♀ | 5.0±1.3 (6) | Thy-1.2 | |
| AKR/ABom ♀ | (AKR/Cum × C3H)F1 ♀ | 55.0±19.6 (6) | Thy-1.2 | <0.05 |
| AKR/ABom ♀ | C3H ♀ | 183.7±75.8 (6) | Thy-1.2 | <0.05 |
| AKR/Cum ♂ | AKR/ABom ♂ | 14.3±3.0 (6) | Thy-1.1 | |
| AKR/Cum ♂ | MA ♂ | 125.5±21.1 (6) | Thy-1.1 | <0.005 |
| AKR/Cum ♀ | AKR/J ♀ | 4.5±1.0 (4) | Thy-1.1 | |
| ARK/Cum ♀ | (AKR/J × MA)F1 ♀ | 240.2±37.1 (6) | Thy-1.1 | <0.005 |
| AKR/Cum ♀ | AKR/J ♀ | 4.6±2.1 (5) | Thy-1.1 | |
| AKR/Cum ♀ | (AKR/J × MA)F1 ♀ | 218.7±39.1 (7) | Thy-1.1 | <0.005 |

*Note*: Immune spleen cells were collected 6 days after primary intravenous immunization with $4 \times 10^7$ donor thymocytes. Target thymus cells were from strain AKR/Cum (lines 1-3), AKR/ABom (lines 4,5), or AKR/J (lines 6-9).

mocytes from the distantly-related strain MA/MyJ or from (AKR/J × MA/MyJ)F1 hybrids are used as immunogen (Table 3, lines 4–9).[3]

Two other requirements of the carrier hypothesis are also fulfilled by this alloantigen system. Physical association between the Thy-1 and "carrier" determinants is required, and the ability of recipient animals to produce augmented responses to the "carrier plus Thy-1" complex is thymus-dependent (Table 4, Lake and Douglas 1978). By using thymocytes from F1 hybrids which had inherited the *Thy-1*$^a$ allele from one parent and one or more genes controlling "carrier" determinants from the other parent, it was possible to show that the increased immunogenicity of Thy-1 determinants on (AKR/J × B10.BR)F1 hybrid thymocytes is not mimicked by mixtures of AKR/J and B10.BR cells. Furthermore, the increased immunogenicity of these F1 thymocytes is not seen in "B" mice which have been thymectomized, irradiated, and reconstituted with fetal liver cells, though it is evident in similarly-treated sham-thymectomized controls (Table 4).

## Secondary Anti-Thy-1 Responses

In keeping with the carrier hypothesis, it would be expected that animals which had been primed with Thy-1 in association with one "carrier" determinant should produce enhanced secondary responses when restimulated with Thy-1 in association

[3]Based on our earlier finding that AKR/Cum anti AKR/J sera characteristically have higher titers than do AKR/J anti-AKR/Cum sera, the weakness of the AKR/Cum anti-AKR/J primary PFC response was surprising. The basis for the different patterns of maturation seen in these two antibody responses has not yet been explored.

**Table 4.** Evidence that Helper Alloantigens Must be on the Cells Expressing the Determinants which are Helped and Thymus-dependence of the Effect.

| Expt 1<br>Thymus donor | Thy-1 phenotype | Anti Thy-1.1<br>PFC per spleen |
|---|---|---|
| AKR/J | Thy-1.1/1.1 | 345 ± 127 |
| B10.BR | Thy-1.2/1.2 | 0 |
| (AKR × B10.BR)F1 | Thy-1.1/1.2 | 4,554 ± 425 |
| AKR + B10.BR[a] | Thy-1.1/1.1 + Thy-1.2/1.2 | 387 ± 72 |
| AKR + B10.BR[b] | Thy-1.1/1.1 + Thy-1.2/1.2 | 186 ± 36 |

| Expt 2<br>Thymus donor | Pre-irradiation treatment | Anti Thy-1.1<br>PFC per spleen |
|---|---|---|
| AKR + B10.BR | Thymectomy | 54 ± 71 |
| (AKR × B10.BR)F1 | Thymectomy | 9 ± 20 |
| AKR + B10.BR | Sham thymectomy | 33 ± 22 |
| (AKR × B10.BR)F1 | Sham thymectomy | 753 ± 252[c] |

*Note*: (AKR/Cum × CBA)F1 mice, in groups of five recipients each, were injected i.v. with $4 \times 10^7$ of the indicated cell suspension except for the cell mixture where in ([a]) $8 \times 10^7$ cells were injected and in ([b]) $4 \times 10^7$ cells were injected. Cells were mixed in a 1:1 ratio. PFC were determined after 7 d. In Experiment 2, (CBA × AKR/Cum)F1 mice were thymectomized or manipulated surgically but not thymectomized. After a recovery interval of 3 weeks, all mice were given 750 rad of $\gamma$-irradiation and $5 \times 10^6$ fetal liver cells from syngeneic mice. The mice were used after an additional 5-week period.

[c]AKR/J thymus cells were used as targets. Portions of these spleens (1/30) were tested on AKR/Cum targets and no PFC were detectable.

*(Source: Lake and Douglas 1978.)*

with the same "carrier." This phenomenon is illustrated in Table 5. It can be seen that AKR/Cum thymocytes, which lack effective "carrier" determinants, can neither prime AKR/ABom recipients for a strong secondary PFC response to Thy-1.2 nor effectively boost recipients which previously have been primed with C3H/HeJ thymocytes.

The analysis of secondary anti-Thy-1.2 PFC responses has also provided direct evidence for the immunological specificity of "carrier" recognition. Rather than comparing a highly-immunogenic donor strain (C3H/HeJ) with a poorly-immunogenic strain (AKR/Cum) as described above, Drs. Edward Clark and Phil Lake have compared two different highly-immunogenic donor strains, CBA and B10.BR. In these two strains the "carrier" determinants for Thy-1.2 differ sufficiently so that CBA-primed AKR/J recipients produce much larger anti-Thy-1.2 secondary PFC responses when challenged with CBA thymocytes whereas B10.BR-primed recipients respond better when challenged with B10.BR cells (Clark and Lake, personal communication).

## Genetic Analysis of "Carrier" Determinants

Because effective "carrier" determinants are expressed in a dominant or codominant manner, it is possible to obtain a direct estimate of the number of genetic factors which control these determinants. Among the backcross progeny of a highly-immunogenic F1 hybrid and its poorly-immunogenic parental strain, the frequency of individuals whose thymocytes are poorly immunogenic should be $(1/2)^n$ where n is equal to the number of independently-segregating "carrier" determinant-controlling loci. Because the density of a given Thy-1 determinant is less on the thymocytes of *Thy-1$^a$/Thy-1$^b$* heterozygotes than on those of the appropriate homozygote (Reif and Allen 1966b), it is necessary to avoid Thy-1 dosage differences among the backcross progeny either by starting out with parental strains homozygous for the same Thy-1 allele or by separating the backcross progeny into two classes according to their zygosity for Thy-1.

The results of such a backcross are shown in Figure 3. When injected into AKR/J recipients, thymocytes from the majority (58/76 = 76%) of (CBA × AKR/Cum)F1 × AKR/Cum backcross donors induced augmented anti-Thy-1.2 primary PFC responses whereas thymocytes from the remaining donors (18/76 = 24%) induced poor responses. Assuming that the "carrier" genes are fully penetrant, this result is most consistent with the presence of two such loci in the CBA genome.

An objection to this analysis is that one of the two genetic factors identified above might not be a "carrier" determinant at all, but might instead reflect the existence of heretofore undiscovered variation among supposedly equivalent *Thy-1$^b$* alleles. Under this hypothesis it is assumed that the variant Thy-1.2 antigen of strain CBA is somehow intrinsically more immunogenic in AKR/J recipients than is the Thy-1.2 determinant of strain AKR/Cum. One of the two apparent "carrier"

**Table 5.** The "Carrier" Effect in Secondary PFC Responses.

| | Donor | | | |
|---|---|---|---|---|
| **Recipient** | **Primary** | **Secondary** | **PFC** | **p** |
| AKR/ABom ♀ | AKR/Cum ♀ | AKR/Cum ♀ | 100 0±25.2 (5) | |
| AKR/ABom ♀ | C3H ♀ | C3H ♀ | 1084.3±191.2 (4) | <0.01 |
| AKR/ABom ♀ | AKR/Cum ♀ | AKR/Cum ♀ | 76 3±11.3 (3) | |
| AKR/ABom ♀ | AKR/Cum ♀ | C3H ♀ | 118 3±38.3 (3) | n.s. |
| AKR/ABom ♀ | C3H ♀ | AKR/Cum ♀ | 60 0±26.5 (5) | n.s. |
| AKR/ABom ♀ | C3H ♀ | C3H ♀ | 899 3±98.9 (4) | <0.005[a] |

*Note*: Recipients were primed by the intravenous injection of $4 \times 10^7$ thymocytes on day 0 and challenged on day 21 (experiment 1) or day 14 (experiment 2) with an intravenous injection of $4 \times 10^7$ thymocytes. Secondary PFC responses were evaluated with AKR/Cum thymus cell targets on the third day after challenge, when the splenic PFC response is maximal (Fuji et al. 1971).

[a]The result of line 4 in experiment 2 also gave a p value of less than 0 005 when compared with the results of lines 2 or 3 in the same experiment.

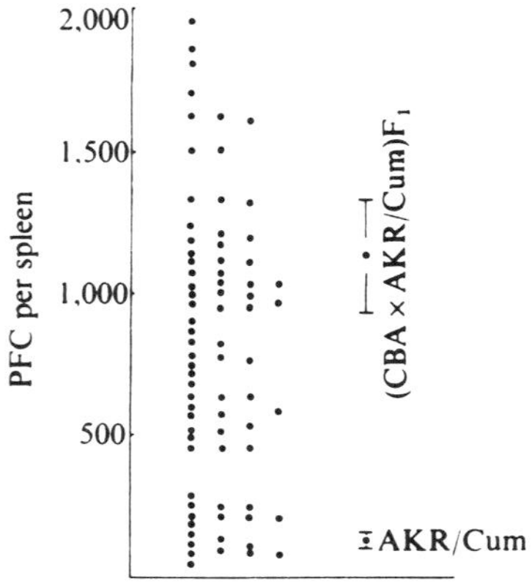


**Figure 3.** Distribution of immunogenicity of thymus cells from individual backcross mice with segregating helper determinants. Evidence for two antigenic "helper genes." A large age-matched pool of AKR/J female mice was randomized and arranged in groups of two or three recipients per backcross donor thymus and in groups of five or six for control thymus suspensions (a pool of several donors). The recipients were immunized with $4 \times 10^7$ (CBA × AKR/Cum)F1 × AKR/Cum backcross thymus cells i.v. and PFC per spleen determined on day 7. Each point represents the mean PFC per spleen of two or three recipients. Vertical bars represent ± 1 standard error of the mean.

SOURCE: *Lake and Douglas 1978.*

loci could then be attributed to the segregation of two distinct Thy-1 alleles which previously had been believed to be equivalent.

The validity of this type of objection can be assessed if segregation data for one or more genetic markers closely linked to Thy-1 are available. Any augmented immunogenicity actually due to differences in Thy-1 alleles should show up as a statistical association between Thy-1 immunogenicity and the Thy-1-linked allele inherited from the highly-immunogenic strain. Recently we have begun to analyze the progeny from an AKR/J × (AKR/J × MA/MyJ)F1 backcross in which alleles for the *Mpi-1* (mannosephosphate isomerase) locus are segregating. This locus, which is located approximately 7 centimorgans distal to Thy-1, provides an easily-typed marker for this region of chromosome 9 (Douglas and Dawson 1979a).

This backcross is also segregating for the marker *Glo-1* (glyoxalase I), which is located approximately 2.4 centimorgans proximal to *H-2K* (Douglas and Dawson 1979b; Rubinstein et al. 1979). It will thus be possible to test whether Thy-1 immunogenicity is being controlled in this backcross by an *H-2*linked factor even though MA/MyJ and AKR/J are both homozygous for the $H\text{-}2^k$ haplotype. Several genetic markers located on chromosomes other than 9 and 17 offer additional possibilities for the genetic mapping of "carrier" loci in this cross.

To date only a small number of AKR/J × (AKR/J × MA/MyJ)F1 backcross progeny have been examined. Assessment of the possible linkage associations of "carrier" loci must await more data, but the high frequency of animals whose thymocytes are poorly immunogenic (6/12 = 50%) indicates that only one or a few such loci are involved.

A second approach to the genetic analysis of "carrier" loci is through the use of congenic strains. Knowledge of the relative immunogenicities of thymocytes from a series of different congenic strains sharing a common genetic background might provide considerable information about the location and identity of Thy-1 "carrier" loci. Making use of this general approach, we have taken advantage of the "natural congenic" situation existing in all inbred mouse strains due to sexual dimorphism. Thymocytes from male donors present Thy-1 determinants in association with the male antigen, H-Y, whereas thymocytes from female donors do not (Králová and Démant 1976; Wachtel 1977). By using Thy-1 incompatible female recipients it is thus possible to judge whether H-Y can serve as a "carrier" determinant for Thy-1.

AKR/J and AKR/ABom females produced weak primary PFC responses against AKR/Cum thymocytes regardless of the sex of the donor (Table 6, lines 1–4). The use of (AKR/Cum × C3H/HeJ)F1 donors resulted in higher overall responses, but still no significant sex effect was observed.

In the reciprocal strain combination, the anti-Thy-1.1 response of AKR/Cum females to thymocytes of AKR/J males was statistically higher than that against AKR/J females in one of two experiments (lines 9 and 10), but this was due largely to the weakness of the control response rather than the strength of the response against male cells. When MA/MyJ donors were employed the overall anti-Thy-1.1 response was stronger (lines 11 and 12), but again no significant sex effect was seen.

The failure of H-Y to serve as an effective "carrier" determinant in the AKR sublines was apparent, but this result could not be generalized due to the low-responder status of $H\text{-}2^k$ mice toward the H-Y antigen (Wachtel 1977). It was therefore of interest to extend these experiments to $H\text{-}2^b$ animals, which have been shown on the basis of skin graft rejection to be high-responders to H-Y (Wachtel 1977). The primary anti-Thy-1.2 PFC response of B6-*Thy-1*$^a$ females[4] to C57BL/6J male thymocytes was significantly greater than that to C57BL/6J female thymocytes in one of two experiments (Table 6, lines 15 and 16), but this result is difficult to interpret with any certainty due to the high control responses seen against female cells. This is probably due to residual genetic differences between these two strains, and may indicate the presence of Thy-1-linked "carrier"-controlling gene in C57BL/6J.

[4]This congenic strain, which is more fully designated as B6.PL-*Thy-1*$^a$/Cy, was produced by Dr. Marianna Cherry at the Jackson Laboratory in Bar Harbor, Maine, who introduced the *Thy-1*$^a$ allele of strain PL/J onto the C57BL/6J background by 10 generations of backcrossing followed by an intercross and selection for *Thy-1*$^a$ homozygotes.

**Table 6.** Effect of Donor's Sex on Thy-1 Immunogenicity.

| Recipient[a] | Donor | PFC | | Target cells: Strain | Target cells: Thy-1 | p |
|---|---|---|---|---|---|---|
| AKR/J ♀ | AKR/Cum ♀ | 8.5± 2.6 | (6) | AKR/Cum ♀ | b | |
| AKR/J ♀ | AKR/Cum ♂ | 12.2± 5.6 | (6) | AKR/Cum ♀ | b | n.s. |
| AKR/ABom ♀ | AKR/Cum ♀ | 3.4± 1.3 | (5) | AKR/Cum ♀ | b | |
| AKR/ABom ♀ | AKR/Cum ♂ | 2.0± 1.4 | (6) | AKR/Cum ♀ | b | n.s. |
| AKR/ABom ♀ | (AKR/Cum × C3H)F1 ♀ | 55.0±19.6 | (6) | AKR/Cum ♀ | b | |
| AKR/ABom ♀ | (AKR/Cum × C3H)F1 ♂ | 75.5 ±26.6 | (6) | AKR/Cum ♀ | b | n.s. |
| AKR/Cum ♀ | AKR/J ♀ | 8.7± 5.3 | (6) | AKR/J ♀ | a | |
| AKR/Cum ♀ | AKR/J ♂ | 5.0± 1.8 | (6) | AKR/J ♀ | a | n.s. |
| AKR/Cum ♀ | AKR/J ♀ | 1.0± 0.3 | (5) | AKR/J ♀ | a | |
| AKR/Cum ♀ | AKR/J ♂ | 15.5± 6.6 | (6) | AKR/J ♀ | a | <0.05 |
| AKR/Cum ♀ | MA ♀ | 88.5±27.2 | (4) | AKR/J ♀ | a | |
| AKR/Cum ♀ | MA ♂ | 142.5± 8.1 | (4) | AKR/J ♀ | a | n.s. |
| B6-*Thy-1^a* ♀ | C57BL/6J ♀ | 260.0±56.7 | (6) | C57BL/6J ♀ | b | |
| B6-*Thy-1^a* ♀ | C57BL/6J♂ | 261.2±67.3 | (6) | C57BL/6J ♀ | b | n.s. |
| B6-*Thy-1^a* ♀ | C57BL/6J ♀ | 65.7±25.3 | (6) | C57BL/6J ♀ | b | |
| B6-*Thy-1^l* ♀ | C57BL/6J ♂ | 163.3±18.9 | (6) | C57BL/6J ♀ | b | <0.025 |
| C57BL/6J ♀ | B6-*Thy-1^a* ♀ | 3.0± 0.8 | (5) | B6-*Thy-1^a* ♂ | a | |
| C57BL/6J ♀ | B6-*Thy-1^a* ♂ | 194.6±55.2 | (6) | B6-*Thy-1^a* ♂ | a | <0.025 |
| C57BL/6J ♀ | B6-*Thy-1^a* ♀ | 18.8± 3.8 | (6) | B6-*Thy-1^a* ♀ | a | |
| C57BL/6J ♀ | B6-*Thy-1^a* ♂ | 95.5±20.0 | (6) | B6-*Thy-1^a* ♀ | a | <0.01 |
| C57BL/6J ♀ | B6-*Thy-1^a* ♂ | 113.8±24.1 | (6) | B6-*Thy-1^a* ♂ | a | <0.01 |
| C57BL/6J ♀ | B6-*Thy-1^a* ♂ | 0.0 | (6) | C57BL/6Tex ♂ | a | n.s. |

[a]Recipients were injected intravenously with $4 \times 10^7$ thymocytes. Primary PFC responses were evaluated on day 6.

The results obtained with C57BL/6J anti B6-*Thy-1^a* immunizations were much more clear-cut.[5] Responses against B6-*Thy-1^a* male cells exceeded those against B6-*Thy-1^a* female cells by more than 60-fold in the first experiment and by more than 5-fold in the second (Table 6, lines 17–20). The demonstration of a donor sex effect was greatly facilitated in this case by the low control response to female thymocytes. Because a shortage of B6-*Thy-1^a* animals forced us to use male target cells in the first experiment, it was necessary to show that the apparently augmented

[5]The inbred strain C57BL/6J was originally classified by Zaleski and co-workers as a low responder to Thy-1.1 on the basis of experiments in which *H-2^b*, *Thy-1^b* mice were immunized with thymocytes from *H-2^k*, *Thy-1^a* donors. Although the early results obtained by this group suggested that anti-Thy-1 responses were not affected by donor genes other than Thy-1 (Fuji et al. 1972; Zaleski and Klein 1974; Zaleski 1975; Zaleski and Klein 1975; Zaleski and Klein 1976), it has been demonstrated subsequently that *H-2* incompatibility between donor and recipient can have strong negative effects on Thy-1 immunogenicity (Lake and Mitchison 1977; Zaleski and Klein 1978; Zaleski et al. 1978). In order to avoid the complicating factor of *H-2* incompatibility in these experiments, we have used only *H-2*-matched donor/recipient combinations.

immunogenicity of Thy-1.1 seen in this experiment was not due to the detection of H-Y-specific PFC. This possibility was clearly ruled out by the results of the second experiment. Male B6-*Thy-1^c^* target cells, which present both H-Y and Thy-1.1 determinants, did not reveal significantly more PFC than did female cells. Furthermore, C57BL/6Tex male thymocytes, which present H-Y in the absence of Thy-1.1, detected no PFC at all. It seems clear, therefore, that H-Y is functioning as an effective "carrier" for Thy-1.1 in this strain combination.

## Concluding Remarks

The transplantation of genetically incompatible cells can potentially induce both cellular and humoral immune responses. In the experiments described above we have focused on the latter, using the genetically polymorphic Thy-1 antigens as a model. The immunogenicity of the Thy-1 antigens present on transplanted thymocytes is dependent upon several genetic factors, all of which are related to the ability of the recipient's immune system to distinguish "self" from "non-self." To provoke a strong anti-Thy-1 response, the transplanted cells must first express Thy-1 determinants that can be recognized as foreign. Second, in most (and possibly all) of the cases examined so far, these cells must express one or more additional alloantigens which can serve as an immunological "carrier" for the otherwise poorly-immunogenic Thy-1 determinants. Finally, the donor cells should not present foreign *H-2* antigens. The usually suppressive effect of *H-2* incompatibility on Thy-1 immunogenicity has been observed in a number of cases (Lake and Mitchison 1977; Zaleski et al. 1978), but the mechanism underlying this phenomenon is not yet fully understood.

Our recent experiments strongly suggest that the male antigen, H-Y, can serve as an effective "carrier" for Thy-1. The ability of H-Y to fulfill this function in the $H$-$2^b$ strain C57BL/6J and possibly in B6-*Thy-1*$^a$, but not in the $H$-$2^k$ strains AKR/J or AKR/Cum, is in accord with other evidence indicating that the recognition of "carrier" determinants for Thy-1 is immunologically specific. We are hopeful that this development, together with others such as the successful demonstration of *in vitro* anti-Thy-1 antibody responses (Fuji and Milgrom 1973; Lake 1976) and the discovery that virus-induced antigens can provide "help" for Thy-1 (Lake and Bromberg 1979), will open up new avenues of research. The improved understanding of cell surface immunogenicity to which these lines of experimentation appear to be leading is of consequence not only to immunogeneticists who are actively working in this area, but also to the much larger circle of researchers and clinicians who are concerned with the transplantation or transfusion of living cells.

ACKNOWLEDGMENTS

We thank Dr. Edward Clark (a second generation member of Ray Owen's academic pedigree) for permission to cite his unpublished results regarding the carrier specificity of secondary anti-Thy-1 PFC responses. Mice of the congenic strain B6.PL-*Thy-1*$^a$/Cy and specific sheep anti-mouse IgM antiserum were gifts from Drs. Marianna Cherry and Georges Köhler, respectively. Dr. Elizabeth Blankenhorn assisted in the recovery of data from some of our original experiments with Thy-1. This work was supported by Grants GM 00086, GM 19513, and AI 15772 from the U.S. National Institutes of Health, Contract AT 04-3-767 from the U.S. Atomic Energy Commission, a National Defense Education Act fellowship, and research funds provided by F. Hoffmann-LaRoche and Co. through the Basel Institute for Immunology.

# References

Acton, R.T. et al. 1973. Variations among sublines of inbred AKR mice. Nature New Biol. 245:8.

Boyse, E.A. and Old, L.J. 1969. Some aspects of normal and abnormal cell surface genetics. Ann. Rev. Genet. 3:269.

Dorf, M.E. and Stimpfling, J.H. 1977. Couples complementation of immune response genes controlling responsiveness to the *H*-2.2 alloantigen. J. Exp. Med. 146:571.

Douglas, T.C. 1972. Occurrence of a theta-like antigen in rats. J. Exp. Med. 136:1054.

Douglas, T.C. and Dawson, P.E. 1979a. Location of the gene for theta antigen in the mouse. III. The position of Thy-1 relative to Lap-1 and *Mpi-1*. J. Hered. 70:250.

Douglas, T.C. and Dawson, P.E. 1979b. The position of the gene for Glyozalase I on chromosome 17 of the mouse. Immunogenetics 8:367.

Dulbecco, R and Vogt, M. 1954. Plaque formation and isolation of pure lines with poliomyelitis viruses. J. Exp. Med. 99:167.

Frelinger, J.A. and Murphy, D.B. 1976. A new alloantigen, Ly-8, recognized by C3H anti-AKR serum. Immunogenetics 3:481.

Fuji, H. and Milgrom, F. 1973. Plaque-forming cells after *in vitro* stimulation with θ-AKR antigen. Cell. Immunol. 7:502.

Fuji, H. et al. 1971. Immune response to alloantigens of thymus studied in mice with plaque assay. J. Immunol. 106:56.

Fuji, H. et al. 1972. Genetic control of immune response to θ-AKR alloantigen. J. Immunol. 108:223.

Kralova, J. and Demant, P. 1976. Expression of the H-Y antigen on thymus cells and skin: Differential genetic control linked to K end of *H-2*. Immunogenetics 3:583.

Krog, H.-H. 1976. Identification of inbred strains of mice, *Mus musculus*. I. Genetic control of inbred strains of mice using starch gel electrophoresis. Biochem. Genet. 14:319.

Lake, P. 1976. Antibody response induced *in vitro* to the cell-surface Allo-antigen Thy-1. Nature 262:297.

Lake, P. and Bromberg, J. 1979. Viruses and alloantigens can act as helper determinants for antibody responses to another surface antigen, Thy-1. In Cell Biology and Immunology of Leukocyte Function. M.R. Quastel, ed. New York: Academic Press.

Lake, P. and Douglas, T.C. 1978. Recognition and genetic control of helper determinants for cell surface antigens. Cold Spring Harbor Symp. Quant. Biol. 41:589.

Raff, M.C. 1971. The use of surface antigenic markers to define different populations of lymphocytes in the mouse. In Cell Interactions and Receptor Antobodies in Immune Responses. O. Mäkelä, A. Cross, and T.U. Kosunen, eds. London: Academic Press.

Reif, A.E. and Allen, J.M.V. 1964. The AKR thymic antigen and its distribution in leukemias and nervous tissues. J. Exp. Med. 120:413.

Reif, A.E. and Allen, J.M.V. 1966a. Mouse nervous tissue isoantigens. Nature 209:523.

Reif, A.E. and Allen, J.M.V. 1966b. Mouse thymic isoantigens. Nature 209:521.

Rubinstein, P. et al. 1979. The location of the C3 and *GLO* (glyoxalase I) loci of the IXth linkage group in mice. J. Immunol. 122:2584.

Schachner, M. and Hämmerling, U. 1974. The postnatal development of antigens on mouse brain cell surfaces. Brain Res. 73:362.

Schlesinger, M. and Hurvitz, D. 1969. Characterization of cytotoxic isoantisera produced in RIII mice. I. Demonstration of antibodies against the θ-C3H isoantigen. Transplantation 7:132.

Shen, F. et al. 1975. Preparation and use of Ly antisera. Immunogenetics 2:591.

Snedecor, G.W. and Cochran, W.G. 1967. Statistical Methods. Ames, Iowa: Iowa State University Press, p. 114.

Snell, G.D. 1971. The histocompatibility systems. Transplant. Proc. 3:1133.

Taylor, G.M. and Bennett, J. 1973. A modified plaque test for the detection of cells forming antibody to alloantigens. J. Immunol. Methodol. 2:213.

Wachtel, S.S. 1977. H-Y antigen: Genetics and serology. Immunol. Rev. 33:33.

Wernet, D. and Lilly, F. 1975. Genetic regulation of the antibody response to *H-2D*$^b$ alloantigens in mice. I. Differences in activation of helper T-cells in C57BL/10 and BALB/c congenic strains. J. Exp. Med. 141:573.

Zaleski, M.B. 1975. Preliminary evidence of genetic control of the immune response to the Thy-1.2 antigen in mice. Immunogenetics 2:21.

Zaleski, M.B. and Klein, J. 1974. Immune response of mice to Thy-1.1 antigen: Genetic control by alleles at the *Ir*-5 locus loosely linked to the *H-2* complex. J. Immunol. 113:1170.

Zaleski, M.B. and Klein, J. 1975. A new locus (*Ir*-5) controlling immune response to Thy-1.1 (θ-AKR) antigen. Transplant. Proc. 7:101.

Zaleski, M.B. and Klein, J. 1976. Immune response of mice to the Thy-1.1 antigen: Intra-*H-2* mapping of the complementary *Ir*-Thy-1 loci. J. Immunol. 117:814.

Zaleski, M.B. and Klein, J. 1978. Genetic control of the immune response to Thy-1 antigens. Immunol. Rev. 38:120.

Zaleski, M.B. et al. 1978. Effect of *H-2* incompatibility between recipient and donor on the magnitude of response to Thy-1.1 antigen. Immunogenetics 6:553.

Hildemann, ed. Frontiers in Immunogenetics

# Function, Structure, and Regulation of the Murine C4/Slp Protein Variants

Donald C. Shreffler

*Department of Genetics, Washington University, School of Medicine, St. Louis, Missouri*

## Introduction

It is a particular pleasure to have the opportunity through this symposium to express to Ray Owen my respect and affection and my gratitude to him for his example of excellence and responsibility as a scientist and a person. This presentation will deal in some detail with the historical development and current status of the murine Ss-Slp serum protein variant system. I think this is especially appropriate on this occasion, because Ray was responsible for its discovery.

The genetic variation in this system was initially recognized when a rabbit antiserum reactive with multiple mouse serum globulins was tested in Ouchterlony immunodiffusion against sera from mice of a number of different inbred strains. Ray Owen recognized, in those immunodiffusion results, the fact that a few inbred strains have very low quantitative levels of one of the several serum proteins recognized by the rabbit antiserum. When the complex rabbit antiserum was absorbed with serum from the mice with low levels of that specific protein, a monospecific antiserum was produced. The specific antiserum made it possible to classify a large number of inbred mouse strains as either Ss-High or Ss-Low. The term Ss, serologically detected serum protein, was applied to the variant protein (Shreffler and Owen 1963). It was also possible to use the Ss antiserum to classify $F_1$, $F_2$, and backcross progeny for their Ss levels and to demonstrate that the observed quantitative differences are due to a single autosomal locus with two additively acting alleles. We then recognized that the controlling locus is linked to the genetic system called at that time the *H-2-locus,* which of course has been defined subsequently as a gene complex with multiple loci. It was observed that all Ss-Low strains have the same, *H-2*$^k$, haplotype. (I am grateful to Dr. Bill Hildemann for

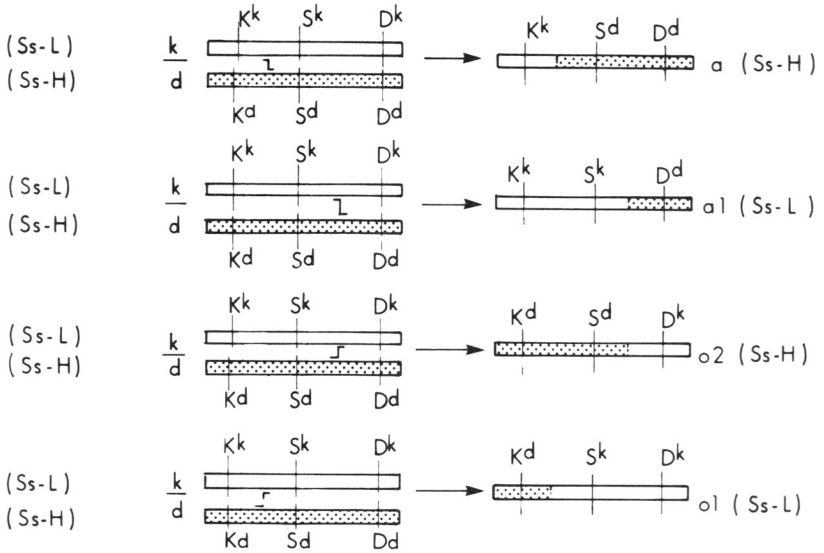

**Figure 1.** An example of the intra-*H-2* recombinants which have mapped the Ss and Slp traits inside the *H-2* complex, to the *S* region.

first raising the question of po sible *H-2* linkage.) Backcross linkage tests then showed a close association between the *H-2* alloantigens and the Ss variation (Shreffler and Owen, 1963; Shreffler 1964).

The recognition of *Ss-H-2* linkage, and the complexity of the *H-2* locus (gene complex) that was emerging from work at that time by Gorer and Mikulska (1959), Hoecker et al. (1959), and Stimpfling and Richardson (1965), prompted a search for genetic recombination in crosses involving differences in both the *H-2* alloantigens and the Ss protein, in order to map the Ss locus with respect to *H-2*. This resulted in the early detection or recognition of four intra-*H-2* recombinants (Figure 1), analyses of which clearly positioned the Ss locus inside the *H-2* complex, between the two alloantigen-determining loci that were eventually named *H-2K* and *H-2D* (Shreffler 1965). These and many recombinants analyzed subsequently thus defined the *S* region of the *H-2* complex (cf. Klein 1975; Shreffler and David 1975).

In 1966, Howard Passmore joined my laboratory and began a search for structural variations in the Ss protein. One approach was to perform alloimmunizations, with serum, among strains differing with respect to Ss level. These studies resulted in the production of alloantisera that defined strain differences in the expression of one specific class or form of the Ss serum protein. Curiously, this protein was expressed only in males of the positive strains (Passmore and Shreffler 1970). Further investigation established that the expression of this allotypic antigen, called Slp (sex-limited protein) because of its male-limitation, is under the control of a single dominant gene which is linked to *H-2* and localized in the same *S* region as the Ss quantitative variation. The sex-limitation was shown to be due to a requirement in the Slp-positive strains for induction by testosterone of the expression of the Slp protein (Passmore and Shreffler 1971).

The availability of the Slp marker made possible the further detailed characterization of the many intra-*H-2* recombinants already defined. These analyses further strengthened the conclusion that the *S* region separates the *H-2K* and *H-2D* loci and clarified a number of ambiguities with respect to previous genetic maps of the *H-2* complex (Shreffler et al. 1971; Stimpfling 1971; Snell et al. 1971). Continuing analyses of intra-*H-2* recombinants have resulted in an exceedingly complex map of the *H-2* gene complex. The map in Figure 2 depicts the multiple loci and functional classes that are represented within the *H-2* complex, and features those loci that are thought to represent genetic duplicates. The concept of genetic duplication within the *H-2* complex was a fundamental element in the clarification of the *H-2* genetic map (Shreffler et al. 1971). Current evidence suggests that at least five, and probably at least several more, duplicate genes determine Class I products, and that there are at least two duplicate genes for each of the two polypeptide subunits of the Class II products or *Ia* antigens. In this map, we further postulate the existence of two discrete structural genes (C4 and Slp) that determine the structures of two discrete classes of Ss proteins, and that have associated with them regulatory elements that mediate Ss quantitative genetic variation and Slp allotype expression. In the remainder of this paper, the evidence for those postulates will be developed.

Before proceeding, however, a brief discussion of notation is necessary. The original Ss serum protein variation was defined by a rabbit antiserum that was specifically reactive with a *class* of serum proteins. The serum protein which is expressed at low level in Ss-Low mice is now known to be the fourth component of murine complement, C4. Ss-Low mice uniformly fail to express Slp. Work

**Figure 2.** A genetic map of the murine *H-2* gene complex depicting loci thought to have derived through gene duplication.

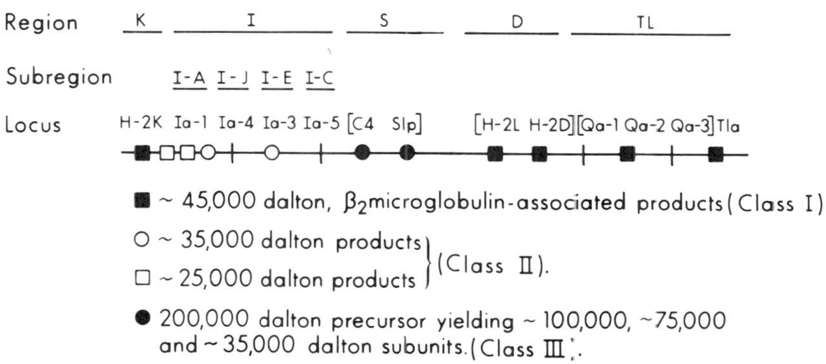

by Howard Passmore and by Ted Hansen in my laboratory demonstrated that the anti-Ss antibodies also react with those molecules that are reactive with the Slp alloantiserum (Passmore and Shreffler 1970; Hansen et al. 1974). In sequential immunoprecipitation analyses, anti-Ss serum precipitated all Slp-reactive molecules, however prior treatment with anti-Slp removed only a fraction of the Ss-reactive molecules. More recent experiments have demonstrated that those molecules responsible for typical C4 functional activity and those molecules reactive with the anti-Slp serum are antigenically and structurally discrete (see below). These results indicate that anti-Ss serum recognizes a *class* of related proteins comprised of at least two distinct subpopulations, one of which is the typical C4 molecule, the other of which is the Slp molecule. Consequently, in the map in Figure 2, the two structural loci are designated as C4 and Slp. In the remainder of this paper, the C4/Slp notation will be utilized for these two related but structurally distinct proteins.

## Function of the Ss Proteins

There was no clue to the biological function of the Ss-Slp proteins until 1973, when Demant et al. demonstrated the existence of *H-2*-linked, *S* region-localized, differences in *total* hemolytic complement activity in mice (Demant et al. 1973). In 1975, Tommy Meo demonstrated that anti-Ss sera cross-react with a component in human serum, which he identified as the fourth component of human complement (C4). He also found that anti-human C4 reagents cross-react with mouse Ss proteins, indicating a close structural similarity of these proteins (Meo et al. 1975). This finding suggested a possible functional homology between the Ss protein and human C4. Concordant observations were subsequently reported from other laboratories (Curman et al. 1975; Lachmann et al. 1975; Goldman and Goldman 1976).

The development of sensitive, specific hemolytic assays for murine C4 in the laboratories of Capra and Nussenzweig (Carroll and Capra 1978; Ferreira et al. 1978) and by my colleague at Washington University, John Atkinson (Atkinson et al. 1980a,b), has made it possible to examine the functional roles of the two Ss proteins. In such an assay system, we have demonstrated three discrete, genetically-determined levels of C4 functional activity (Table 1). One is associated with $H\text{-}2^k$ haplotype, which has low Ss levels and low C4 hemolytic activity, a second with the $H\text{-}2^{w7}$ haplotype, which has high Ss levels but intermediate C4 functional activity. All other *H-2* haplotypes examined determine high Ss levels and high C4 functional activity. Analyses of multiple intra-*H-2* recombinants have shown that these quantitative differences in C4 levels are determined by the *S* region of the *H-2* complex. In addition to these variations in functional C4 levels, different *H-2* haplotypes can also be discriminated on the basis of expression or nonexpression of the Slp antigen and, further, on the basis of differences in quantitative levels of expression of the Slp antigen (Table 1).

The $H\text{-}2^{w7}$ haplotype is also of particular interest because it determines the highest levels of Ss and Slp found thus far, and because in strains carrying this haplotype both *males* and *females* express the Slp protein. The work of Hansen (Hansen and

**Table 1.** Ss, Slp and C4 Levels in Plasmas From Male Mice of Congenic Strains With Standard *H-2* Haplotypes.

| | | Level of: | | | | |
|---|---|---|---|---|---|---|
| | | Ss | | Slp | | C4 |
| **Congenic strain** | ***H-2* haplotype** | **H or L** | **Conc.**[a] | **+ or −** | **% of Ss** | **Units/ml**[b] |
| B10 | b | H | 0.72 | − | 0 | 3380 ± 758 |
| B10.D2 | d | H | 1.00 | + | 20-30 | 4313 ± 846 |
| B10.M | f | H | 1.01 | − | 0 | 4687 ± 1104 |
| B10.K | k | L | 0.07 | − | 0 | 410 ± 79 |
| B10.Q | q | H | 0.81 | − | 0 | 4529 ± 1434 |
| B10.S | s | H | 0.93 | + | 5-10 | 4085 ± 1785 |
| B10.WR | w7 | H | 1.24 | + | 50-60 | 1158 ± 212 |

[a]Expressed in arbitrary units—1.0 equals the level in a pool of B10.D2 male mice. Taken from data published by Hansen and Shreffler (1976).

[b]The mean ± SEM for 5 to 27 mice between 6 and 12 weeks of age for each strain. Taken from data of Atkinson et al. (1980b).

Shreffler 1976) indicated that the *S* region of such mice carries a control element that determines simple dominant expression of the Slp protein *without* any significant regulation by male hormone. This "constitutive" expression of Slp is further discussed below.

The high Ss levels, but low C4 functional levels, associated with the $H\text{-}2^{w7}$ haplotype have been of particular interest. The simplest explanations for this observation are either that the C4 molecule of the $H\text{-}2^{w7}$ haplotype has a greater susceptibility to proteolytic inactivation or that it has a reduced C4 functional activity. An alternative explanation was that it might have reduced activity due to interference with C4 functional activity by the high levels of the Slp protein expressed in the serum of such animals, since previous results had suggested that the Slp protein is functionally inactive in C4 hemolytic assays (Ferreira et al. 1978). Data bearing on this point are presented in Table 2. They demonstrate: (1) that, since anti-Ss totally depletes C4 functional activity, Ss-reactive proteins include all functional C4 molecules, and (2) that, since depletion of all Slp-reactive molecules

**Table 2.** Effects of Depletions by Anti-Ss and Anti-Slp Sera on C4 Functional Activity.[a]

| | Residual C4 units | | Residual C4 units | |
|---|---|---|---|---|
| **Congenic strain** | **Control** | **Ss-depleted** | **Control** | **Slp-depleted** |
| B10.M | 5361 | 0 | 5247 | 5712 |
| B10.D2 | 4107 | 0 | 4076 | 4123 |
| B10.WR | 786 | 0 | 963 | 979 |

[a]Pools of three males, 6-9 weeks of age.

with anti-Slp does not at all influence C4 functional hemolytic activity, the Slp molecules are functionally inactive, at least in this assay system. Since the C4 functional activity in mice with the $H$-$2^{w7}$ haplotype is unchanged after Slp depletion, the low C4 functional activity of these animals cannot be attributed to interference or competition by Slp molecules. A structural difference in the α-chain of the C4 molecule determined by the $H$-$2^{w7}$ haplotype has been defined (see below), and we believe that this structural difference is most likely responsible for the reduced C4 functional activity of these mice (Atkinson et al. 1980a).

Other data from our laboratory suggest that the Slp molecules may indeed exhibit at least some aspects of C4 functional activity, since they can be bound to antibody-sensitized sheep erythrocytes in a manner directly comparable to that of C4 molecules. This binding can be demonstrated by the agglutination of such indicator erythrocytes by anti-Slp antibodies. It is possible that the current C4 assay system, which utilizes C4-deficient guinea pig serum, does not detect functional activity of the Slp molecule because of incompatibilities between murine and guinea pig components. It is also possible that the Slp molecule has an alternative function that does not involve the lytic complement pathway. The functional activity of the Slp molecule is a question of continuing interest and investigation in our laboratory. The potential to examine such questions more thoroughly now exists, because of the development of methodology for the structural characterization of the C4 and Slp proteins.

## Structural Studies of the C4 and Slp Proteins

The development by my graduate student, Marleen Roos, of the methodology for *in vitro* radiolabeling and immunoprecipitation of the C4 and Slp proteins made possible some significant advances in our understanding of the structures of these molecules (Roos et al. 1978). Briefly, this method involves the culture of resident peritoneal macrophages for periods of 1 to 24 hours in the presence of radiolabeled amino acids or sugars. Immunoprecipitations are performed, at equivalence, on the culture supernatants and macrophage lysates, in the presence of carrier plasma, first with anti-Slp (when this protein is present), followed by anti-Ss to precipitate residual C4 molecules. The precipitates are separated on SDS-polyacrylamide gels, which are subjected to autoradiography for visualization of the radiolabeled polypeptides. The labeled materials may then be recovered from the SDS gels for peptide mapping or microsequencing.

Analyses by this method demonstrated that the cultured macrophages secrete, into the culture supernatant, antigenically distinct C4 and Slp molecules, which can be separated by the sequential immunoprecipitation procedure. The surprising finding was made by Roos that, while both the C4 and Slp molecules have the expected α, β, and γ subunits with molecular weights of approximately 100,000, 75,000, and 35,000, as previously found for human and guinea pig C4, the precise molecular weights of the C4 and Slp subunits differ by several thousand daltons. This implied that the two populations of molecules are the products of discrete structural genes.

An observation in the guinea pig (Hall and Colten 1977), suggesting that the α, β, and γ subunits may be derived from a single polypeptide precursor, led us to examine the Ss- and Slp-reactive intracellular materials from lysates of the cultured macrophages. The lysate precipitates revealed the presence of two discrete single chain polypeptides of approximately 200,000 molecular weight, which could be separated by the sequential precipitation procedure. Our interpretation of these results was that duplicate, discrete structural genes for the C4 and Slp precursors exist, and that mutational divergence of these genes has resulted in precursors that are processed somewhat differently, to yield α, β, and γ subunits of differing molecular weights.

These initial observations led us to postulate a general model for the genetic control of the biosynthesis of the C4 and Slp proteins, shown in Figure 3. More recent investigations have been directed toward the resolution of several specific questions about this model. The evidence bearing on these questions, deriving primarily from the work of a graduate student, Keith Parker, is summarized in the following sections.

**Figure 3.** A model for the genetic control and biosynthesis of the murine C4 and Slp proteins. The heavy segments at the left side of the C4 and Slp structural genes are intended to represent regulatory elements.

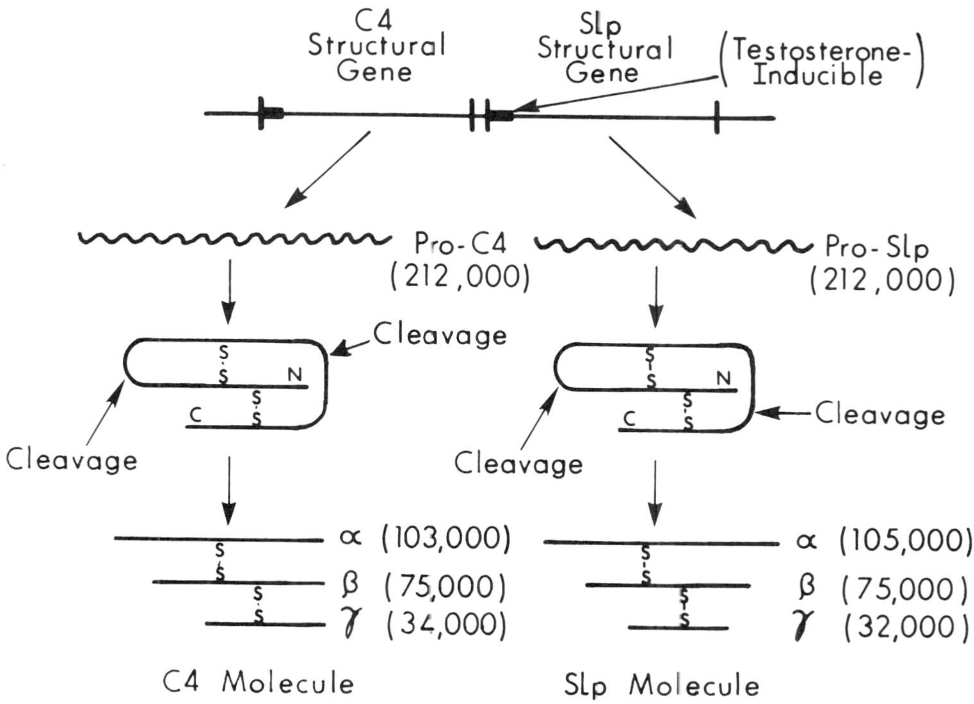

| | | | | | | 5 | | | | | 10 | | |
|---|---|---|---|---|---|---|---|---|---|---|---|---|---|
| Human | C4 α-chain | Asn | Val | Asn | Phe | Gln | Lys | Asn | Ile | Asn | Glu | Lys | Leu |
| Murine | C4 α-chain | | | | Phe | | Lys | | | | | Lys | Leu |

| | | | | | | 5 | | | | |
|---|---|---|---|---|---|---|---|---|---|---|
| Human | C4 β-chain | Lys | Pro | Arg | Leu | Leu | Leu | Phe | Val | Pro |
| Murine | C4 β-chain | Lys | | | Leu | Leu | Leu | Phe | | |
| Murine | C4 precursor | Lys | | | Leu | Leu | Leu | Phe | | |

| | | | | | | 5 | | | | | 10 | | |
|---|---|---|---|---|---|---|---|---|---|---|---|---|---|
| Human | C4 γ-chain | Glu | Ala | Pro | Lys | Val | Val | Glu | Glu | Gln | Glu | Ser | Arg |
| Murine | C4 γ-chain | | | | Lys | | | | | | | | |

**Figure 4.** Results of partial amino-terminal sequencing of murine C4 α-, β-, and γ-chains and precursor, and comparison with human C4.

## *The Precursor-Subunit Relationship*

The first question asked was whether the high-molecular weight single polypeptide intracellular molecules precipitated by anti-Slp and anti-Ss are indeed the precursors of the three-subunit molecules found in the culture supernatants. This question was first approached by pulse-chase experiments in which a one-hour pulse of $^{35}S$-methionine was shown to transfer in the succeeding three hours from the two discrete intracellular polypeptides into the α, β, and γ subunits of C4 and Slp. Secondly, by comparing peptide maps of the radiolabeled C4 and Slp precursors with the individual subunits of both the C4 molecules and Slp molecules, it was demonstrated in all comparisons that all peptides present in the subunits were also present in the corresponding precursor (Parker et al. 1979). Recently, through collaboration with Dr. J. Donald Capra, Texas Southwestern Medical Center, partial microsequencing of the C4 precursor and subunits has been done. These results, depicted in Figure 4, clearly confirm the homology of murine and human C4 and further demonstrate that the C4 precursor shares it amino-terminal sequence with that of the C4 β-chain (Parker et al. 1980b). This result indicates that the β-chain subunit is indeed related to the precursor and is located at the amino-terminal of the precursor. Less extensive, but entirely concordant, results have been obtained for comparisons between the Slp precursor and subunits.

## *The C4-Slp Structural Relationship*

Our next question concerned the postulate that the C4 and Slp precursors and subunits differ in their primary structure, i.e., in amino acid sequence. In peptide map comparisons between the α-chains and β-chains of these two populations of molecules, multiple shared and multiple discrete peptides were observed (Parker et al. 1979). Approximately 50% of peptides were shared between the two molecules. This is approximately the level of sharing observed in comparisons of different *H-2K* or *H-2D* allelic products. It suggests a substantial sequence homology, with approximately 80 to 90% identical residues. The extent of peptide dissimilarities argues against some post-translational processing mechanism, such as differential glycosylation or differential proteolytic cleavage of a *common* C4/Slp precursor. The peptide map differences thus strongly imply that the C4 and Slp precursors are the products of *discrete* structural genes.

### *Location of the C4 and Slp Structural Genes*

We have postulated that the C4 and Slp *structural* genes are located in the *S* region, in association with control elements which modulate their expression. To demonstrate that the structural genes for these proteins are located in the *S* region, it was necessary to demonstrate that the C4 and Slp products of different *H-2* haplotypes exhibit genetically determined variations in structures. Two lines of evidence on the C4 protein are consistent with this postulate. Both involve comparisons of the C4 product of the $H\text{-}2^{w7}$ haplotype with the products of other haplotypes. First, a single peptide map difference is seen in comparisons of the β-chains from the $H\text{-}2^{w7}$ C4 molecule with C4 produced by strains of other *H-2* haplotypes (Parker et al. 1980a). Secondly, a difference of approximately 5,000 daltons in the apparent molecular weight on SDS-polacrylamide gels of the α-chains of the $H\text{-}2^{w7}$ C4 molecule, relative to the C4 α-chains of all other haplotypes examined, implied a structural difference in that chain as well (Roos et al. 1978). A peptide map difference has also been observed in comparisons of the $H\text{-}2^{w7}$ precursor with the precursors of other haplotypes (D. Karp, unpublished). In animals heterozygous for the $H\text{-}2^{w7}$ haplotype and other haplotypes, the two α-chains of different molecular weights are both expressed. The codominant expression of these chains argues in favor of a primary structural difference, rather than some post-translational modification mechanism, to explain the molecular weight differences (Parker et al. 1980a). Carroll and Capra (1979) have also defined a single peptide difference among the C4 β-chains from different *H-2* haplotypes by the Cleveland-Laemmli, V8 protease mapping procedure and have localized this difference to the *S* region.

Preliminary results with the Cleveland-Laemmli method applied to unlabeled Slp molecules from $H\text{-}2^{w7}$ and $H\text{-}2^{a}$ haplotypes have revealed a single peptide difference in the β-chains. In males heterozygous for these two haplotypes, both peptides are expressed in about equal quantities, once again arguing against a post-translational mechanism. It is of particular interest that in females heterozygous for these two haplotypes, one of which ($H\text{-}2^{w7}$) determines *constitutive* expression of Slp and the other of which ($H\text{-}2^{a}$) determines *sex-limited* expression of Slp, only the constitutive form is expressed, indicating a *cis-dominant* regulation of Slp expression by the $H\text{-}2^{w7}$ haplotype. (Parker et al. 1981). This exemplifies the ways in which the availability of structural markers for these two proteins should make it possible to examine in greater detail the many interesting regulatory variations in the C4/Slp system.

## Regulatory Variations in C4 and Slp Expression

The first variation recognized in this system was the quantitative Ss-High vs Ss-Low difference, which we now know is due to a difference in the C4 protein. To date, we have been unable to detect structural differences between the C4 products

**Table 3.** Regulatory Variations in Slp Expression.[a]

| | Nature of expression: | | |
|---|---|---|---|
| **Property** | **Sex-limited** | **Constitutive** | **Permissive** |
| Expressed in | ♂♂ only | ♂♂ and ♀♀ | ♂♂ and ♀♀ |
| Slp levels | Variable | ♂ ≥ ♀ | ♂ ≫ ♀ |
| Genetic control of expression | *S* region, dominant | *S* region, dominant | *S* region, plus 2 non-*H-2* (*rsl*) genes, recessive |
| Effect of male castration | Eliminates | Minimal reduction | Reduces to ♀ level |
| Effect of testosterone in female | Induces | Minimal increase | Increases to ♂ level |
| Effect of *Tfm* (testicular feminization | Eliminates | No effect | Reduces to ♀ level |
| Developmental appearance | Sexual maturity | Before birth | Sexual maturity |

[a]Based upon data of Passmore and Shreffler (1971); Hansen (1975); Hansen and Shreffler (1976); Brown and Shreffler (1980); Brown (1980).

of the $H\text{-}2^k$ haplotype and the products of other, SS-High *H-2* haplotypes. Although the quantitative difference could be the result of a difference in the C4 structural gene influencing rate of transcription, rate of translation, stability of the C4 product, etc., we have interpreted this difference as reflecting genetic variation in a cis-acting control element associated with the C4 structural gene (Hansen 1975). Further structural comparisons of these proteins are in progress.

A number of very interesting regulatory variations in Slp expression have now been defined. These variations, summarized briefly in Table 3, make this system of great potential interest for the examination and definition of mammalian regulatory mechanisms. Three forms of regulatory control of Slp expression have been recognized. The original *sex-limited* expression requires testosterone induction in animals carrying those *H-2* haplotypes that are capable of expressing Slp protein. *Constitutive* expression of Slp is determined by the $H\text{-}2^{w7}$ haplotype, with both males and females expressing Slp protein in essentially complete concordance with their expression of C4 protein (Hansen and Shreffler 1976). In mice of this type, there is minimal influence by testosterone. Recently, a third variation involving Slp expression was recognized when we were sent a Japanese strain, FM, for *H-2* typing. This strain was found to carry the $H\text{-}2^d$ haplotype, which normally is associated with sex-limited expression of the Slp protein. However, female mice of this strain also express Slp, although at significantly lower levels than males. Examination of additional inbred strains not previously classified for Slp revealed that the NZB/BlJ, PL/J, and LG/J strains, which carry *S* regions derived from the $H\text{-}2^d$ haplotype, all have Slp-positive females. Genetic studies to date indicate that all four of these strains exhibiting *permissive* female expression of Slp do so *via* the same genetic mechanisms. Permissive expression requires an *S* region that is capable of determining the Slp antigen, i.e., an *S* region from $H\text{-}2^d$, $H\text{-}2^s$, etc., but also requires positive alleles of at least two non-*H-2* genes, which have been tentatively denoted *rsl* (regulator of sex-limitation) (Brown and Shreffler 1980).

Our analyses suggest that, in those strains exhibiting permissive female expression of Slp protein, the typical testosterone induction mechanism still operates in the males. These males have much higher levels of Slp than females, but castration eliminates the testosterone-inducible increment of Slp expression and reduces the levels to those of the females. Administration of testosterone to females induces additional Slp expression and increases levels to those of the males. The testicular feminization gene *(tfm)* reduces the level of expression to those typical of females. Thus, the data suggest that *both* mechanisms of regulation are operating in these strains, i.e., both males and females express a basal level of Slp, this expression mediated by the *rsl* genes, but the males express an additional increment of Slp protein, due to induction by testosterone. Our findings suggest that the two mechanisms of regulation operate essentially independently (Brown 1980). This might reflect differential mechanisms of Slp induction in two different cell types, one testosterone-induced, the other *rsl*-induced, or it might reflect the existence of *two Slp* structural genes in the *S* regions of those strains which express Slp, one potentially testosterone-inducible, the other potentially *rsl*-inducible. Obviously, the resolution of these questions will require extensive examination, in mice exhibiting these various regulatory variations, of possible regulatory mechanisms at the levels of translation and transcription, and probably at the level of DNA sequence organization. It seems clear that the molecular tools are becoming available to approach these questions. This should be a highly interesting system for such investigations.

## Associations of Complement Components with the Major Histocompatibility Complexes

With the recognition that complement variations were associated with *H-2* complex, many other MHCs were examined for possible linkage of complement components. The current status of such associations, summarized in Table 4, reveals two points

**Table 4.** Variations in Complement Components Linked to the Major Histocompatibility Complexes of Five Species.

| | | | |
|---|---|---|---|
| *Mouse (H-2)* | | *Guinea Pig (GPLA)* | |
| C2 | Quantitative | B4 | Electrophoretic |
| C3 | Quantitative and electrophoretic | C2 | Deficiency and electrophoretic |
| C4 (Slp) | Quantitative and electrophoretic | C4 | Deficiency and electrophoretic |
| *Man (HLA)* | | *Rhesus (RhLA)* | |
| Bf | Electrophoretic | Bf | Electrophoretic |
| C2 | Deficiency and electrophoretic | | |
| C4 | Deficiency and electrophoretic | *Chicken (B)* | |
| | (Duplicate genes) | Total Complement | |

of particular interest. First, it has been observed that quantitative differences in total complement activity are associated with the *B* locus of the chicken, implying that complement genes may be linked to the *MHC* in both major classes of higher vertebrates and thus suggesting that complement genes are a consistent feature of *MHCs*. Secondly, in two mammalian species—man and the guinea pig—the structural genes for components C2 and Factor B (Bf) are linked to the *MHC*, in addition to the C4 structural genes. It is also of interest that in man the C4 structural genes are duplicated, at least on some chromosomes.

The linkage of C2 and Bf to other *MHC's* predicts that linkage of these genes also might be found with the *H-2* gene complex. A search for Bf variants has thus far been unsuccessful. However, my colleague John Atkinson has developed a functional assay for murine C2 hemolytic activity, and defined quantitative variations in C2 functional titers among congenic strains differing in *H-2* haplotypes. These range from 1600 for the $H\text{-}2^k$ haplotype, to 1000 for $H\text{-}2^d$, to 750 for $H\text{-}2^s$, and 500 for $H\text{-}2^u$. Differences between the $H\text{-}2^k$ and $H\text{-}2^d$ haplotypes and between the $H\text{-}2^k$ and $H\text{-}2^s$ haplotypes have been mapped to the *S* region (Gorman et al. 1980). Thus far, no evidence for C2 *structural* variations in these strains has been obtained, but these quantitative variations at least suggest potential sources of structural variation. Further investigations of these differences are in progress.

ACKNOWLEDGMENTS

My own role in this story is, to a substantial degree, that of historian. The system was discovered by Ray Owen, who generously allowed me to work on it. During the ensuing 20 years, I have mostly watched with fascination and admiration as a series of gifted students and fellows, Howard Passmore, Ted Hansen, Tommy Meo, Marleen Roos, Keith Parker, and Laura Brown, and colleagues, John Atkinson and Don Capra, have advanced it to its present state. I look forward with great anticipation to the next 20 years of progress on this system, and to further occasions to honor Ray Owen.

Supported in part by National Institutes of Health Research Grant AI 12734 and Program Project Grant AI 15353.

# References

Atkinson, J.P., McGinnis, K., Brown, L.J., Peterein, J., and Shreffler, D.C. 1980a. A murine C4 molecule with reduced hemolytic activity. J. Exp. Med. 151:492–497.

Atkinson, J.P., McGinnis, K., and Shreffler. D.C. 1980b. Development and characterization of a hemolytic assay for mouse C4. J. Immunol. Meth. 33:351–368.

Brown, L.J. 1980. Genes regulating the expression of the *H-2*-linked sex-limited protein. Ph.D. Thesis, Washington University, St. Louis, Mo.

Brown, L.J. and Shreffler, D.C. 1980. Female expression of the *H-2*-linked sex-limited Protein (Slp) due to non-*H-2* genes. Immunogenetics 10:19–29.

Carroll, M.C. and Capra, J.D. 1978. Studies on murine Ss protein: Demonstration that Ss protein is functionally the fourth component of complement. Proc. Natl. Acad. Sci. U.S.A. 75:2424–2428.

Carroll, M.C. and Capra, J.D. 1979. Studies on murine Ss protein: Demonstration that *S* locus encodes structural gene for fourth component of complement. Proc. Natl. Acad. Sci. U.S.A. 76:4641–4645.

Curman, B., Ostberg, L., Sandberg, L., Malmheden-Eriksson, I., Stalenheim, G., Rask, L., and Peterson, P.A. 1975. *H-2* linked Ss protein is C4 component of complement. Nature 258:243–245.

Demant, P., Capkova, J., Hinzova, E., and Voracova, B. 1973. The role of the histocompatibility-2-linked Ss-Slp region in the control of mouse complement. Proc. Natl. Acad. Sci. U.S.A. 70:863–864.

Ferreira, A., Nussenzweig, V., and Gigli, I. 1978. Structural and functional differences between the *H-2* controlled Ss and Slp proteins. J. Exp. Med. 148:1186–1197.

Goldman, M.B. and Goldman, J.N. 1976. Relationship of functional levels of early components of complement to the *H-2* complex of mice. J. Immunol. 117:1584–1588

Gorer, P.A. and Mikulska, Z.B. 1959. Some further data on the *H-2* system of antigens. Proc. R. Soc. (Lond.) B 151:57–69.

Gorman, J.C., Jackson, R.J., DeSantola, J.R., Shreffler, D.C., and Atkinson, J.P. 1980. Development of a hemolytic assay for mouse C2 and determination of its genetic control. J. Immunol. 125:344–351.

Hall, R.E. and Colten, H.R. 1977. Cell-free synthesis of the fourth component of guinea pig complement (C4): Identification of a precursor of serum C4 (Pro-C4). Proc. Natl. Acad. Sci. U.S.A. 74:1707–1710.

Hansen, T.H., Krasteff, T.N., and Shreffler, D.C. 1974. Quantitative variations in the expression of the mouse serum antigen Ss and its sex-limited allotype Slp. Biochem. Genet. 12:281–293.

Hansen, T.H. 1975. Studies of regulatory and functional aspects of the Ss serum protein system in the mouse. Ph.D. thesis. University of Michigan, Ann Arbor.

Hansen, T.H. and Shreffler, D.C. 1976. Characterization of a constitutive variant of the murine serum protein allotype, Slp. J. Immunol. 117:1507–1513.

Hoecker, G., Counce, S., and Smith, P. 1959. The antigens determined by the *H-2* locus: A rhesus-like system in the mouse. Proc. Natl. Acad. Sci. U.S.A. 40:1040–1051.

Klein, J. 1975. Biology of the Mouse Histocompatibility-2 Complex. New York: Springer-Verlag.

Lachmann, P.J., Grennan, D., Martin, A., and Demant, P. 1975. Identification of Ss protein as murine C4. Nature 258:242–243.

Meo, T., Krasteff, T., and Shreffler, D.C. 1975. Immunochemical characterization of murine *H-2* controlled Ss (serum substance) protein through identification of its human homologue as the fourth component of complement. Proc. Natl. Acad. Sci. U.S.A. 72:4536–4540.

Parker, K.L., Roos, M.H., and Shreffler, D.C. 1979. Structural characterization of the murine fourth component of complement and sex-limited protein and their precursors: Evidence for two loci in the *S* region of the *H-2* complex. Proc. Natl. Acad. Sci. U.S.A. 76:5853–5857.

Parker, K.L., Atkinson, J.P., Roos, M.H., and Shreffler, D.C. 1980a. Genetic and structural characterization of *H-2* controlled allelic forms of murine C4. Immunogenetics 11:55–63.

Parker, K.L., Capra, J.D., and Shreffler, D.C. 1980b. Partial amino acid sequences of the murine fourth component of complement (C4): Demonstration of homology with human C4 and identification of the amino-terminal subunit in Pro-C4. Proc. Natl. Acad. Sci U.S.A. 77:4275–4278.

Parker, K.L., Carroll, M.C., Shreffler, D.C., and Capra, J.D. 1981. Detection of *H-2*-controlled allelic forms of the murine sex-limited protein (Slp). J. Immunol., in press.

Passmore, H.C. and Shreffler, D.C. 1970. A sex-limited serum protein variant in the mouse: Inheritance and association with the *H-2* region. Biochem. Genet. 4:351–365.

Passmore, H.C. and Shreffler, D.C. 1971. A sex-limited serum protein variant in the mouse: Hormonal control of phenotypic expression. Biochem. Genet. 5:201–209.

Roos, M.E., Atkinson, J.P., and Shreffler, D.C. 1978. Molecular characterization of the Ss and Slp (C4) proteins of the mouse *H-2* complex: Subunit composition, chain size polymorphism, and an intracellular (Pro-Ss) precursor. J. Immunol. 121:1106–1115.

Shreffler, D.C. 1964. A serologically detected variant in mouse serum: Further evidence for genetic control by the histocompatibility-2 locus. Genetics 49:973–978.

Shreffler, D.C. 1965. The Ss system of the mouse—a quantitative serum protein difference genetically controlled by the *H-2* region. In Isoantigens and Cell interactions. J. Palm, ed. Philadelphia: Wistar Institute Press. pp. 11–19.

Shreffler, D.C. and David, C.S. 1975. The *H-2* major histocompatibility complex and the *I* immune response region: Genetic variation, function, and organization. Adv. Immunol. 20:125–195.

Shreffler, D.C., David, C.D., Passmore, H.C., and Klein, J. 1971. Genetic organization and evolution of the mouse *H-2* region: A duplication model. Transplant. Proc. 3:176–179.

Shreffler, D.C. and Owen, R.D. 1963. A serologically detected variant in mouse serum: Inheritance and association with the histocompatibility-2 locus. Genetics 48:9–25.

Snell, G.D., Cherry, M., and Demant, P. 1971. Evidence that *H-2* private specificities can be arranged in two mutually exclusive systems possibly homologous with two subsystems of HL-A. Transplant. Proc. 3:183–186.

Stimpfling, J.H. 1971. Recombination with a histocompatibility locus. Ann. Rev. Genet. 5:121–142.

Stimpfling, J.H. and Richardson, A. 1965. Recombination within the histocompatibility-2 locus of the mouse. Genetics 51:831–846.

# SECTION III:

# Immunodifferentiation and Development

Hildemann, ed. Frontiers in Immunogenetics

# Macronuclear Assortment and Structure in *Tetrahymena thermophila:* A Cytogenetic Approach Using Immunogenetic Markers

R.M. Preparata, F.P. Doerder, and D.L. Nanney

*Department of Genetics and Development, University of Illinois, Urbana, Illinois*

The genetic organization of the ciliate macronucleus is a long-standing puzzle that is only now beginning to yield to a combination of genetic and molecular analyses. Our purpose here is to report an exploration of macronuclear structure in *Tetrahymena thermophila* that uses a combination of cytogenetic and immunogenetic techniques.

The genetic system employed is the *H* serotype system, first characterized by Owen and his associates at Caltech in the late 1950's (Loefer, Owen and Christensen 1958; Margolin, Loefer and Owen 1959; Nanney and Dubert 1960). The *H* locus is one of a set of loci that controls alternative forms of a cell-surface protein, the immobilization or i-antigen. This set of loci, though unlinked, is associated into a system of mutual exclusion; only one locus is ordinarily expressed at any one time. We need not be concerned here with the other loci because under the conditions of the experiments only the *H* locus is usually expressed.

The *H* locus is polymorphic in natural populations, and three of its distinctive alleles have been used: $H^{A}$, $H^{D}$, and $H^{E}$, or according to more recent terminology, *serH-1, serH-3,* and *serH-4*. The serotype of a cell is readily defined by means of antisera prepared against whole cells, cilia or purified i-antigens (Bruns 1971). The antisera immobilize the cells at high dilutions, and if necessary can be rendered essentially monospecific by cross-absorption.

The alleles at the *H* locus manifest "allelic assortment" in heterozygous clones, and indeed provided the first example of this phenomenon (Nanney and Dubert 1960) though mating type assortment with similar kinetic characteristics had been reported earlier (Allen and Nanney 1958). Nearly all loci in this species manifest allelic assortment, and all examples studied show about the same rates of production of phenotypically pure sublines (see Sonneborn 1974). The very few cases of apparent non-assortment may reflect a severe selective disadvantage of one allele during or after macronuclear development rather than a failure of assortment to occur. When assortment is observed, and particularly when no selective differential is seen between alleles, the "equilibrated" rate of production of pure lines is about 0.0113 per cell generation in rapidly dividing cultures.

The current interpretation of allelic assortment (Nanney and Preparata 1979) is that the alleles in question are multiplied in the formation of the macronucleus following conjugation (possibly differentially) and that they are subsequently replicated precisely once in each cell cycle. At cell division, each daughter receives only approximately half of the DNA (and allelic components) (Cleffmann 1968; Doerder 1979), but the components received are random with respect to kind (Orias and Flacks 1975). Under these conditions the total number of assorting units (N) may be calculated from Schensted's (1958) formula

$$R_f = \frac{1}{2N\text{-}1}$$

where $R_f$ is the probability of producing a "pure" macronucleus at any fission in an equilibrated population of cells. The calculation indicates that the total number of assorting units is about 45, which is also the number of haploid genomes estimated from the amount of macronuclear DNA (Woodard et al. 1972; Doerder et al. 1977). The kinetic behavior appears to provide a reliable guide to the number of genetic units assorting in the macronucleus. This relationship is central to the interpretation of the experiments to be discussed.

The assortment of *H*-serotypes in heterozygous diploids has been extensively studied (Nanney and Dubert 1960; Nanney et al. 1964), but the opportunity has only recently become available to construct triallelic macronuclei (Preparata and Nanney 1977) and to examine their assortment patterns. Triploid tetrahymenas may be selected by isolating the rare triplet conjugants observed in mixtures of two mating types; such triplets commonly yield clones of diverse karyotype, one haploid, one diploid, and one triploid. The triploid cell is generated by the transfer of migratory pronuclei from the two cells of the same mating type into the single cell of the other type. If the cells of one type are homozygous for a serotype allele not found in the cells of the other type, their triploid progeny will receive two alleles of one kind and one allele of the other. Of greater interest are crosses in which three strains representing three different genotypes but only two mating types are mixed. Some fraction of the triplets in such crosses will be composed of three genotypes, and their triploid progeny are triallelic. The triallelic clones can be identified by immobilization tests, and the assortment of pure lineages of the three kinds can be studied.

Triallelic clones with a different karyotypic base can be constructed from triploids. A triploid can be crossed to a diploid to produce karyotypically diversified progeny, ranging from diploid to triploid, but generally trisomic for one or more chromosomes. Clones triallelic for serotype markers can be selected by immobilization tests, and their micronuclear karyotypes can be assessed by staining their meiotic nuclei. Again the assortment of markers from triallelic clones may be studied to determine if trisomic clones behave the same way that triploids behave.

We report here for the first time the detailed results of these experiments, but some of the conclusions from the earlier studies were briefly summarized (Nanney and Preparata 1979).

## Materials and Methods

Three homozygous strains of *T. thermophila* provided the three serotype alleles employed in the studies: strain C3 for *serH-1*, strain B for *serH-3*, and B3 for *serH-4*.

The strains were maintained and crossed in monoxenic culture using *Klebsiella pneumoniae* as the bacterial food source. The bacteria were grown at 37°C in 1% proteose peptone and the plateau cultures were stored at 4°C until used; at the time of use they were diluted 1/80 with sterile deionized water. In the later experiments, crosses were made in Cerophyl (Cerophyl Laboratories, Kansas City, Missouri) infusions (1.5 g/liter) because triplet conjugants seem to be more common in this medium.

Bacterized medium was used instead of the more commonly employed axenic medium (1% proteose peptone), because of the large number of single cell isolations required. The cells must be isolated by microscopic manipulation using micropipettes. The isolation cultures are inevitably subject to a small hazard of contamination by air-borne bacteria or molds. The bacteria can be controlled by antibiotics in the media, but with the possibility of side effects on the tetrahymena. Neither bacterial nor fungal contaminants are serious problems in experiments using media already exhausted by bacteria.

The antisera against strains manifesting the three *H* alleles were prepared in rabbits by the usual procedures (Nanney and Dubert 1960). Immobilization tests were carried out in serological depression slides with 1 drop of antiserum and 1 drop of culture; each culture was tested with all the relevant antisera at concentrations near the threshold of detection of the homologous types. In most cases each antiserum was used in at least two concentrations. Observations for immobilization or retardation were made after 40–60 minutes. When in a series of serial isolations a culture tested negative for a particular allelic type for three transfers in a row, the lineage was considered to have become "pure" with respect to that specificity at the time it first failed to manifest a positive response. In some experiments, adequately controlled, purity was defined on the basis of only two "pure" tests in sequence. This practice is somewhat arbitrary (because "false" negatives do occasionally express a positive response even after three transfers), but it is justified so long as all the lineages studied within an experiment are treated in the same manner.

The cell lines were reinitiated by single cell isolations in 3-spot depression slides two or three times per week; a rigid schedule was not maintained, because the growth rates of the cultures were not uniform from time to time. The irregular growth rates may have been caused in part by temperature fluctuations in the laboratory. These environmental variations were considered of little consequence because of the presence of internal controls of normal diploid heterozygotes in the experiments. In no cases were new cultures started until at least ten cell divisions had occurred in the previous culture. The maximum number of divisions in 3/4 ml of bacterized medium is about 13 (i.e., 8–10,000 cells), and most cultures had exhausted the medium and were beginning to starve at the time of testing and reinitiation. Because they were necessary in the later computations, the lower rates of growth were always recorded.

The rate of stabilization per transfer ($R_t$) for a particular specificity was calculated by summing the subcultures showing a first negative response to a particular antiserum (and destined to show a negative response for two more transfer generations in most cases) and dividing that total by the number of new cultures initiated at that transfer generation from cultures with positive (or reversible) responses. The rate of stabilization per transfer was converted into the rate of stabilization per fission ($R_f$) by dividing $R_t$ by the number of cell generations in the previous growth interval.

The triallelic triploids were selected after mixing strains B(VI), C3(V), and B3(VI). From these mixtures were isolated triplet conjugants, and the three participants were reisolated at the end of conjugation. The exconjugant clones were tested for sexual maturity by mixing samples with mature tester strains; all clones manifesting the ability to mate were discarded. The remaining clones were subjected to immobilization tests with antisera against the three parental strains. The ideal result expected was one monoallelic, one diallelic, and one triallelic exconjugant clone from each triplet analyzed, but this result was not always obtained. One or more of the exconjugant clones often failed to survive. Nevertheless, all the expected classes of exconjugant clones were observed among the progeny of triplets. These were examined cytologically, using the Feulgen technique, and the expected three size classes of micronuclei were observed even though systematic studies of nuclear size were not undertaken at this time.

For further study, a triallelic clone with large micronuclei was expanded into several isolation lines and these were serotyped. One subline with near equal response to the three parental antisera was expanded again into thirty or more sublines, and these were followed through serial isolations with regular testing of all "left-over" cultures after the next isolations had been made.

The reliability of the estimated rate of assortment depends importantly upon the number of events sampled. If only 30 sublines are initiated, and if no replacement of stabilized lines is undertaken, the calculated rate has a very large standard error. This problem is compounded by the fact that the initial rate of stabilization in a cluster of subclones is markedly dependent upon the balance in the originating macronucleus. If the ratio of macronuclear subunits is highly skewed, the initial rate of production of pure types will be very high; the $R_t$ will only approach its characteristic level as the ratio of subnuclear types in the remaining population of macronuclei moves toward equality. Schensted's (1958) simulations showed that 20–30 cell divisions are required for "equilibration," and by this time a large fraction of a sample of sublines from an asymmetric clone will have stabilized. The solution to the problem of an adequate sample size is the replacement of sublines that have stabilized with new sublines from the lineages still manifesting mixed responses. In this way an experiment may be continued more or less indefinitely, until an adequate sample of fixation opportunities has accumulated.

The triallelic trisomics were selected from progeny of crosses of triploid clones *(serH-1/serH-1/serH-4)* to diploid clones *(serH-3/serH-3)*. These crosses (see below) produce high frequencies of viable progeny, and these can be screened for immaturity (to avoid lines with retained macronuclei) and for immobilization responses to the critical antisera. The detection of three allelic specificities in the macronucleus strongly indicates the presence of three *H*-bearing chromosomes in the precursor (synkaryon) of both the macronucleus and the micronucleus, but the micronuclear chromosomes are adequately examined only during the first meiotic division. Since the macronuclear assortment must be studied before alleles have been lost, the assortment analysis was started with immature clones, and these were karyotyped only later. The later quantitative cytochemical studies were in some cases carried out after a year or more of laboratory culture. Since spontaneous changes in micronuclear karyotypes occur, the deferred analyses are less critical than the karyotype studies undertaken soon after maturity was reached.

The DNA contents of the macronuclei with slow assortment kinetics were measured by fluorescence cytophotometry (Doerder and DeBault 1975, 1978). Briefly, fast exponential cells were harvested, fixed, stained with decolorized basic fuchsin, and mounted. Individual G2 macronuclei were identified in predivision cells recognized by micronuclear or macronuclear division figures and cytokinesis. They were measured with a Leitz MPV2 microspectrophotometer equipped with Ploem vertical illumination (Leitz filter system M). The arbitrary fluorescence units read from the photomultiplier output were converted into haploid equivalents (C) using the G2 micronucleus of a diploid control as a 4C standard (Doerder and DeBault 1975).

The computer program to examine the assortment kinetics expected in triallelic clones was in the form of a subroutine added to a previously written Fortran program in which macronuclear assortment and division were simulated (Doerder 1979). The main program simulates macronuclear division according to "Model II" regulation (Doerder and DeBault 1978; Doerder 1979) and allows the user to stipulate the numbers of each of up to four types of assorting units as well as the total number of clones, In the present instance the numbers of three types of units, representing the three alleles of a triallelic clone, were specified and the specially written subroutine monitored the transition from a triallelic to a diallelic condition. The simulation was based on a mean of 45 assorting units in a G1 macronucleus. The Fortran program was executed on the University of Pittsburgh's DEC10A computer.

# Results

## *Serotype Assortment in a Triallelic Triploid*

The analysis of serotype assortment in a triallelic triploid clone began with a depression slide culture derived from an exconjugant that had been involved in a three-genotype, two-mating type *ménage à trois* (see Materials and Methods). Because most of the cells in the culture were immobilized by each of the parental antisera, the genotype *serH-1/serH-3/serH-4* was assigned to the clone, and it was assumed to be triploid. A set of 15 subclones was initiated from the original clone by single cell isolations, and each of these was again tested for serotypes. One of these subclones was then chosen on the basis of its balanced responses to the parental antisera to be the source for the major experimental sublines; 48 sublines were established and serial transfers were reinitiated two or three times per week from each transfer. The left-over cultures were tested for immobilization responses.

The loss of one of the three immobilization responses occurred very quickly in the serial transfer lineages, and any of the alleles might disappear. Rarely two alleles would disappear in the same transfer generation. The observed rate of loss ($R_t$) was 107/295, greater than a third of the isolations made from triallelic cultures. Since cultures were replaced only after a loss was confirmed in two sequential subcultures, the supply of triallelic stem-lines declined quickly. The transfers were made after about 13 fissions so that the rate of loss of an allele per cell generation ($R_f$) is about 1/13 of $R_t$ when $R_f$ is low, but more complicated treatment is required when multiple losses can occur often in the same culture. We will consider the significance of this value later.

Once one of the alleles disappears from a triallelic lineage, that lineage becomes a diallelic lineage, qualitatively similar to an ordinary heterozygous diploid line, but three different classes of diallelic triploids are recovered: that which is apparently *serH-1/serH-3,* that which seems to be *serH-3/serH-4,* and that which acts as if it were *serH-1/serH-4*. The question at issue is whether the diallelic triploids behave quantitatively the same as their diploid analogues. The answer is obtained by expanding well-balanced diallelic cultures into enough sublines to measure the rates of assortment.

The results of the experiment are summarized (Table 1) according to the transfer generation from the initiation of the series. According to previous experiments, and in agreement with Schensted's (1958) simulations, the rates of allelic loss during the first few transfer generations are highly variable and dependent upon the allelic ratios in the progenitor cultures. As expected, given the deliberate attempt to select for balanced diallelic cultures as progenitors, the rate of loss in the early transfer generations was low in all the series (Mean $R_f$ = 0.0048 vs the expected rate of 0.0113 after equilibration). In the second and third transfer intervals (6–10 and 11–15), the rates rose to the expected level ($P \simeq .50$), and the rates were similar in the three series ($P = 0.19$ in a chi square homogeneity test).

Had the experiment terminated at this point, about 200 cell divisions beyond the first expansion, nothing anomalous would have been noted. In the next five transfers,

**Table 1.** Assortment Rates in Ditypic Sublines of a Triallelic Triploid Clone of *Tetrahymena Thermophila*.

| Transfer interval | Alleles assorting | Fraction stabilized | Fissions/ transfer | $R_f$ | Mean $R_f$ |
|---|---|---|---|---|---|
| 1-5 | 1-3 | 9/227 | 13 | 0.0030 | |
| | 3-4 | 14/213 | 13 | 0.0051 | 0.0048 |
| | 1-4 | 17/210 | 13 | 0.0062 | |
| 6-10 | 1-3 | 21/154 | 13 | 0.0105 | |
| | 3-4 | 22/127 | 13 | 0.0133 | 0.0101 |
| | 1-4 | 13/157 | 13 | 0.0064 | |
| 11-15 | 1-3 | 10/141 | 10 | 0.0071 | |
| | 3-4 | 13/141 | 10 | 0.0128 | 0.0115 |
| | 1-4 | 26/138 | 13 | 0.0145 | |
| 16-20 | 1-3 | 6/163 | 11 | 0.0033 | |
| | 3-4 | 7/154 | 11 | 0.0041 | 0.0049 |
| | 1-4 | 12/127 | 13 | 0.0073 | |
| 21-23 | Pooled | 19/284 | 13 | 0.0051 | |

however, the rate of allelic loss fell in all series, back to a level close to that in the first transfer interval. To test the persistence of the reduced rate of assortment, the experiment was continued for an additional three transfers with very similar results. This previously unobserved depression of assortment rate, occurring after a long period of subculturing, we refer to as "assortment depression." We will consider possible mechanisms for it later.

### *Serotype Assortment in Triallelic Aneuploids*

Several triallelic trisomics were constructed by crosses of triploids and diploids and their assortment behavior was examined in serial transfers. The first experiment was undertaken (Experiment 1, Table 2) before the antisera had been adequately cross-absorbed and before our cytological techniques were well developed. Uncertainty about the specificity of the immobilization reactions left doubtful the initial allelic constitutions of both the clones studied. Unquestionably at least one subline of clone 6 and one of 17 were assorting serotypes *serH-1* and *serH-3*. As in the diallelic triploid lines, the initial assortment rates (in transfers 1-6) were lower than the standard equilibrated rate, but by the second transfer interval had reached the expected level. In the third transfer interval, the rates were still reasonably high and, because of the sample size, indistinguishable from the normal rate. In the final transfer interval, however, the assortment rate dropped in both series to a significantly low level ($P = >.0001$ for the combined data), less than a third of the expected rate.

The cytological preparations of meiotic chromosomes in crosses of clones 6 and 17 to normal lines were not entirely satisfactory. The number of chromosomes present in both lines was clearly above the 10 chromosomes (5 pairs) present in the normal stocks. Most of the chromosome counts indicated that twelve chromosomes

**Table 2.** Assortment Rates in Ditypic Sublines of Aneuploid Clones of *T. Thermophila*.

| | Transfer interval | Alleles assorting | Clone no. | Fraction stabilized | $R_f$ | Mean $R_f$ |
|---|---|---|---|---|---|---|
| Exp. 1 | 1-6 | 1-3 | 6 | 13/138 | 0.0072 | 0.0072 |
| | | 1-3 | 17 | 13/139 | 0.0072 | |
| | 7-12 | 1-3 | 6 | 12/75 | 0.0123 | 0.0112 |
| | | 1-3 | 17 | 11/84 | 0.0101 | |
| | 13-17 | 1-3 | 6 | 6/44 | 0.0105 | 0.0097 |
| | | 1-3 | 17 | 6/52 | 0.0089 | |
| | 19-25 | 1-3 | 6 | 4/77 | 0.0040 | 0.0033 |
| | | 1-3 | 17 | 4/117 | 0.0026 | |
| Exp. 2 | 1-8 | 1-3-4 | E | 17/297 | 0.0044 | |
| | | 1-3 | F | 32/222 | 0.0111 | 0.0084 |
| | | 3-4 | G | 32/226 | 0.0109 | |
| | | 1-4 | H | 26/232 | 0.0086 | |
| | 1-8 | 1-3-4 | L | 23/292 | 0.0061 | |
| | | 1-3 | M | 57/289 | 0.0152 | 0.0097 |
| | | 3-4 | N | 30/254 | 0.0091 | |
| | | 1-4 | O | 26/243 | 0.0082 | |
| Exp. 3 | 1-16 | 1-4 | K (Diploid control) | 60/388 | 0.0119 | |
| | 1-16 | 1-3 | FF | 78/400 | 0.0150 | |
| | | 3-4 | GG | 62/502 | 0.0095 | 0.0116 |
| | | 1-4 | HH | 69/487 | 0.0109 | |
| Exp. 4 | 1-12 | 3-4 | (Diploid control) | 63/376 | 0.0129 | |
| | 1-10 | 1-4 | K-40 (Diploid) | 26/202 | 0.0099 | |
| | 1-11 | 3-4 | GG-14 | 29/220 | 0.0101 | 0.0093 |
| | | 3-4 | GG-33 | 26/246 | 0.0081 | |

were present in both clones 6 and 7, but occasional figures seemed to have thirteen chromosomes. Because of uncertainties about the presence of a third allelic specificity, we do not know whether three or only two *serH* chromosomes were present. We do know that both clones 6 and 17 are aneuploid, and that the *proportion* of *serH* chromosomes to the total chromosome number is atypical. Yet the assortment kinetics are normal until after the 15th transfer, when the same kind of assortment depression occurs as in the triploid triallelics.

Three other similar experiments were carried out but not for so long a time. Two triallelic trisomics were obtained by crossing a triploid and a diploid clone. One of the triallelic clones was expanded into four different subclones (E, F, G, and H) which were themselves expanded into multiple lineages. At maturity these lineages were crossed and stained, and found to contain 11 micronuclear chromosomes. The other triallelic clone was treated similarly and expanded into subclones L, M, N, and O. At maturity it was found to contain 12 micronuclear chromosomes. Each of the subclones was followed in multiple lineages through eight single cell transfer generations, and the assortment rates were calculated (Table 2). Although the subclones showed considerable variability in assortment rate, as is expected for lineages not fully "equilibrated," the total assortment rate is not significantly different from that observed in diallelic diploids.

For Experiment 3, the trisomic with 11 chromosomes in Experiment 2 was selected, after a period of starvation, for more extensive analysis, and three newly expanded subclones were studied through 16 additional transfer generations. These sets of clones were followed in parallel with a set of 42 sublines of a newly generated heterozygous diploid. These sets of clones showed less variability than did those in the previous experiment, mainly because of the longer interval of observations. The total rate of assortment is indistinguishable from that of the diploid diallelic control.

Experiment 4 was a continuation of Experiment 3, again after a period of starvation. Two sublines (GG-14 and GG-33) of series GG that had not stabilized in the 17 transfers of the previous experiment were expanded and followed for an additional 11 transfers. A diploid subline (K-40) with similar stability characteristics was also chosen for further study. A new diploid control was also developed. The basis for this experiment was the suspicion that these long term diallelics might have "stabilized" as permanent diallelics. As can be seen (Table 2), however, the new series assorted, and only slightly more slowly than did the diploid control.

These studies establish that aneuploid diallelics assort with essentially the same kinetics as do triploid diallelics. After equilibration the rate of assortment in both instances is that observed in diploids, i.e., 0.0113. In both trisomics and (especially) triploids assortment depression may set in after 15-20 transfer generations, with constant selection for non-assorted sublines. Significantly, we were unable to recover "stable" diallelics, as might be expected on the basis of Allen's (1971) observations on acid phosphatase assortment (see also Orias 1973).

Whether assortment depression also occurs in diploid diallelics has not been fully explored. In the presently reported experiments, no such depression was observed in diploid, but the diploids were not followed long enough to yield significant depression even if it occurs as regularly as in triploids and trisomics. Summarizing the data at hand (including that in Table 2), the stabilizations in diploid controls for transfers 1-6 give an $R_f$ of 0.0123 (95 stabilizations/593 opportunities). For transfers 6-12, the $R_f$ was 0.0120 (63/400), and for transfers 13-16, the $R_f$ 0.0112 (29/199). We suspect that assortment depression may occur in clones with any initial karyotype, but we have no convincing evidence for it yet in diploids.

## *The Effect of Starvation on Depressed Sublines*

An interesting question concerning the lineages with depressed assortment rates concerns the stability of the depression. One test of that stability was carried out on diallelic tubed cultures from the last transfers in the triploid study. The cultures were allowed to starve for two weeks. Such a starvation is severe, but it does not usually lead to a detectable loss of cell density, nor to inviability of cells isolated into nutrient medium. Single cells were isolated from several different diallelic cultures (to avoid some of the complications of equilibrating from a culture with a narrow range of allelic ratios). Of the first 73 isolation cultures tested, 18 were pure for one of the serotypes. The parental cultures were estimated to have undergone a total of about 18 cell divisions from their previous isolations—13 divisions in the depression slide and an additional 5 divisions in the tube—and then to have starved nearly two weeks. The $R_t$ for this sample is 18/73 = 0.247; the $R_f$ was 0.014. These reisolation cultures were continued in series and stabilizations scored for the next two transfers. A total of 22 stabilizations in 88 opportunities gave an $R_t$ of 0.25 and an $R_f$ of 0.019. Obviously the depressed rate of assortment did not persist through the tube culture experience, but returned to at least the usual rate.

The generality of reversal by starvation was explored in one further experiment (Table 3) in which two sublines (14 and 33) from Experiment 4, assumed to be depressed, were tubed and starved while unstarved sublines were scored as controls. Neither of the clones selected was severely depressed; one showed an $R_f$ of 0.008 and the other a rate of 0.010. In both instances, the isolation lines studied after a 2-week starvation interval showed faster assortment but the differences between the starved and non-starved lineages were not significant ($P \simeq .20$). Assortment depression may be readily reversible by starvation, but only the data from Experiment 1 provide fully acceptable evidence.

### *The DNA Content of the Macronuclei in Lines With Assortment Depression*

The slow rate of assortment in selected lines, presumably in selected lines of any initial karyotype, must reflect some change in the macronucleus. Generally speaking, the slowly assorting macronuclei must differ from "normal" macronuclei either in the organization of their genetic elements, or in their numbers. The simplest hypothesis to test is that assortment depression is a consequence of selecting sublines with larger macronuclei.

We first must consider briefly the relationship between the karyotype of the

**Table 3.** The Effect of Starvation on the Assortment Rates in Lineages of Trisomic Showing Assortment Depression.

| | Transfer interval | Clone | Alleles assorting | Fraction stabilized | $R_f$ |
|---|---|---|---|---|---|
| Exp. 4 | 1-11 | 33-depressed | 3-4 | 26/246 | 0.0081 |
| | 1-10 | 33-starved | 3-4 | 29/193 | 0.0112 |
| Exp. 4 | 1-11 | 14-depressed | 3-4 | 29/220 | 0.0101 |
| | 1-10 | 14-starved | 3-4 | 27/183 | 0.0113 |
| | 14 + 33 | depressed | | 55/466 | 0.0091 |
| | 14 + 33 | starved | | 55/376 | 0.0113 |

macronuclear primordium and the DNA content of the mature macronuclei. This question has been examined by Seyfert and Preparata (1979) who find that the total DNA content of mature macronuclei is the same, i.e., equivalent to about 45 haploid chromosome sets, in all clones examined, regardless of whether their macronuclei are derived from haploid, diploid, triploid, or aneuploid primordia. The mechanism of regulating the size of the macronucleus (see Cleffmann 1974) is apparently insensitive to the DNA content of the primordium, but regulates the DNA to the same level in spite of discrepancies in initial DNA amounts. The time and mode of the regulation has not been established.

The macronuclear DNA amount is not very precisely regulated in individual cells, however. Macronuclear division is often referred to as "amitotic," and the daughters are only approximately equal (Cleffmann 1968; Doerder 1979). Since DNA replication appears to be all-or-none (Cleffman 1975), the variability arising at one cell division is not compensated at the next, but continues to accumulate up to a point. Adjustments are achieved, however, by sensors of DNA amount that may either trigger an additional *S* phase prior to cytokinesis (when the DNA level falls below some threshold), or trigger a cell division before *S* phase (when the DNA level reaches an upper threshold). Other minor adjustments may be important under some circumstances, as when chromatin is extruded at cell division (Cleffman and Jauker 1968; Doerder 1979).

In any case, considerable variability in DNA content is observed within a culture. That variability should be correlated with assortment rate; the larger macronuclei should be less likely to yield "pure" progeny. A constant selection of lines that have not stabilized might enrich for lines with large macronuclei, providing that macronuclear size is "hereditary." The current interpretation of macronuclear regulation assumes that the thresholds for cell cycle bypasses are uniform within a population. If this assumption is correct, the selection of large macronuclei could have at best a very short-range effect.

One can readily imagine, however, mechanisms whereby bypass thresholds could vary, and show hereditary differences. A somatic mutation affecting a threshold sensor, for example, might reduce its sensitivity to detect a DNA overload, or might reduce its ability to effect a cell cycle bypass. In fact, one would expect to recover such mutants whenever strong selective pressure for macronuclear size could be exerted. At issue are two questions: First, is the selection for unassorted macronuclei in the serotype system of sufficient magnitude to identify such mutants? Second, are the selected lines in fact lines with increased DNA contents? Actually, the answer to the second question provides an answer to both. If the slowly segregating lines have high DNA contents, the selective pressure necessary to enrich for hereditary variants for high DNA content must have been adequate. In fact, evidence for high DNA content was not obtained.

Macronuclear DNA amounts in cells of four slowly-assorting clones are shown in Table 4. Although as in previous studies (Doerder and DeBault 1978; Doerder 1979) considerable variation was observed within the samples, the macronuclear DNA amounts in the slowly-assorting clones were clearly not significantly larger

**Table 4.** DNA Contents in Clones Manifesting Slow Assortment of Serotype Alleles.

| Clone type | Code | Cells counted | Mean DNA content (C) | Coefficient of variation (%) | Range of sample means[a] |
|---|---|---|---|---|---|
| Normal diploid control | C3 | 158 | 106 | 25.0 | (91-124,5) |
| Slow trisomics (28th transfer) | GG-33-4 | 133 | 100 | 21.6 | (89-114,6) |
| | GG-14-6 | 160 | 108 | 22.6 | (90-120,6) |
| | GG-33-7 | 22 | 97 | 15.8 | (97,1) |
| Slow diploid | K-40 | 182 | 98 | 20.2 | (93-107,5) |

[a]Multiple samples of each clone were taken on different days and fixed for cytofluorimetry. The ranges of the sample means and the numbers of samples are shown in parentheses.

than the control. They were not, moreover, as large as would be predicted from the slow rate of assortment by the Schensted formula. At the levels of compoundness we are concerned with, the assortment rate is linearly but inversely related to the number of assorting units. If the assortment rate is reduced to half, the number of assorting units must be doubled in order to explain it. In the moderately depressed clones subjected to analysis, we expect a DNA content of about 120 compared to 100 in the controls. The total DNA content are not significantly changed. Slow assortment is apparently not a consequence of an increase in total DNA content, but more severely depressed lineages need to be studied in order to strengthen this conclusion.

### *The Expected Assortment Rates of Triallelic Macronuclei*

The assortment properties of triallelic macronuclei may be grasped intuitively—at least in a qualitative way. If the total number of assorting units in a triallelic macronucleus is the same as in a diallelic macronucleus, the rate of loss of an allele will be higher from the triallelic nucleus simply because the mean number of each allelic type is smaller. How much higher is not so apparent. To investigate this matter, we simulated the assortment pattern by a computer program (see Materials and Methods), postulating a total of 45 initial units distributed among three classes in a ratio of 5:15:25. The initial input ratio is not expected to have a major effect on the equilibrated rates. The results from two simulations, after a nine fission equilibration interval, are summarized in Table 5. From the 10th fission onward the rate of assortment was essentially invariant, except for sampling fluctuations. The mean rate, 0.0375, is about 3 times the rate of loss of an allele from a diallelic macronucleus, 0.0113.

This result has not been rationalized, but it provides a demonstration of, and an explanation for, the rapid initial allele loss in our experiments. We were unable to measure the rate of first loss accurately because it occurs so rapidly. An allele was observed missing from a triallelic nucleus in 107 cases in 295 opportunities (0.3627),

**Table 5.** Estimates of Rates of Loss of the First Allele From a Triallelic Macronucleus, Based on a Computer Simulated Assortment of a Macronucleus with 45 Components and an Initial Composition of 5:15:25.

| Fission interval | Trial 1 | | | Trial 2 | | | Total rate |
|---|---|---|---|---|---|---|---|
| | Losses | Opportunities | Rate | Losses | Opportunities | Rate | |
| 10-19 | 156 | 3579 | 0.044 | 118 | 3376 | 0.035 | 0.0394 |
| 20-29 | 77 | 2425 | 0.032 | 97 | 2246 | 0.043 | 0.0373 |
| 30-39 | 72 | 1687 | 0.043 | 52 | 1517 | 0.034 | 0.0387 |
| 40-49 | 32 | 1151 | 0.028 | 43 | 1048 | 0.041 | 0.0341 |
| 50-59 | 28 | 845 | 0.033 | 22 | 717 | 0.031 | 0.0320 |
| Totals | 365 | 9687 | 0.0377 | 333 | 8904 | 0.0374 | 0.0375 |

measured as isolation lines derived from a 13-fission culture initiated with a triallelic progenitor. The expected number of such losses based on the computer simulation is easily derived. Within such a culture the probability of remaining triallelic after one cell division is 1-0.0375, or 0.9625. The fraction of cells still triallelic after the second division is $(0.9625)^2$, after the third division it is $(0.9625)^3$, after thirteen divisions it is $(0.9625)^{13}$, or 0.608. The expected fraction of cells *lacking* one or more alleles is therefore 1-0.608, or 0.392. The observed value of 0.363 must be considered well within the permitted range of variation.

On the other hand, a similar computer simulation with a macronucleus containing 60 units (in a ratio of 5:20:35) yields a rate of first allele loss not very different from that of a macronucleus with 45 units. The simulated loss rate (658 losses in 19,733 opportunities) was 0.0333, compared with the 0.0375 value for the smaller macronucleus. The expected fraction of cells lacking an allele under these conditions is 0.334, again indistinguishable from the observed value of 0.363. The first-loss data with samples of the size available cannot adequately measure the macronuclear multiplicity.

## Discussion

The studies presented here need to be considered in conjunction with previous observations concerning the structure and behavior of the genetic elements in the macronucleus. We summarize the conclusions derived from such studies, and then consider how they may be integrated. We should emphasize that the conclusions are based on observations of one particular species in the *Tetrahymena pyriformis* complex, i.e., *T. thermophila,* and should not be generalized casually.

1. Haploid, diploid, triploid, and aneuploid macronuclear primordia give rise to functional macronuclei with no demonstrable differences in mean DNA content (Seyfert and Preparata 1979).
2. Diploid, triploid, and aneuploid (trisomic) macronuclei show allelic assortment rates consistent with a content of 45 genetic elements of each kind. Triallelic nuclei assort in two stages: The rapid loss of one allele is followed by the slow loss of a second allele, equivalent to that in a diallelic diploid.
3. The DNA content of a G1 macronucleus is equivalent to about 45 haploid micronuclear genomes (Gorovsky 1973; Doerder et al. 1977), but its composition is somewhat different from that of micronuclear DNA. Specifically, the rDNA is amplified (Gall 1974; Engberg et al. 1974), certain middle repetitive sequences are underrepresented (Yao and Gall 1979; Iwamura et al. 1979), and simple repeated sequences are organized very differently (Yao and Gall 1979).
4. Genes at loci found to be linked in meiotic analysis show independent allele assortment in the macronucleus (Allen 1964; Doerder 1973). No close linkages are yet available in Tetrahymena; "somatic coupling" of loci at distances less than 5 meiotic recombination units cannot be excluded.

5. The size of the DNA components of the macronucleus is not certain. The pieces are certainly not as small as the gene-sized pieces found in many hypotrich macronuclei, but they may have a mean size as small as 1/40 of a chromosome (Preer and Preer 1979, using sedimentation methods), or as large as whole chromosomes (Williams et al. 1978, using viscoelastometric procedures).
6. After prolonged growth without starvation, but with selection for diallelic cells, heterozygous clones of any origin may produce sublines with assortment rates only 1/3 to 1/2 the normal assortment rate. The slowly-assorting diallelic lines examined do not have atypical DNA contents. The slow assortment may be reversed by starvation. Stable diallelic lineages are never observed for serotypes, though lineages that might be so interpreted have been reported for other loci (Allen 1971; Orias 1973).

These observations do not lead to a unique or universally acceptable interpretation of macronuclear structure. The macronucleus is clearly not a "polyploid" structure, with simple multiples of each micronuclear chromosome. The chromatin of the macronucleus is a highly edited version of the micronuclear chromatin. This processed DNA may also be fragmented into a larger number of kinds of elements than occur in the micronucleus.

The real puzzle of the macronucleus comes from the conflict between the evidence for its unorganized fragmentation, and the evidence for its genetic integrity and continuity. The macronucleus of *T. thermophila* is essentially immortal, and it shows little evidence of segregational imbalance. Inviable sublines do not appear in adequate numbers to suggest random chromosomal loss. All genetic markers studied by allelic assortment show a constant mean G1 content of 45 elements. After a systematic examination of models of random assortment the Preer's (1979) conclude "that some regulatory or nonrandom segregational mechanism must operate to maintain balance."

At issue then are two classes of "nonrandom" mechanisms that might be responsible for the conservation of genetic balance. The oldest model under consideration is that of the *genomic subnucleus,* the idea that a complete set of genetic elements is physically associated during assortment. Imprecision in the distribution of whole genomic units would not lead to genetic imbalance. Against this interpretation is the evidence for a drastically edited macronuclear genome, and strong indications of fragmentation. No genomic units have been convincingly demonstrated in the tetrahymena macronucleus. Nevertheless, the genomic subnucleus cannot be dismissed categorically. One might imagine, for example, that the genomic unit is a temporary structure, constructed only as a unit of assortment. It might be constructed at the time of macronuclear division by the association of recognition sequences at the ends of chromatinic elements, and so provide for the distribution of whole genomes to daughter cells. Its dissolution after cytokinesis could account for the absence of somatic coupling of loosely linked alleles, as well as the small DNA pieces reported.

The *ad hoc*ery of such interpretations leads to an alternative model, particularly to a model of independent regulation for each essential genomic element. The model is derived from observations on the amplified rDNA elements. These are clearly different from the vast majority of chromatic components. They are present in some 200× the frequency of the other genes, and they are replicated under a separate control system. The cell can measure the bulk DNA of the cell and regulate its amounts by means we need not consider here. It can also measure and regulate the amounts of rDNA, quite independently of the bulk DNA. The hypothesis of independent regulation suggests that the cell has more than two independent regulatory systems; indeed it suggests as many regulatory systems as there are different genetic components. If the chromosomes persist intact in the macronucleus (see Seyfert 1979), only five systems of regulation would be required, in addition to that for rDNA. If each chromosome is fragmented into 20–40 pieces, a hundred or two hundred different systems would be required.

We do not know how the quantities of rDNA are sensed and controlled. Hence we are in no position to evaluate whether the mechanism could be extended to a large number of separate components. The amount of rDNA is probably not regulated, however, by a precise control of its assortment at cell division, but by compensatory replication (Preer's 1979, Model I). In contrast, the remainder of the DNA appears to be replicated in an all-or-none mode (Cleffmann 1975), with excesses and deficiencies compensated by extra *S* phases, or extra divisions (Preer's Model II; see Doerder 1979). Preer argues, however, that the amount of independent replication required for maintenance of balance is very small, and would be difficult to detect.

Both of the macronuclear models are thus unsatisfactory in some ways. Both become less plausible as the numbers of genetic elements increase—as for example in the hypotrich ciliates. A few thousand specific telosynapses are almost as implausible as are a few thousand separate controls of DNA replication. But perhaps we do not need to encompass all the ciliates at this point; immortal hypotrichs are not known, and their mortality may well be a consequence of their excessive genetic fragmentation.

We need finally to direct attention briefly to item 6. Does assortment depression cast any light on the organization of the macronucleus? It certainly is a consequence of a modification of the macronucleus, either of its organization or of its composition. The slow rate of assortment could be a consequence of a larger number of assorting elements. Since the number of assorting elements is inversely proportional to the assortment rate, depressed assortment would require more than the normal number of assorting units. Gross DNA measurements show no detectable increase in mean DNA amounts in slowly assorting sublines. Additional measurements are required on more severely depressed lineages, but present indications are that slow assortment is not the consequence of selection for large macronuclei.

If a single chromosome type were differentially increased in selected lines, the increase in some kinds of genetic elements could be achieved without a corresponding increase in total DNA. If one of the five chromosome types were doubled in amount, the total DNA would be increased only 20%. Because of the high variance of DNA content (a consequence of Model II regulation), even this increase is difficult to exclude. The data suggest no such increase, of course. But if the genophore differentially replicated were only 1/40 of the size of a chromosome, we would have no hopes of detecting it in terms of total DNA.

The aberrant assortment in selected lines may, however, reflect not primarily the quantities of DNA, but their organization. One might imagine, for example, that the associations of genomic elements might occasionally bring together in a genomic complex two, instead of one, "allelic" units. One might postulate the formation of inappropriate termini by illegitimate exchanges. Such diallelic genomes could easily cause slower assortment rates, even if they are inherently unstable themselves. Detailed models of such organizational variants could be provided, but are unwarranted in our present state of ignorance. Genetic and molecular studies have provided much information concerning the organization of the ciliate macronucleus. That information has not yet, however, provided a satisfactory increase in our understanding.

ACKNOWLEDGMENTS

Work supported by Grants from the National Science Foundation to F.P. Doerder (PCM 77-25401, PCM 80-00714) and from the National Institute of Health to D.L. Nanney (AG-00010 and GM-07779).

## References

Allen, S.L. 1964. Linkage studies in variety 1 of *Tetrahymena pyriformis:* A first case of linkage in ciliated protozoa. Genetics 49:617–627.

Allen, S.L. 1971. A late-determined gene in Tetrahymena heterozygotes. Genetics 68:415–433.

Allen, S.L. and Nanney, D.L. 1958. An analysis of nuclear differentiation in the selfers of Tetrahymena. Am. Naturalist 92:139–160.

Bruns, P.J. 1971. Immobilization antigens of *Tetrahymena pyriformis*. I. Assay and extraction. Exp. Cell Res. 65:445–453.

Cleffmann, G. 1968. Regulierung der DNS-Menge bei Tetrahymena. Exp. Cell Res. 50:193–207.

Cleffmann, G. 1974. The cell cycle. In Actualites Protozoologiques. P. de Puytorac and J. Grain, eds. Fourth International Congress Clermontterrand, Vol. 1. Clermontterrand University, pp. 315–325.

Cleffmann, G. 1975. Amount of DNA produced during extra *S* phases in Tetrahymena. J. Cell Biol. 66:204–209.

Cleffmann, G. and Jauker, F. 1968. Die Regulierung der DNS-Menge nach der Amitose. Hoppe-Seyler's Z. Physiol. Chem. 349–1243.

Doerder, F.P. 1973. Regulatory serotype mutations in *Tetrahymena pyriformis*. Genetics 74:81–106.

Doerder, F.P. 1979. Regulation of macronuclear DNA in *Tetrahymena thermophila*. J. Protozool. 26:28–35.

Doerder, F.P. and DeBault, L.E. 1975. Cytofluorometric analysis of nuclear DNA during meiosis, fertilization and macronuclear development in the ciliate *Tetrahymena pyriformis*, syngen 1. J. Cell Sci. 17:471–493.

Doerder, F.P. and DeBault, L.E. 1978. Life cycle variation and regulation of macronuclear DNA content in *Tetrahymena thermophila*. Chromosoma 69:1–19.

Doerder, F.P., Lief, J.H., and DeBault, L.E. 1977. Macronuclear subunits of *Tetrahymena thermophila* are functionally haploid. Science 198:946–948.

Engberg, J., Christiansen, G., and Leick, J.V. 1974. Autonomous rDNA molecules containing single copies of the ribosomal RNA genes in the macronucleus of *Tetrahymena pyriformis.) Biochem. Biophys. Res. Commun. 59:1356–1365.*

Gall, J.C. 1974. Free ribosomal genes in the macronucleus of Tetrahymena. Proc. Natl. Acad. Sci. U.S.A. 71:3078–3081.

Gorovsky, M. 1973. Macro- and micronuclei of *Tetrahymena pyriformis:* A model system for studying the structure and function of eukaryotic nuclei. J. Protozool. 20:19–25.

Iwamura, Y., Sakai, M., Mita, T., and Muramatsu, M. 1979. Unequal gene amplification and transcription in the macronucleus of *Tetrahymena pyriformis*. Biochemistry 24:5289–5294.

Loefer, J.B., Owen, R.D., and Christensen, E. 1958. Serological types among 31 strains of the ciliated protozoan *Tetrahymena pyriformis*. J. Protozool. 5:209–217.

Margolin, P., Loefer, J.B., and Owen, R.D. 1959. Immobilizing antigens of *Tetrahymena pyriformis*. J. Protozool. 6:207–215.

Nanney, D.L. and Dubert, J.M. 1960. The genetics of the *H* serotype system in variety 1 of *Tetrahymena pyriformis*. Genetics 45:1351–1358.

Nanney, D.L., Nagel, M.J.,and Touchberry, R.W. 1964. The timing of *H* antigenic differentiation in Tetrahymena. J. Exp. Zool. 155:25–42.

Nanney, D.L. and Preparata, R.M. 1979. Genetic evidence concerning the structure of the *Tetrahymena thermophila* macronucleus. J. Protozool. 26:2–9.

Orias, E. 1973. Alternative interpretation of the molecular structure and somatic genetics of acid phosphatase-1 in *Tetrahymena pyriformis*. Biochem. Genet. 9:87–90.

Orias, E. and Flacks, M. 1975. Macronuclear genetics of *Tetrahymena pyriformis,* syngen 1. Genetics 79:187–206.

Preer, J.R., Jr. and Preer, L.B. 1979. The size of macronuclear DNA and its relationship to models for maintaining genic balance. J. Protozool. 26:14–18.

Preparata, R.M. and Nanney, D.L. 1977. Cytogenetics of triplet conjungation in Tetrahymena: Origin of haploid and triploid clones. Chromosoma 60:49–57.

Schensted, I.V. 1958. Model of subnuclear segregation in the macronucleus of ciliates. Am. Naturalist. 92:161–170.

Seyfert, H.M. 1979. Evidence for chromosomal macronuclear substructures in Tetrahymena. J. Protozool. 26:66–74.

Seyfert, H.M. and Preparata, R.M. 1979. The regulation of amounts and proportions of genetic elements in the macronuclei of *Tetrahymena thermophila* strains of diverse karyotype. J. Cell Sci. 40:111–123.

Sonneborn, T.M. 1974. *Tetrahymena pyriformis*. In Handbook of Genetics, Vol. 2. R.C. King, ed. New York: Oxford University Press. pp. 433–467.

Williams, J.B., Fleck, E.W., Hellier, L.E., and Uhlenhopp, E. 1978. Viscoelastic studies on Tetrahymena macronuclear DNA. Proc. Natl. Acad. Sci. U.S.A. 75:5062–5065.

Woodard, J., Kaneshiro, E.S., and Gorovsky, M.A. 1972. Cytochemical studies on the problem of macronuclear subnuclei in Tetrahymena. Genetics 70:251–260.

Yao, M.C. and Gall, J.G. 1979. Alteration of the Tetrahymena genome during nuclear differentiation. J. Protozool. 26:10–13.

Hildemann, ed. Frontiers in Immunogenetics

# Mouse Teratocarcinoma 402AX Growth in Syngeneic and Allogeneic Hosts

Suzanne Ostrand-Rosenberg

*University of Maryland Baltimore County (UMBC), 5401 Wilkens Avenue, Catonsville, Maryland*

## Introduction

Recent studies in this laboratory have been aimed at defining the genetic and cellular basis of resistance and susceptibility in mice to the 402AX teratocarcinoma tumor. Teratocarcinomas have been considered by a number of workers as model systems for developing mammalian embryos because of their ability to give rise to differentiated cell types from undifferentiated stem cells both *in vivo* and *in vitro* (Stevens 1958; Kleinsmith and Pierce 1964), as well as their expression of various enzymes characteristic of embryonic cell types (Sherman 1979), and their expression of cell-surface antigens shared with preimplantation mouse embryos (Edidin et al. 1971; Artzt et al. 1973). From an immunological viewpoint teratocarcinomas are interesting because the undifferentiated stem cells of the tumor do not express the major histocompatibility antigens and show varied *in vivo* growth patterns. This article will attempt to describe recent studies in this laboratory involved in understanding teratocarcinoma tumor cell growth in syngeneic and allogeneic hosts. The results presented demonstrate genetic control of tumor resistance and susceptibility and indicate that resistant hosts have the ability to turn on *H-2* antigen expression on the otherwise *H-2* negative teratocarcinoma cells. Additional studies indicate there are a number of serologically defined 402AX teratocarcinoma antigens that potentially could serve in conjunction with *H-2* antigens as target antigens for effector lymphocytes in cell-mediated immune responses. Specifically, the following topics will be discussed: (1) A brief overview of teratocarcinoma biology; (2) the genetic basis of teratocarcinoma 402AX resistance and susceptibility; (3) two gene control of resistance and susceptibility to the 402AX teratocarcinoma tumor; (4) *H-2* linkage of one of the genes controlling 402AX susceptibility; (5) modulation of *H-2* antigens on teratocarcinoma cells passaged in genetically resistant hosts; (6) cell-mediated immunity to the 402AX teratocarcinoma; (7) serological characterization of 402AX tumor antigens; and (8) biochemical characterization of some of the 402AX defined antigens.

## Teratocarcinoma Biology

Teratocarcinomas are malignant tumors of the testes or ovaries which consist of metastatic embryonal carcinoma cells and non-tumorigenic differentiated cells which are derived from the three embryonic germ layers. They resemble very closely the multipotential cells of early embryos in that the embryonal carcinoma cells can give rise to a multitude of differentiated tissues (Damjanov and Solter 1974, Stevens 1967). A single embryonal carcinoma cell will give rise *in vivo* to tumors whose cells are derivatives of all three germ layers (Kleinsmith and Pierce 1964). In addition, teratocarcinoma cells can participate in normal fetal development and give rise to normal adult tissue when implanted into allogeneic mouse blastocysts (Brinster 1975; Illmensee and Mintz 1976, Papaioannou et al. 1975).

A number of different teratocarcinoma lines have been described all derived from 129 strain mice. These include the OTT6050 tumor, (Illmensee and Mintz 1976), the F9 teratocarcinoma (Artzt et al. 1973), and the 402AX teratocarcinoma (Stevens 1958). Although these tumors are all derived initially from the same mouse strain and hypothetically all from embryonic germ layers, they display considerable variation in their properties with respect to growth characteristics, cell-surface antigens, tumorgenicity, and morphology. These differences probably result because the various teratocarcinomas reflect expanded cell populations derived from slightly different embryonic stages and/or embryonic germ layers. Despite the many variations between the teratocarcinoma cell lines, several common properties are known. One of these characteristics is the lack of major histocompatibility antigens (*H-2* antigens) on the undifferentiated, malignant cells of the tumor (Artzt and Jacob 1974; Isa 1976; Forman and Vitetta 1975; Ostrand-Rosenberg, unpublished). However, when tumor cells differentiate they have been shown to become positive for *H-2* antigens (Artzt and Jacob 1974; Stern et al. 1975; Nicolas et al. 1976).

## Genetic Basis of Teratocarcinoma 402AX Resistance and Susceptibility

In order to study the *in vivo* growth of the 129 ($H\text{-}2^b$) derived 402AX teratocarcinoma, numerous inbred strains of mice were injected intraperitoneally with $7 \times 10^6$ 402AX cells. The mice were observed over a period of up to six months for their resistance or susceptibility to the tumor. If they were tumor-free after this period, they were considered resistant to the tumor. If they died during this period and upon autopsy ascites fluid was found containing tumor cells, the hosts were considered susceptible to the tumor. As shown in Table 1, of the eight inbred strains of mice tested, seven were completely susceptible to the tumor showing mean

**Table 1.** Mean Survival Times of Various Inbred Strains of Mice Injected with Teratocarcinoma 402AX.

| Tumor host | *H-2* haplotype | Dead/total injected | MST (days) |
|---|---|---|---|
| 129/SvS1 | $H\text{-}2^b$ | 20/20 | 18 ± 2 |
| C57BL/10 | $H\text{-}2^b$ | 0/20 | >200 |
| C3H.SW | $H\text{-}2^b$ | 5/5 | 39 ± 27 |
| DBA/2J | $H\text{-}2^d$ | 19/19 | 17 ± 3 |
| C3H/HeJ | $H\text{-}2^k$ | 14/14 | 27 ± 4 |
| AKR/J | $H\text{-}2^k$ | 18/18 | 25 ± 9 |
| SWR/J | $H\text{-}2^q$ | 15/15 | 30 ± 9 |
| SJL/J | $H\text{-}2^s$ | 15/15 | 30 ± 18 |

survival times (MST ± standard deviation) ranging from 18 to 39 days post-injection of teratocarcinoma cells. One strain (C57BL/10) is apparently completely tumor resistant. If tumor rejection in this system were based on *H-2* incompatibility between the host and tumor, then one would expect non-$H\text{-}2^b$ hosts to be resistant to the tumor and $H\text{-}2^b$ hosts to be susceptible to the tumor. As shown in Table 1, however, many non-$H\text{-}2^b$ strains are completely susceptible, while C57BL/10 mice which are $H\text{-}2^b$ are fully resistant. These studies have also been performed using various doses of inoculating teratocarcinoma cells. In all cases, susceptible strains and the resistant strain behave the same, regardless of the number of tumor cells given. Because of the absence of correlation of tumor resistance with *H-2* haplotype, it appears that rejection in the 402AX teratocarcinoma system is not based on tumor-host *H-2* incompatibility. (Ostrand-Rosenberg et al. in press).

### *Resistance and Susceptibility to the 402AX Teratocarcinoma Tumor are Under the Control of Two Genes*

In order to determine the genetic basis of 402AX resistance/susceptibility, susceptible (SWR) females were crossed with resistant (C57BL/10) males. The resulting F1 mice were tested for tumor susceptibility to $7 \times 10^6$ 402AX cells given intraperitoneally. 100% (25/25) of the F1's were completely susceptible showing mean survival times (26 ± 6 days) comparable to the susceptible parental strain. F1's of the reciprocal cross (C57BL/10 female × SWR male) were also 100% susceptible (11/11) showing a mean survival time of 33 ± 4 days. These F1 crosses demonstrate a genetic basis for 402AX susceptibility and suggest that the gene(s) controlling susceptibility is dominant to the gene(s) controlling resistance. In order to determine the number of genes involved in 402AX susceptibility, F1 mice have been backcrossed to the recessive C57BL/10 parent and the resulting offspring challenged with a tumor inoculum of $7 \times 10^6$ 402AX cells. Of 42 injected (SWR × C57BL/10)F1 × C57BL/10 backcross mice, 74% (31 mice) were fully susceptible to the tumor, while 26% (11 mice) were tumor free at 110 days post-injection. F2 crosses of (SWR × C57BL/10) F1's result in 6% tumor resistant mice. These data are compatible with tumor resistance and susceptibility being under the control of two genes.

### *H-2 Linkage of One of the Genes Controlling 402AX Teratocarcinoma Susceptibility*

The possible involvement of the *H-2* gene complex in 402AX resistance was tested by inoculating various B10 congenic strains of mice with varying doses of 402AX tumor cells. As shown in Table 2 for a tumor dose of $7 \times 10^6$ cells, most of the congeneics are only partially resistant to the tumor. Because the B10 congeneics are partially resistant, tumor susceptibility is probably influenced by a gene(s) in the B10 background. However, the B10 background alone is not sufficient to prevent tumor growth in all hosts. Therefore, a gene(s) other than the resistance gene(s) in the B10 background is implicated in resistance to 402AX. The full tumor resistance of C57BL/10 mice ($H$-$2^b$) suggests that resistance is also controlled by a gene(s) closely linked to the $H$-$2^b$ complex. Because the F1, F2, and backcross studies indicate that resistance is under the control of two genes, it is probable that one of these genes resides in the B10 background and that the second gene is closely linked to the *H-2* complex.

## Modulation of H-2 Antigens on Teratocarcinoma Cells Passaged in Genetically Resistant Hosts

In order to determine whether cell surface antigens of the 402AX tumor cells were modulating in tumor susceptible hosts, *in vitro* and *in vivo* passaged cells have been compared by indirect immunofluorescence. Cultured cells and cells passaged in susceptible (SWR × C57BL/10) F1 mice are both strongly positive (100%) with a syngeneic 129-anti-402AX serum and a xenogeneic rabbit anti-402AX serum. Both populations of cells are negative (4% and 10% fluorescent cells, respectively) for *H-2* antigens as detected by a panel tested congeneic anti-*H-2* serum (C3H anti-C3H.SW). *In vitro* tumor cells and cells passaged *in vivo* in susceptible hosts therefore show no obvious indications of surface antigen modulation. However, if one compares *in vitro* cultured cells and cells taken from the peritoneal cavity of genetically resistant hosts, the situation is quite different. Peritoneal exudate cells (principally small lymphocytes, 402AX tumor cells, and macrophages) are removed from mice that have been injected five to nine days earlier with the standard 7

**Table 2.** Mean Survival Times of Congeneic B10 Mice Injected with Teratocarcinoma 402AX.

| Tumor host | Total mice injected | Dead | MST (days) | Alive | MST (days) |
|---|---|---|---|---|---|
| B10.M | 19 | 3 | 31 ± 19 | 16 | > 100 |
| B10.PL | 15 | 7 | 72 ± 9 | 8 | > 100 |
| B10.A(2R) | 20 | 8 | 68 ± 56 | 12 | > 180 |
| B10.129 (6M) | 6 | 0 | | 6 | > 150 |
| B10.129(12M) | 9 | 6 | 53 ± 24 | 3 | > 120 |

$\times 10^6$ tumor cell dose. Macrophages are largely removed by allowing them to plate out onto plastic; the teratocarcinoma cells, lymphocytes, and other miscellaneous cell types are largely non-adherent to plastic. The remaining cells are then tested for *H-2* antigens using a congeneic C3H anti-C3H.SW antiserum which is specific for *H-2* complex antigens. Peritoneal exudate cells have been monitored by indirect immunofluorescence using goat-anti-mouse-IgG coupled to tetramethylrhodamine isothiocyanate (GAMIgG-TMR) or GAMIgG coupled to fluorescein isothiocyanate (GAMIgG-FITC), or by complement dependent dye exclusion microcytotoxicity as previously described (Ostrand-Rosenberg et al. 1977a,b). 402AX teratocarcinoma cells are readily distinguishable from other cells in the peritoneal cavity because of their distinctive morphology and size under the phase microscope. In addition, the teratocarcinoma cells immunogluoresce with a specific syngeneic 129-anti-402AX serum and GAMIgG-FITC, and hence double-staining experiments can be performed to specifically detect the *H-2* labeling status of the *in vivo* passaged teratocarcinoma cells. As shown in Table 3, those strains that are fully susceptible to the tumor (SJL, 129/SvS1, C3H.SW, and SWR) show relatively few *in vivo* passaged 402AX cells that are *H-2* antigen positive by either immunofluorescence or microcytotoxicity. 402AX cells carried in SWR mice are typically more *H-2* positive than teratocarcinoma cells carried in other susceptible strains.

However, almost 100% of tumor cells from resistant mice are strongly positive for *H-2* complex antigens. The limited number of B10 congeneics that are partially resistant and that have been tested show intermediate values for *H-2* antigen expression. That is, *in vivo* passaged 402AX cells from certain individuals show relatively high percentages of *H-2* positive cells, while other individuals show relatively low percentages of *H-2* positive cells.

*In vivo* passaged 402AX tumor cells from many of the strains shown in Table 3 have also been tested for *H-2* antigen expression with the NIH D series antiserum D-2, which is an anti-D end of H-2 antiserum ($K^bD^d \times K^rD^r$ anti-$K^bD^b$). All cells

**Table 3.** H-2 Expression on *In Vivo* passaged 402AX Teratocarcinoma Cells.

| | | **% *H-2* positive 402AX** | |
|---|---|---|---|
| **Strain** | **402AX susceptibility** | **Immunofluorescence** | **Cytotoxicity** |
| SJL | susceptible | 0, 0, 0, 0, 0 | |
| 129/SvSl | susceptible | 4, 14, 0, 0, 0, 0 | |
| SWR | susceptible | 37, 41, 23, 55, 53 | 38, 28 |
| C3H.SW | susceptible | 13, 18, 15 | 32, 24 |
| C57BL/10 | resistant | 100, 100, 96, 100, 57, 96 | 100, 95 |
| BI0.SM | resistant | 100, 100, 100, 100, 100 | |
| BI0.129(6M) | resistant | | 43, 86 |
| BI0.PL | partial | 25, 16, 44, 60 | |
| BI0.A (2R) | partial | 100, 100, 100 | |

that tested positive with the C3H-anti-C3H.SW serum were also positive with the D-2 antiserum. To determine whether K end, D end, and/or *la* antigens are produced on the tumor cells, C57BL/10 passaged 402AX cells were also tested with the NIH A.TH anti-A.TL serum, which detects *la* 1, 2, 3, 7, by indirect immunofluorescence. The 402AX cells were largely negative with this antiserum (14% positive).

Because of recent reports of alien histocompatibility antigens on tumor cells (Garrido et al. 1976; Nowinski and Klein 1975; Meschini et al. 1977) we have monitored *H-2* positive C57BL/10 passaged teratocarcinoma cells to determine whether they have turned on for genetically unexpected *H-2* antigens in addition to their turn-on for $H\text{-}2^b$ antigens. The NIH D series D-17 antiserum (anti-$K^qD^q$) and D-3 antiserum (anti-$K^sD^s$) are both non-reactive with $H\text{-}2^b$ haplotype lymphocytes, and hence should be negative on C57BL/10 passaged 402AX cells unless the tumor cells express non-$H\text{-}2^b$ *H-2* antigens. By indirect immunofluorescence C57BL/10 passaged 402AX cells are non-reactive with these antisera (10%, 0% fluorescent cells respectively).

402AX teratocarcinoma cells passaged in resistant hosts therefore appear to turn-on *K* and *D* end *H-2* antigens of the haplotype expected, based on their genotypic origin (129, $H\text{-}2^b$), and do not turn-on *la* antigen expression.

The time course of turn-on of *H-2* antigens on teratocarcinoma cells passaged *in vivo* in genetically resistant hosts has also been studied. $7 \times 10^6$ 402AX cells were given intraperitoneally to C57BL/10 hosts and peritoneal exudate cells removed and tested by indirect immunofluorescence and/or complement dependent microcytotoxicity at 24-hour intervals post-injection. At 24-hours post-injection, the teratocarcinoma cells are essentially *H-2* negative (6% positive); by 48 hours, the tumor cells have begun to turn on *H-2* (68% positive), and at 72 hours all of the 402AX cells found in the peritoneal cavity are *H-2* positive (100%). 402AX cells have been found to be 100% *H-2* positive for as long as 15 days post-injection. By 15 days post-injection, the resistant hosts have cleared most of the 402AX tumor cells from their peritoneal cavity.

*H-2* antigen turn-off following removal of antigen positive cells from resistant hosts has also been examined. Peritoneal exudate cells are removed sterilly from resistant (usually C57BL/10) hosts and placed in culture in their standard minimal essential medium supplemented with 5% calf serum, 1% penicillin-streptomycin, and 1% L-glutamine (GIBCO). Cells are then maintained in a high humidity, 5% $CO_2$, 37°C incubator and checked periodically for *H-2* antigen expression as monitored by immunofluorescence or microcytotoxicity. As shown in Figure 1, C57BL/10 passaged teratocarcinoma cells loose their *H-2* antigens rapidly after they are removed from the resistant host and placed in culture. Because the doubling time of 402AX cells in culture is approximately 24 hours, the loss of *H-2* antigens cannot be explained as merely a loss due to dilution by cell division.

The relatively rapid turn-on (within 2–3 days *in-vivo* following inoculation) and turn-off (within approximately 24 hours of removal from resistant hosts) of *H-2* antigens on 402AX cells passaged *in vivo* in resistant hosts indicates a strong

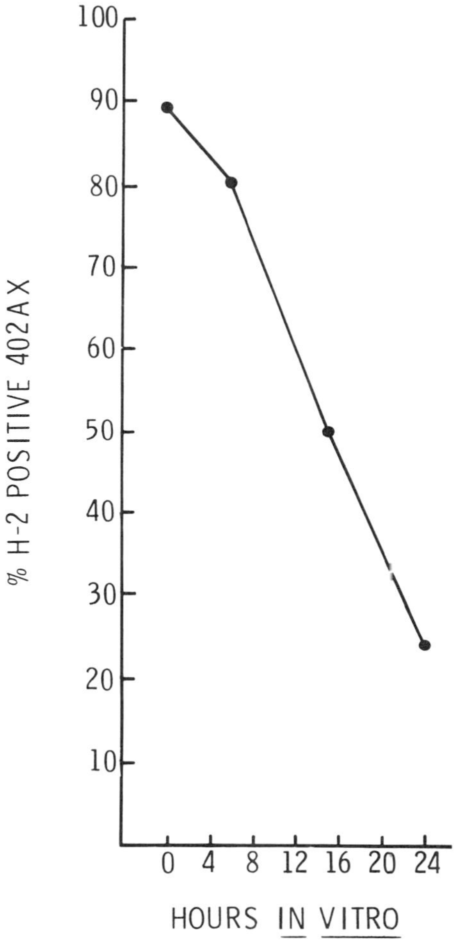


**Figure 1.** Loss of *H-2* antigens from C57BL/10 passaged *H-2* positive 402AX teratocarcinoma cells in culture. *In vivo* passaged 402AX cells were removed aseptically from the peritoneal cavity of C57BL/10 hosts and grown *in vitro*. Aliquots were removed at intervals from the cultures and tested with a congeneic anti-*H-2* serum plus GAMIgG-TMR by indirect immunofluorescence for *H-2* antigens.

interaction between the host and the tumor cells. Turn-on and maintainence of *H-2* expression is apparently an active process and requires the continued presence of some as yet unidentified host cell and/or factor. Studies are currently in progress to identify the cell population and/or factor required to stimulate *H-2* expression in 402AX cells and to determine its role in host resistance. Because of the known association between *H-2* positive teratocarcinoma cells and the differentiated state (see introductory section for details) studies are also in progress to determine whether *H-2* expression in the resistant hosts represents differentiation of the teratocarcinoma cells.

The strong correlation between *H-2* positive teratocarcinoma cells in those strains that are genetically resistant to the tumor and the relatively low number of *H-2* positive tumor cells in genetically susceptible individuals, suggests that *H-2* turn-on *in vivo* may play a role in host strain resistance. Studies in various systems including *in vitro* assays using virally infected cells (Zinkernagel and Doherty 1974; Gardner et al. 1974) and trinitrophenyl modified cells (Shearer 1974), as well as *in vivo* systems using adoptive transfer and virally infected cells (Doherty and Zinkernagel 1975) have demonstrated a requirement for *H-2* compatibility between effector T-cells and target cells. The finding reported here, that *H-2* negative teratocarcinoma tumor cells are converted to *H-2* positive cells in resistant hosts, may reflect a direct *in vivo* requirement for *H-2* antigen expression on target tumor cells for effective host cell-mediated cytotoxicity against resident tumor cells.

## Cell-Mediated Immunity to the 402AX Teratocarcinoma

Earlier reports (Forman and Vitetta 1975; Golstein et al. 1976) failed to detect cell-mediated killing against *H-2* negative teratocarcinoma cells *in vitro*. This negative result was attributed to the lack of *H-2* antigens on the tumor cells and the argument was made that the major histocompatibility antigens were necessary on target cells for effector lymphocyte recognition of the targets. In a more recent report (Wagner et al. 1978). T-cell-mediated killing was reported against the *H-2* negative F9 teratocarcinoma cell line, however, a subsequent paper (Golstein et al. 1978) claimed that the activity was directed against absorbed heterologous serum proteins rather than specific teratocarcinoma tumor antigens. Experiments in this laboratory (Cohn and Ostrand-Rosenberg, unpublished) indicate that specific cell-mediated killing can be obtained in an *in vitro* chromium-51 release assay (Brunner et al. 1976), provided one obtains the appropriate primed effector cells. Such effector cells are only inducible in the genetically resistant mouse strains (e.g., C57BL/10) and are found almost exclusively in the peritoneal cavity of hosts bearing ascites teratocarcinomas. Table 4 shows the percent chromium release from radiolabled *in vitro* cultured (and hence *H-2* negative) 402AX cells in the presence of varying numbers of peritoneal exudate cells from C57BL/10 mice inoculated thirteen days earlier with $7 \times 10^6$ 402AX cells. No control experiment using peritoneal exudate cells from susceptible mice is shown because, at 13 days post-injection of tumor cells, only tumor cells are present in their peritoneal cavity. The values shown in Table 4 are misleadingly low, however, because the effector population of peritoneal exudate cells has unlabeled teratocarcinoma cells mixed in with it. Hence, the ratios shown are the ratios of peritoneal exudate cells to chromium-51 labeled 402AX cells. The true ratio of lymphocytes to targets, however, in this experiment was 5:1. Hence, the normalized killing is 24% at a lymphocyte to target ratio of 5:1. Attempts to locate primed effector cells in the spleens of sensitized hosts have

**Table 4.** Cell-Mediated Immunity to the 402AX Teratocarcinoma Grown *in Vitro*.

| Peritoneal exudate cells: teratocarcinoma cells | % 51-Cr release |
|---|---|
| 100:1 | 24 |
| 50:1 | 24 |
| 25:1 | 17 |

Peritoneal exudate cells were obtained from 14 day *in vitro* primed C57BL/10 donors and included unlabeled 402AX cells at a ratio of 5:1 PEC:402AX. Hence the actual ratios in this experiment are 5:1 PEC:402AX. Therefore it is probable that a much higher % CR-51 release will be found at higher ratios of PED:402AX (see text for a more detailed discussion). The chromium release assay is a modified version of the Brunner et al. (1976) technique.

shown very low levels of specific effector cells, demonstratable only at high lymphocyte to target ratios (i.e., 200:1) in the *in vitro* chromium-51 release assay.

The results already discussed with respect to turn-on of *H-2* antigens on 402AX cells in resistant hosts, suggest that more efficient cell-mediated lysis may be found using *H-2* positive 402AX targets as opposed to the *H-2* negative 402AX targets used in the experiment shown in Table 4. Studies are currently in progress to determine whether such *H-2* positive targets are indeed more readily killed by specifically sensitized effector cells as compared to *H-2* negative teratocarcinoma cells. Greater lysis of *H-2* positive 402AX cells as compared to *H-2* negative tumor cells would support the contention that host resistance is enhanced by *H-2* antigen expression on the target cell, and would be further evidence supporting the requirement for effector-target cell histocompatibility.

## Serologically Defined Cell-Surface Antigens of 402AX Teratocarcinoma Cells

Several laboratories have produced antisera (syngeneic and xenogeneic) directed against teratocarcinoma plasma membrane antigens (Jacob 1977; Hogan 1977; Stern et al. 1975; Dewey et al. 1977; Gooding and Edidin 1974). A comparison of the various sera produced indicates that the different teratocarcinoma cell lines appear to define serologically distinct antigens (Gachelin 1978). Earlier studies (Gooding and Edidin 1974; Gooding et al. 1976; Edidin et al. 1971) using a xenogeneic (rabbit) anti-402AX teratocarcinoma serum defined a minimum of three antigens on 402AX cells: Antigen I is shared with many mouse and human tumor cells and with preimplantation mouse embryos; Antigen II is restricted to a mouse hepatoma cell line, the immunizing 402AX cells, and preimplantation mouse embryos; and Antigen III is specific for 402AX cells. Studies in this laboratory using a syngeneic 129-anti-402AX antiserum demonstrate a minimum of five antigens that appear to be different from the three antigens defined by the xenogeneic antiserum. Attempts have been made to further characterize these antigens both biochemically and serologically because of their possible role as target moieties for effector lymphocytes in cell-mediated immunity against the 402AX tumor.

### *Serological Characterization of 402AX Tumor Antigens*

The syngeneic 129 anti-40AX serum (SR-2) was produced by eight weekly injections of between $5 \times 10^5$ and $4 \times 10^6$ 5000R irradiated (cesium 137 source) 402AX cells intraperitoneally into male 129/SvS1 recipients followed by weekly injections and bleedings. SR-2 is negative on normal mouse tissue, including sperm (0-5% labeled cells) by indirect immunofluorescence. As shown in Table 5, however, the serum is positive with a large variety of established cell lines. Indirect immunofluorescence with GAMIgG-TMR or GAMIgG-FITC shows the presence of 402AX defined antigens on such diverse cell types as mouse blastocyst derived cell lines (MB2, MB21, MB31, and MB4; Sherman 1975a,b) and human teratocarcinoma cells (tera 2; Ostrand-Rosenberg et al. 1977b). Although uninfected mouse primary fibroblasts (129/SvS1) and an established mouse muscle cell line (BALB/c) were both unreactive with the antiserum, 48 hours after infection with SV40 virus both of these cell types were strongly positive with SR-2 on their plasma membranes and stained internally for the SV40 T antigen. SV40 infected tissue culture lines (i.e., SV3T3 and 11A8) are also plasma membrane positive with SR-2. The antiserum therefore appears to define an antigen shared with SV40 infected cells. Recent studies in other laboratories have demonstrated the presence of a host encoded antigen in SV40 infected cells that is also found in F9 teratocarcinoma cells (Linzer and Levine 1979; Segal et al. 1979). The SV40-teratocarcinoma antigen described

**Table 5.** Indirect Immunofluorescence of Anti-40AX Teratocarcinoma Antiserum (SR-2) on Various Target Cells.

| | % Fluorescent cells | | | | |
|---|---|---|---|---|---|
| **Target cells** | **SR-2** | **SR-2[MB2]** | **SR-2[MB31]** | **SR-2[F9]** | **SR-2[SV3T3]** |
| 402AX | 97 | 98 | 97 | 44 | 98 |
| SV40 infected BALB/c muscle | 100 | | | | 0 |
| SV3T3 | 100 | 11 | 0 | 0 | 0 |
| 11A8 | 97 | | | | 4 |
| MB2 | 98 | 11 | 92 | 100 | 98 |
| MB21 | 86 | | | | 0 |
| MB31 | 87 | 0 | 4 | 100 | 80 |
| MB4 | 94 | | | | 0 |
| C11D | 81 | | | | 0 |
| VA2 | 63 | | | | 0 |
| Tera 1 | 22 | | | | 2 |
| Tera 2 | 70 | | | | 0 |
| F9 | 100 | 11 | 22 | | 66 |
| Mel | 9 | | | | 0 |
| Pys-2 | 100 | 0 | 92 | | 0 |
| P815 | 68 | | | | 0 |
| EL-4 | 76 | 0 | 90 | 0 | 0 |

here for the 402AX teratocarcinoma is apparently not the same protein as the F9-SV40 antigen. (The biochemical data supporting this statement will be discussed in the following section: Biochemical Characterization of 402AX Antigens.)

Absorption of the anti-402AX serum with SV3T3 cells produces a reagent that is reactive with a more limited panel of cells. Two of the mouse blastocyst cell lines (MB2 and MB31), the F9 teratocarcinoma, and the immunizing 402AX cells are still reactive. It is apparent that most of the cells that are positive with the anti-402AX serum are expressing the SV40-teratocarcinoma antigen, rather than a teratocarcinoma specific antigen. This group includes the two human teratocarcinoma cell lines tera 1 and tera 2, and the teratocarcinoma derived parietal endoderm line pys-2, all of which have been previously described as expressing teratocarcinoma specific antigens (Ostrand-Rosenberg 1977b; Artzt et al. 1976; Holden et al. 1977). The antiserum can be further fractionated by absorption with the F9 teratocarcinoma (see Table 5). This absorption produces a reagent that retains some activity (44%) for 402AX, indicating that F9 and 402AX share some antigen(s) and that 402AX has its own specific antigens as well. The 402AX specific antibodies also react strongly with two of the mouse blastocyst cell lines (MB2 and MB31), indicating that these cells share the 402AX antigens not found on the F9 teratocarcinoma. Absorption with MB2 cells removes most of the activity of SR-2, including the activity against MB31 cells. Absorption with MB31 cells, however, leaves intact the anti-MB2 activity. This result suggests that MB2 and MB31 cells share at least one 402AX specific antigen, and that MB2 cells have at least one additional 402AX antigen not found on MB31 cells.

Complement dependent cytotoxicity experiments on random bred CD-1 strain preimplantation mouse embryos using unabsorbed and absorbed anti-402AX are shown in Table 6. The antiserum clearly defines teratocarcinoma antigens that are shared with fertilized ova through blastocyst stage preimplantation mouse embryos. The SV3T3 absorbed antiserum still retains its activity for embryos, and hence it cannot be determined whether the SV40-teratocarcinoma antigen is expressed on early embryos. The lack of reactivity with blastocyst stage embryos and the presence of reactivity with fertilized ova, 2-cell, and 4-8 cell embryos with SR-2 absorbed with F9 cells, suggests that the 402AX teratocarcinoma carries at least two antigens shared with preimplantation mouse embryos. One of these antigens is also shared with F9 cells and is present at the blastocyst stage and possibly at earlier stages. The second antigen is not found on the F9 teratocarcinoma and is expressed on fertilized ova through 4–8 cell stage embryos. This observation agrees with the serological fractination data presented in Table 5 for F9 absorbed SR-2. The anti-402AX absorptions with MB2 and MB31 cells indicate that reactivity to antigens other than the MB cell defined embryonic antigens is present in the anti-402AX antiserum. Further absorptions are necessary to determine at which stage these antigens are expressed.

Serological analysis therefore indicates there are at least five antigenic determinants detected by the syngeneic anti-402AX serum as assayed on primary and

**Table 6.** Complement-Dependent Cytotoxicity of Anti-402AX Teratocarcinoma Antiserum (SR-2) on Preimplantation CD-1 Mouse Embryos.

| | Dead/total embryos tested | | | | | |
|---|---|---|---|---|---|---|
| **Target embryo** | **SR-2** | **SR-2[MB2]** | **SR-2[MB31]** | **SR2[F9]** | **SR-2[SV3T3]** | **MNS** |
| Fertilized ova | 9/10 | 5/5 | 5/5 | 5/5 | 8/8 | 2/9 |
| 2-cell | 4/5 | | | 5/5 | | 1/5 |
| 4-8-cell | 3/3 | | | 4/4 | | 0/3 |
| Blastocyst | 6/6 | | | 0/5 | 5/5 | 2/8 |

established cell lines, and at least 2 antigenic moieties detected on preimplantation mouse embryos. It is unclear at present exactly what the relationship is between the embryo and cultured cell antigens. Additional experiments using embryos for absorptions will be necessary to determine the correspondence.

## Biochemical Characterization of Some of the 402AX Defined Antigens

In collaboration with Dr. Daniel Simmons of the University of Delaware, immunoprecipitation experiments have been performed to identify biochemically some of the serologically defined 402AX antigens. Cells were labeled with either tritiated leucine or S-35 methionine in culture, extracted with sodium deoxycholate, immunoprecipitated with antiserum, electrophoresed on SDS-PAGE, and fluorographed as previously described (Simmons et al. 1980; Ostrand-Rosenberg, O'Neill, and Simmons, submitted). Immunoprecipitation of 402AX cells with syngeneic anti-402AX shows a major band at approximately 99K molecular weight and minor bands at 200K and greater than 200K that are absent from normal mouse serum immune precipitates. The SV40 transformed cell line 11A8 shows the 200K protein, as does an immune precipitate from BHK (baby hamster kidney) cells, although to a lesser extent. The immunofluorescence data (Table 5), however, showed no plasma membrane fluorescence of BHK cells and strong reactivity with 11A8 cells. If the 200K protein is the teratocarcinoma antigen that is shared with SV40 transformed cells, then one must explain its apparent conflicting presence in the untransformed BHK cells. Two possibilities can be suggested: (1) In BHK cells the 200K antigen is found in the cytoplasm and is not present in the plasma membrane, hence it is not detected by indirect immunofluorescence of live cells, but is found by immunoprecipitation using solubilization techniques that extract the entire cell contents. (2) The quantity of the antigen on BHK plasma membranes is insufficient to be detected by immunofluorescence. Based on the densities of the 200K bands from 11A8 and BHK cells, this latter hypothesis seems unlikely. It is also possible, however, that the SV40-teratocarcinoma antigen is another molecule not detectable under these conditions (i.e., it is lipid or carbohydrate, or does not contain leucine or methionine).

As was mentioned in the previous section, other studies have demonstrated shared antigens between the F9 teratocarcinoma and SV40 infected cells (Linzer and Levine 1979; Segel et al. 1979). Immunoprecipitation experiments in the F9 system showed this antigen to be a host encoded protein of 54K-56K molecular weight. In order to determine whether the SV40-teratocarcinoma antigen defined in the 402AX system was the same 54K protein, 402AX, F9, and 11A8 cells were immunoprecipitated with serum from a hamster bearing an SV40 induced tumor (Ostrand-Rosenberg, O'Neill, and Simmons, submitted). This serum immunoprecipitates from the SV40 transformed 11A8 cells and the F9 cells exhibiting the 56K middle T or tau antigen. No 56K antigen is seen in 402AX precipitates. Also, no 54-56K protein is seen in 402AX cells immunoprecipitated with the anti-402AX serum. Therefore, the SV40-teratocarcinoma antigen defined by the 402AX teratocarcinoma is a molecule distinct from the 54-56K antigen shared between F9 and SV40 transformed cells.

Additional studies are currently in progress to identify biochemically the antigenic moieties detected by the various absorptions shown in Table 5 and 6, and to determine how these antigens are related to the 100K and 200K 402AX antigens detected by immunoprecipitation.

## Summary

Host immune response to the *H-2* negative 402AX teratocarcinoma is apparently under the genetic control of two genes, one of which is closely linked to the major histocompatibility complex of the mouse. Full resistance to the tumor requires homozygosity at both loci and resistance is recessive to tumor susceptibility. The finding that 402AX cells modulate to become *H-2* positive in resistant individuals suggests that *H-2* antigen expression may be necessary on target cells for efficient host cell-mediated immunity directed against the tumor. Studies are currently in progress to determine the efficiency of effector lymphocytes against *H-2* positive and *H-2* negative 402AX cells. A number of antigens have been serologically defined on 402AX teratocarcinoma using a syngeneic anti-402AX serum. These antigens include a determinant shared with SV40 infected cells and many other malignant cells including human teratocarcinomas, which is different from the 54-56K protein shared between the F9 teratocarcinoma and SV40 infected cells. In addition the antiserum detects antigens shared with preimplantation mouse embryos, mouse blastocyst cell lines and the F9 teratocarcinoma. At present it is not clear which antigens serve as the targets on the tumor cells for effector lymphocytes.

ACKNOWLEDGMENTS
I thank the following people for contributing to these studies: Cindy Ackrill, Sharon Bodmer, Vicky Cohan, Allen Cohn, Tami Rider, and Alex Twarowski. The very capable secretarial help of Susan Schneider and Carol Ferrigno is much appreciated. This study was supported by NIH Grant CA14910.

## References

Artzt, K., Dubois, P., Bennett, D., Condamine, H., Babinet, C., and Jacob, F. 1973. Surface antigens common to mouse cleavage stage embryos and primitive teratocarcinoma cells in culture. Proc. Natl. Acad. Sci. U.S.A. 70:2988–2992.

Artzt, K. and Jacob, F. 1974. Absence of serologically detectable *H-2* on primitive teratocarcinoma cells in culture. Transplantation 17:632–634.

Artzt, K., Hamburger, L., Jakob, H., and Jacob, F. 1976. Embryonic surface antigens: A quasi-endodermal teratoma antigen. Dev. Biol. 51:152–157.

Brinster, R.L. 1975. Can teratocarcinoma cells colonize the mouse embryo? In Teratomas and Differentiation. M.I. Sherman and D. Solter, eds. New York: Academic Press, pp. 51–58.

Brunner, K.T., Engers, H.D., and Cerottini, J. 1976. The $^{51}Cr$ release assay as used for the quantitative measurement of cell-mediated cytolysis *in vitro*. In *In Vitro* Methods in Cell-Mediated and Tumor Immunity. B.R. Bloom and J.R. David, eds. New York: Academic Press.

Damjanov, I. and Solter, D. 1974. Experimental teratoma. Curr. Top. Pathol. 59:69–130.

Dewey, M., Gearhart, J., and Mintz, B. 1977. Cell-surface antigens of totipotent mouse teratocarcinoma cells grown *in vivo:* Their relation to embryo, adult, and tumor antigens. Dev. Biol. 55:359–374.

Doherty, P.C. and Zinkernagel, R.M. 1975. Capacity of sensitized thymus derived lymphocytes to induce fatal lymphocytic choriomeningitis is restricted by the *H-2* gene complex. J. Immunol. 114:30–33.

Edidin, M., Patthey, H.L., McGuire, E.J., and Sheffield, W.D. 1971. An antiserum to embryoid body tumor cells that reacts with normal mouse embryos. In Proceedings of the First Conference and Workshops on Embryonic and Fetal Antigens in Cancer. N.G. Anderson and H.H. Coggin, eds. Oak Ridge, Tennessee: Oak Ridge National Lab, pp. 239–248.

Forman, J. and Vitetta, E.S. 1975. Absence of *H-2* antigens capable of reacting with cytotoxic T-cells on a teratoma line expressing T/t locus antigen. Proc. Natl. Acad. Sci. U.S.A. 72:3661–3665.

Gachelin, G. 1978. The cell-surface antigens of mouse embryonal carcinoma cells. Biochim. Biophys. Acta 516:27–60.

Gardner, I., Bowern, N.A., and Blanden, R.V. 1974. Cell-mediated cytotoxicity against ectromelia virus-infected target cells. Eur. J. Immunol. 4:63–67.

Garrido, F., Schirrmacher, V., and Festenstein, H. 1976. *H-2* like specificities of foreign haplotypes appearing on a mouse sarcoma after vaccinia virus infection. Nature 259:228–229

Golstein, P., Kelly, F., Avner, P., and Gachelin, G. 1976. Sensitiyity of *H-2*-less target cells and role of *H-2* in T-cell-mediated cytolysis. Nature 262:693–695.

Golstein, P., Luciani, M., Wagner, H., and Rollinghoff, M. 1978. Mouse T-cell-mediated cytolysis specifically triggered by cytophilic xenogeneic serum determinants: A caveat for the interpretation of experiments done under "syngeneic" conditions. J. Immunol. 121 2533–2538.

Gooding, L.R. and Edidin, M. 1974. Cell-surface antigens of a mouse testicular teratoma. J. Exp. Med. 140:61–78.

Gooding, L.R., Hsu, Y., and Edidin, M. 1976. Expression of teratoma-associated antigens on murine ova and early embryos. Dev. Biol. 49:479–486.

Hogan, B.L.M. 1977. Teratocarcinoma cells as a model for mammalian development. In International Review of Biochemistry, Vol. 15. J. Paul, ed. Baltimore: University Park Press, pp. 333–376.

Holden, S., Bernard, O., Artzt, K., Whitmore, W.F., and Bennett, D. 1977. Human and mouse embryonal carcinoma cells in culture share an embryonic antigen. Nature 270:518–520.

Illmensee, K. and Mintz, B. 1976. Totipotency and normal differentiation of single teratocarcinoma cells cloned by injection into blastocysts. Proc. Natl. Acad. Sci. U.S.A. 73:549–553.

Isa, A.M. 1976. Lack of demonstrable *H-2* antigens on the surface of teratocarcinoma 402AX of the mouse maintained *in vivo*. Transplantation 21:196–198.

Jacob, F. 1977. Mouse teratocarcinoma and embryonic antigens. Immunol. Rev. 33:2–32.

Kleinsmith, L.J. and Pierce, G.B. 1964. Multipotentiality of single embryonal carcinoma cells. Cancer Res. 24:1544–1548.

Linzer, D.I.H. and Levine, A.J. 1979. Characterization of a 54K dalton cellular SV40 tumor antigen present in SV40-transformed cells and uninfected embryonal carcinoma cells. Cell 17:43–52.

Meschini, A., Invernizzi, G., and Parmiani, G. 1977. Expression of alien *H-2* specificities on a chemically induced BALB/c fibrosarcoma. Int. J. Cancer 20:271–283.

Nicolas, J.F., Avner, P., Gaillard, J., Guenet, J.L., Jakob, H., and Jacob, F. 1976. Cell lines derived from teratocarcinomas. Cancer Res. 36:4224–4231.

Nowinski, R.C. and Klein, P.A. 1975. Anomalous reactions of mouse alloantisera with cultured tumor cells. II. Cytotoxicity is caused by antibodies to leukemia viruses. J. Immunol. 115:1261–1268.

Ostrand-Rosenberg, S., Hammerberg, C., Edidin, M., and Sherman, M.I. 1977a. Expression of histocompatibility-2 antigen on cultured cell lines derived from mouse blastocysts. Immunogenetics 4:127–136.

Ostrand-Rosenberg, S., Edidin, M., and Jewett, M.A.S. 1977b. Human teratoma cells share antigens with mouse teratoma cells. Dev. Biol. 6:11–19.

Ostrand-Rosenberg, S., Rider, T., and Twarowski. 1980. Susceptibility of allogeneic mice to teratocarcinoma 402AX. Immunogenetics, in press.

Papaioannou, V.E., McBurney, M.W., Gardner, R.L., and Evans, M.J. 1975. Fate of teratocarcinoma cells injected into early mouse embryos. Nature 258:70–73.

Segal, S., Levine, A.J., and Khoury, G. 1979. Evidence for non-spliced SV40 RNA in undifferentiated murine teratocarcinoma stem cells. Nature 280:335.

Shearer, G.M. 1974. Cell-mediated cytotoxicity to trinitrophenyl-modified syngeneic lymphocytes. Eur. J. Immunol. 4:527–533.

Sherman, M.I. 1975a. The culture of cells derived from mouse blastocycts. Cell 5:343–349.

Sherman, M.I. 1975b. Long-term culture of cells derived from mouse blastocycts. Differentiation 3:51–67.

Sherman, M.I. 1979. Developmental biochemistry of preimplantation mammalian embryos. Ann. Rev. Biochem. 48:443–470.

Simmons, D.T., Martin, M.A., Mora, P.T., and Chang, C. 1980. Relationship among tau antigens isolated from various lines of Simian virus 40-transformed cells. J. Virol., in press.

Stern, P., Martin, G.R., and Evans, M.J. 1975. Cell-surface antigens of clonal teratocarcinoma cells at various stages of differentiation. Cell 6:455–465.

Stevens, L. 1958. Studies on testicular teratomas of strain 129 mice. J. Natl. Cancer Inst. 20:1257–1276.

Stevens, L. 1967. The biology of teratomas. Adv. Morphol. 6:1–31.

Wagner, H., Starzinski-Powitz, A., Rollinghoff, M., Golstein, P., and Jakob, H. 1978. T-cell-mediated cytotoxic immune responses to F9 teratocarcinoma cells: Cytolytic effector T-cells lyse *H-2*-negative F9 cells and syngeneic spermatogonia. J. Exp. Med. 147:251–264.

Zinkernagel, R. and Doherty, P. 1974. Restriction of *in vitro* T-cell-mediated cytotoxicity in lymphocytic choriomeningitis within a syngeneic or semi-allogeneic system. Nature 248:701–702.

Hildemann, ed. Frontiers in Immunogenetics

# Fetal Membrane Antigens in Normal Development and Neoplasia

Bob G. Sanders

*Department of Zoology, The University of Texas at Austin, Austin, Texas*

It is indeed a pleasure to present studies on chicken fetal antigens (CFA) at a symposium dedicated to Ray D. Owen. This pleasure stems from my association with Ray as a postdoctoral fellow at the California Institute of Technology, and because Ray's long standing interest in gene expression during development and his encouragement and helpful suggestions over the years have played a much appreciated role in shaping and maintaining my interest in fetal antigens.

Ray has always had a keen interest in gene expression during development. When Ray first arrived in California, he noticed that the sea gulls along the Pacific Coast had two distinct feather patterns. Being unable to discern a Mendelian pattern of inheritance for the two feather patterns, he soon concluded that he was observing differential gene expression during development since the brown feather pattern of the juvenile sea gull eventually developed into the mature adult white feather pattern. Ray's observational interests led to laboratory studies which resulted in the first published report on chicken fetal antigens in 1954. In this first report, Ray described a fetal antigen localized to the red blood cell membrane of embryonic chickens but not found on the membrane of red blood cells obtained from adult chickens. Ray's initial observations on CFA were at the forefront of onco-developmental studies in general and laid the cornerstone for the studies that I will report on here.

The objectives of this paper are five-fold: (1) To give an overview of research on chicken fetal antigens; (2) to report on the expression of CFA in normal hematopoietic-lymphoid cellular differentiation; (3) to explain how CFA is useful as a model for investigating the cellular differentiation blockage hypothesis of cancer; (4) to explore the possibilities that CFA is serving as cell-cell communication molecules; and (5) to report on CFA as a viral binding site.

It has been known for over a hundred years that fetal and neoplastic cells share several common features. Both undergo rapid cell division, migrate, invade and colonize tissue at great distances, exhibit similar emzymatic patterns, and exhibit similar, if not identical, membrane glycoproteins. The first evidence that fetal markers were relevant to cancer arose from the observations that alpha fetoprotein (AFP) occurred in high levels in the sera of mice and humans in early development, and that patients or mice with cancer of the liver also exhibited high levels of AFP (Abelev et al. 1963; Tatarinov 1964). Finding elevated levels of AFP in the sera of neonates and adults with primary hepatomas, but not in non-cancerous adults led to the hypothesis that fetal gene products were being "reexpressed" in certain cancers. Gold and Freedman (1965) demonstrated the presence of another fetal antigen, carcinoembryonic antigen (CEA), which was present in elevated levels in the sera during early embryonic development, and occurred in elevated levels in adult humans with adenocarcinoma of the colon. Gold and Freedman (1966) postulated that genes coding for fetal proteins were derepressed in certain cancerous conditions. Studies on AFP and CEA in humans gave support to the hypothesis that fetal gene products were reexpressed in certain cancers and opened up a rapidly developing field of research on onco-fetal markers.

### *Terminology: Fetal—Onco-Fetal—Onco-Developmental*

Procedures for detecting fetal membrane antigens usually involve immunizing suitable animals, such as rabbits, with fetal tissue and adsorbing the resulting antisera with adult tissue. An adsorbed antiserum that gives a positive reaction with fetal tissue and a negative reaction with adult tissue is defined as being capable of detecting fetal-specific antigens.

Fetal antigens are usually transcient antigens that are expressed for only a brief period of time at some specific stage of development from zygote to birth (Table 1). By definition, onco-fetal antigens are expressed only during embryonic development and under cancerous conditions. Not all fetal antigens are reexpressed in cancerous condition. Sensitive assays for onco-fetal antigens have revealed "onco-fetal" antigens to be present on normal tissues of non-cancerous adults. Such antigens are referred to as onco-developmental antigens. Onco-developmental antigens are present in relatively high concentrations during fetal development, in lower

**Table 1.** Fetal-Cancer-Normal Antigenic Relationships.

| | Antigen expression | | |
|---|---|---|---|
| **Terminology** | **Zygote-birth** | **Birth-adult** | **Cancer** |
| Fetal specific | ++ | – | – |
| Cancer specific | – | – | + |
| Onco-fetal | ++ | – | + |
| Onco-developmental | ++ | + | + |

concentrations on normal tissue after birth and are found in elevated amounts in certain cancers. Most studies with fetal antigens have demonstrated a general progression in our understanding from fetal to onco-fetal to onco-developmental. The fact that "fetal" antigens are often times expressed by normal tissues has made the goal of identifying cancer specific markers tantamount to impossible.

## Overview of CFA

### *Discovery of CFA*

Chicken fetal antigens (CFA) were first described by Ray D. Owen when he reported in the California Institute of Technology 1954 Biology Annual Report that:

> "Among the sidelights that have developed in this study has been the recognition of antigenic specificities found in the red cells of embryonic chicks, which disappear during later development. Antisera produced by injecting the blood of embryo-chicks into rabbits, when absorbed by adult chicken red cells, were shown to contain antibodies that lyse the cells of young but not of mature chickens. The chicks lose this 'embryonic' characteristic six weeks after hatching."

### *Fetal Nature of CFA*

CFA is not exclusively fetal or embryonic in nature for while it is first detectable on the circulating red blood cells of a two and one-half-day-old embryo it is gradually lost from peripheral red blood cells of chickens over a 60-day post-hatch period.

### *Onco-Fetal Nature of CFA*

The onco-fetal nature of CFA was established when it was demonstrated that peripheral red blood cells from adult chickens infected with avian myeloblastosis virus (AMV) or avian erythroblastosis virus (AEV) expressed CFA (Teplitz et al. 1974; Sanders et al. 1975). It came as a surprise that the peripheral red blood cells from AMV-infected chickens possessed CFA since AMV induces a cancer of myeloid rather than erythroid cells. Not all of the red blood cells expressed CFA, only 5-25%. Nor did all of the AMV-infected leukemic chickens exhibit CFA positive peripheral red blood cells. In these two regards, CFA resembles the expression of other known onco-fetal antigens. For instance, while 70% of patients with primary hepatomas show elevated levels of AFP, 30% do not and elevated levels of CEA are not present in some patients with adenocarcinoma of the colon (Booth et al. 1974). Even more troublesome is that AFP and CEA have been reported in elevated levels in some non-cancerous controls (Von Kleist, 1976).

Closer inspection of the peripheral blood from the AEV-infected chickens showed that CFA was being expressed only on the more immature erythroid cell types. These studies established CFA as an onco-fetal antigen and suggested that CFA might be present on erythroid cells of normal adults.

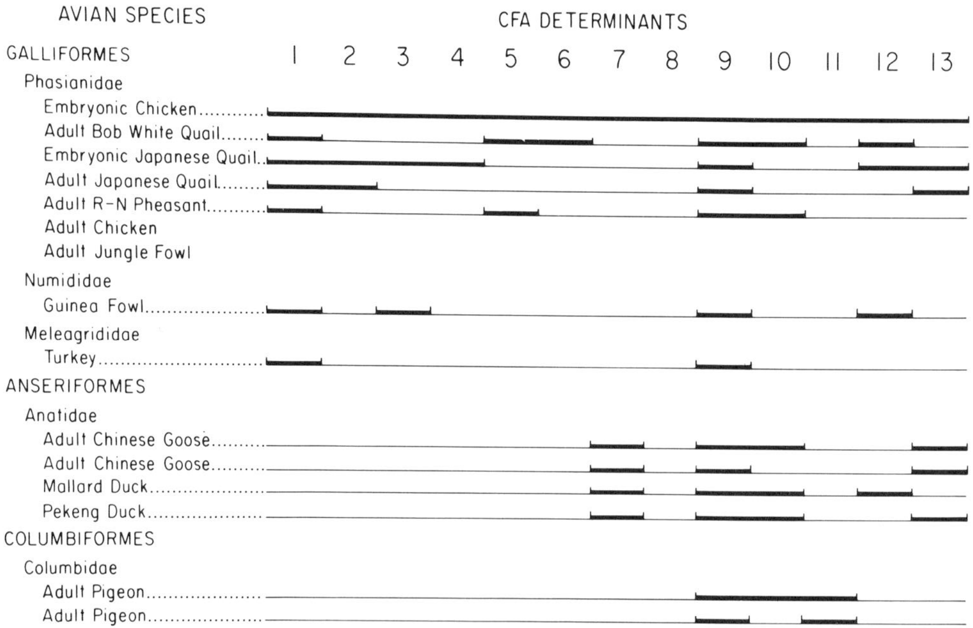


**Figure 1.** CFA expression on peripheral red blood cells of avians is depicted by the horizontal bar graphs. For example, red blood cells from the embryonic chicken express CFA determinants 1-13, while red blood cells from adult chickens are CFA negative. CFA expression on goose and pigeon peripheral red blood cells show genetic polymorphism. Goose red blood cells express either CFA determinants 7, 9, 10, 12 or CFA determinants 7, 9, 12; whereas, pigeon red blood cells express CFA determinants 9, 10, 11 or CFA determinants 9, 11.

### *Onco-Developmental Nature of CFA*

After showing the onco–fetal nature of CFA, research focused on establishing the genetic basis for the reexpression of fetal antigens in cancers. One clue to the question of whether fetal gene expression required the derepression of turned-off fetal genes came when it was shown that adult chickens made anemic with phenylhydrazine-HC1 exhibited reticulocytes in circulation that were positive for CFA (Sanders and Kline 1975). Furthermore, anti-CFA, adsorbed with spleen and bone marrow obtained from adult chickens, is unable to react with test cells positive for CFA indicating that normal adult splenic and bone marrow cells possessed CFA. Finding CFA on erythroid cells undergoing cellular differentiation in the bone marrow established CFA as onco-developmental in nature rather than fetal specific or onco-fetal.

### *Serologically Complex Nature of CFA*

CFA expression on peripheral red blood cells in chickens is universal. That is to say, no chicken strain thus far examined has been found that doesn't express CFA on its red blood cells during early development. Phylogenetic analyses of CFA expression on the peripheral red blood cells obtained from a variety of avians demonstrated CFA to be present in all avians tested with one major and important exception. Anti-CFA adsorbed with red blood cells from non-chicken avians did not result in completely adsorbed antisera. This indicated that there was more than one CFA and has led to the dissection of anti-CFA sera so that thirteen distinct antigens are now detectable (Figure 1). CFA is not greatly different from other onco-fetal markers in this regard; for instance, a total of six distinct CEA antigens have been reported (Von Kleist 1976).

As can be seen in Figure 1, analyses of CFA determinants among several avians again showed the non-fetal nature of CFA in that certain CFA determinants are expressed throughout the lifetime of all avians except chickens and Jungle fowl. Figure 1 also illustrates the distinct phylogenetic expression of CFA. Finding differential expression of CFA in avians now permits one to dissect anti-CFA sera through differential adsorptions and elutions from red blood cells with known CFA determinants (Figure 2). Adsorption-elution procedures with specific combinations of red blood cells now permit the dissection of anti-CFA into thirteen specific reagents (Sanders et al. 1980).

Finding the differential expression of CFA among related avians not only permitted the dissection of anti-CFA, but permits limited breeding experiments via interspecific hybrids (Dietert and Sanders 1978). For example, adult hybrid offspring from turkey-chicken crosses (phurkeys) always express the CFA determinants of the non-chicken avian. The developmental profile of CFA determinant expression in the phurkey hybrid is currently under investigation.

Analyses of CFA expression on different cells and tissues of the two and one-half-day-old chick embryo show CFA to be expressed only by hematopoietic-lymphoid cells (Figure 3). At this writing, CFA is best described as a serologically

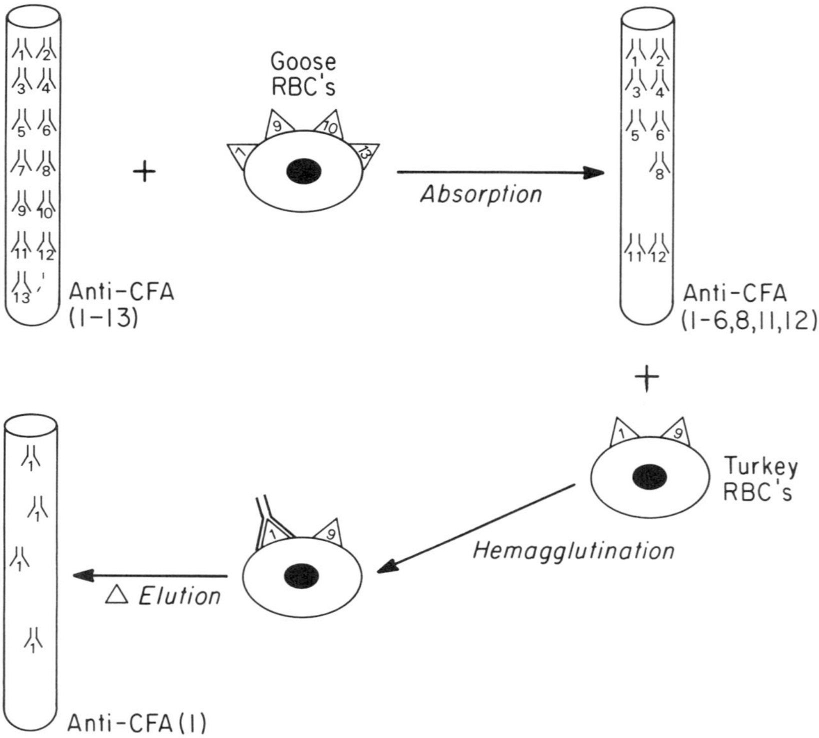


**Figure 2.** Production of an antibody reagent that specifically detects CFA determinant 1 is accomplished by first adsorbing anti-CFA (1-13) with goose red blood cells (goose red blood cells express CFA determinants 7, 9, 10, 13) in order to remove antibodies to CFA determinant 9. Next, the adsorbed antisera is reacted with turkey red blood cells (turkey red blood cells express CFA determinants 1 and 9). The agglutinated turkey red blood cells with anti-CFA-9 antibodies bound to CFA determinant 9 are washed thoroughly to remove any trapped antibodies, then anti-CFA-1 is eluted from the turkey red blood cells by gently agitating the red blood cell-antibody complexes at 58°C for 20 minutes. Other adsorption-elution combinations permit one to dissect anti-CFA-sera into thirteen antibody reagents specific for the 13 CFA determinants.

complex membrane glycoprotein localized to hematopoietic-lymphoid tissues of chickens.

## Expression of CFA on Erythroid and Lymphoid Cells of Normal Chickens

Hematopoietic-lymphoid tissues continually proliferate and differentiate throughout the life time of an animal in order to renew themselves. Thus, erythroid and lymphoid cell lines serve as good models for studying cellular differentiation.

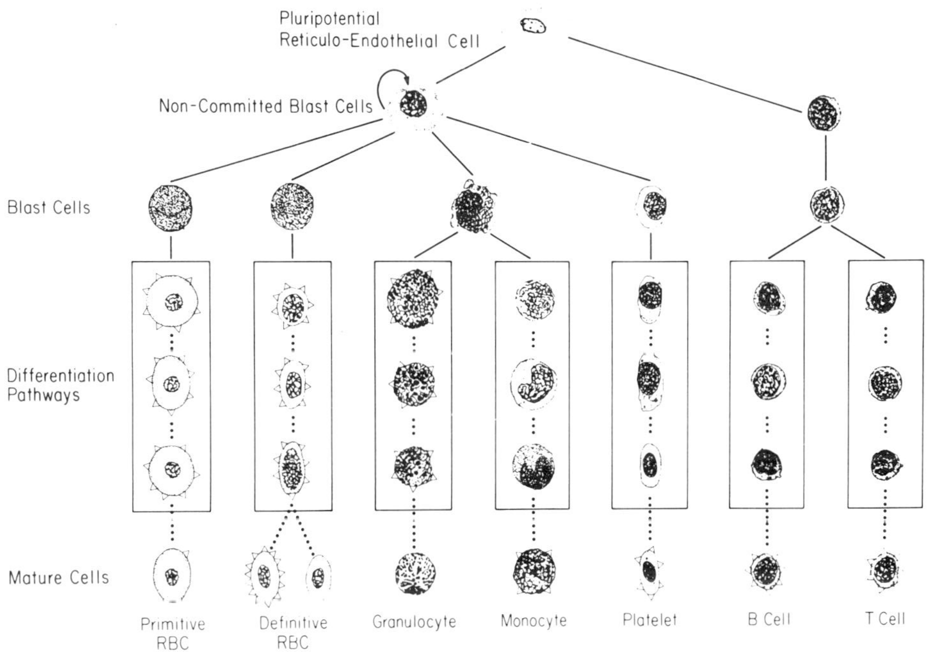


**Figure 3.** CFA's as hematopoietic-lymphoid specific membrane glycoproteins are depicted. CFA expression by cells is depicted by spikes (e.g., note the erythroid series). Cells, including the pluripotential stem cells as well as the differentiating cells, that do not show CFA spikes projecting from their membranes, have not been studied. Mature cells not expressing CFA have been studied and have been found to be CFA negative.

## *Erythroid Cells*

In chickens, the erythroid cell line can be readily studied at all ages of chicken development and such studies are enhanced by the fact that cells in the erythroid cell series can be distinguished by several criteria such as: (1) Morphology (Lucas and Jamroz 1961); (2) biochemical expression of different fetal and adult hemoglobins; (3) distinct patterns of DNA and RNA synthesis (Williams 1972); (4) chromatin condensation differences (Sung 1977), and (5) phosphorylation of erythrocyte specific histone (H5) which becomes progressively phosphorylated with cellular differentiation and which becomes completely dephosphorylated at the terminal stage of cellular maturation (Sung 1977; Sung and Freedlender 1978).

Erythroid cells in the chicken are derived from two cell series, the primitive erythroid series and the definitive erythroid series. The primitive and definitive cell series are thought to represent two distinct cell lineages. Cells in both series undergo cellular differentiation, with each differentiation stage identifiable by distinct morphological characteristics (Lucas and Jamroz 1961).

Cells of the primitive erythroid cell series comprise the earliest circulating red blood cells in a developing chick. The primitive erythrocytes are located in blood islets and synthesize embryonic hemoglobins (Mahoney et al. 1977). They undergo rather synchronous cell division, thereby enabling one to obtain relatively pure (greater than 70%) populations of cells which represent cellular differentiation stages from erythroblast to mature erythrocyte. The primitive erythrocytes are the only circulating erythrocytes present throughout the first six days of circulation and they are almost completely gone, being gradually replaced by the definitive erythrocytes, by the tenth day of embryonic development.

Definitive erythrocytes are first detected between six and eight days of embryonic development, and constitute the only erythroid cell series expressed throughout the remainder of embryonic development and adult life. Thus, the chicken with its special advantages for studying early chick embryos has permitted the examination and identification of CFA expression. This applies to erythroid cells undergoing maturation in the embryo and bone marrow of developing chickens as well as CFA expression on circulating red blood cells throughout chicken development.

## *CFA Expression On Circulating Primitive Erythroid Cells*

Chick embryoes from two and one half days to ten days old have been examined for the presence of individual CFA determinants on erythroblast, early-mid-late polychromatic erythrocytes, reticulocytes, and mature erythrocytes of the primitive cell series, utilizing antiserum specific for each CFA determinant. All CFA determinants are present on the erythroblast; however, the determinants are lost in a sequential manner with the mature primitive cells exhibiting only CFA determinant #9 (Figure 4; left panel).

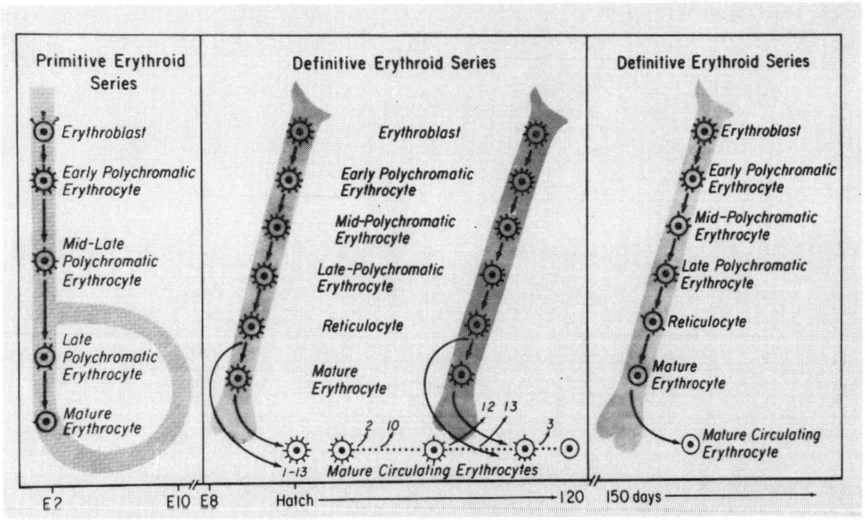


**Figure 4.** CFA expression on differentiating primitive and definitive erythroid cells at various developmental ages are depicted. The left panel shows CFA loss from circulating primitive erythroid cells undergoing cellular differentiation. Only CFA determinant 9 is found on mature primitive red blood cells. CFA expression on the definitive erythroid cells is depicted in the middle and right panels. The middle panel shows that the loss of CFA with development may occur in the circulating peripheral blood, or the loss of CFA that is observed in the peripheral blood may be reflective of CFA loss from erythroid cells differentiating in the bone marrow. The right panel depicts CFA loss with cellular differentiation in the bone marrow giving rise to only CFA negative circulating peripheral red blood cells.

### *CFA Expression on Circulating and Non-Circulating Definitive Erythroid Cells*

CFA expression on cells of the definitive erythroid cell series is much more complicated than CFA expression on cells of the primitive erythroid cell series. The pattern of CFA expression differs on cells undergoing erythropoiesis in different aged chickens (Figure 4, middle panel). At hatching, cells in all stages of erythroid differentiation express all of the CFA determinants including circulating mature red blood cells. The number of circulating mature red blood cells positive for CFA gradually diminishes with post-hatch development until by 50 days post-hatch, hemagglutination analyses no longer detect CFA positive red blood cells in the circulation. From 60 days post-hatch development on throughout adulthood, CFA is sequentially lost during erythropoiesis in the bone marrow giving rise to only CFA negative mature red blood cells for release into the circulation (Figure 4, right panel).

Analyses of single determinant expression by circulating mature red cells from hatch to 50 days post-hatch reveals the sequential loss of CFA determinants (Figure 4, middle panel) (Dietert et al. 1980). Whether this sequential loss of CFA from mature red blood cells is: (1) occurring in the circulation after release from the bone marrow, (2) occurring during erythropoiesis in the bone marrow or (3) is a combination of both mechanisms has not been fully resolved but differences in regulation of erythroid differentiation in different aged chickens is suspected to be involved. Regulation of erythropoiesis includes such factors as proliferation of a pluripotent stem cell, committment of hematopoietic stem cells to erythropoiesis, erythroid cellular differentiation processes, terminal differentiation steps, and release of cells into circulation (Quesenberry and Levitt 1979). The terminal stages of erythroid cellular differentiation involves discrete morphological and chemical changes which include: Chromatin condensation, terminal cell division, accumulation of globulin mRNA, increase in heme synthesis, synthesis of characteristic erythrocyte enzymes and, the appearance of erythrocyte-specific membrane antigen and other proteins such as spectrin (Marks 1978).

Morphologically mature erythrocytes from one-day-hatched chickens do not exhibit condensed chromatin whereas mature erythrocytes from adult chickens do. Erythrocytes from adult chickens exhibit an adult antigen which is not present on peripheral red blood cells from newly hatched chickens. Blanchet demonstrated two erythrocyte plasma membrane antigens, one specific for embryoes and the other specific for adults (Blanchet 1976a,b). Blanchet observed three types of antigen expression among peripheral blood erythrocytes with development: Embryonic only; both embryonic and adult; and adult only. Studies in our lab have also demonstrated the presence of an adult antigen in the peripheral blood as well as in the bone marrow of adult chickens (unpublished data).

To account for his observations of embryonic and adult specific antigens, Blanchet postulated (1) a single stem cell that sequentially gives rise to all three (embryonic, embryonic and adult, and adult) antigenically distinct erythrocyte populations or

(2) several independent stem cells which give rise to the three antigenically distinct populations of erythrocytes (Blanchet 1976a,b). Our studies support the first hypothesis. One supportive observation is that CFA is present on all erythroid cells in the early stages of cellular differentiation in the bone marrow of all aged chickens (Nelson et al. 1980).

Bone marrow reconstitution studies performed by Sanders and Wiley (1971) also support the first hypothesis. When donor bone marrow cells from one-day hatched chickens were injected into X-irradiated adult chickens, the donor one-day hatched erythrocytes in the adult peripheral blood were CFA negative. When donor bone marrow cells from adult chickens were injected into one-day hatched chicks, the donor adult erythrocytes in the peripheral blood of the developing chicks were CFA positive. These studies suggest that the status of the bone marrow rather than several stem cell populations control the expression of CFA on peripheral red blood cells (Figure 5).

Blanchet et al. (1976) transplanted bone marrow from adult chickens into X-irradiated 23-day-old chickens and observed that the transplanted bone marrow cells

**Figure 5.** A model describing CFA expression on erythroid cells in the bone marrow and circulating peripheral blood is depicted. Up to ten days post-hatch, erythroid cells undergoing cellular differentiation in the bone marrow express CFA and release CFA positive erythroid cells into the peripheral blood. The status of CFA on erythroid cells undergoing cellular differentiation in the bone marrow changes with development from positive to negative. This change is reflected in the peripheral blood. At approximately 60 days post-hatch, all cells being released into the peripheral blood are CFA negative. Erythroid cells at some differentiation stage(s) express CFA, independent of the age of the chicken. As cells expressing CFA decrease, cells expressing an adult antigen increase. Cells undergoing cellular differentiation may concurrently express CFA and adult antigen at some stage.

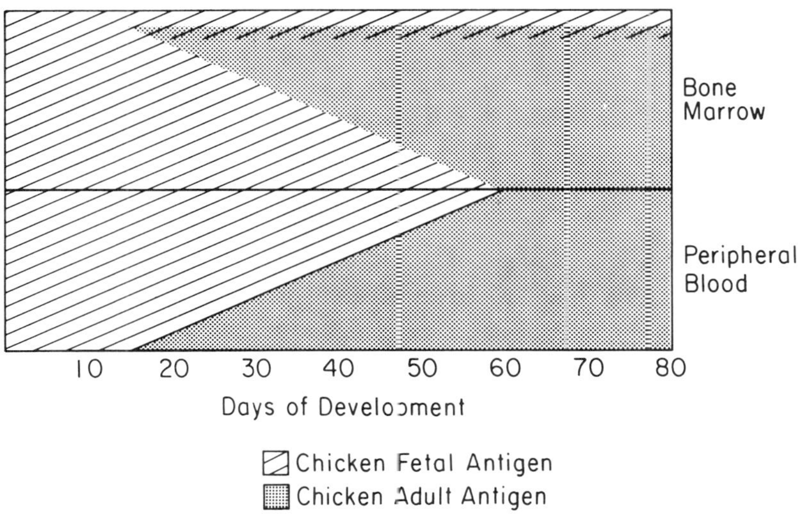

gave rise to only embryonic antigen negative peripheral red blood cells. According to the model in Figure 5, one would have expected donor peripheral blood erythrocytes both positive and negative for the embryonic antigen, in 23-day post-hatched chickens. Not finding embryonic positive erythrocytes of donor origin may indicate other restrictions in addition to the microenvironment of the bone marrow or may be interrupted as supportive of the second hypothesis. A third possibility is that our anti-CFA and Blanchet's anti-embryonic erythrocyte antigen sera are detecting different embryonic antigens.

CFA expression varies both qualitatively and quantitatively. Sequential loss of CFA determinants is observed in differentiating primitive erythroid cells (Patel et al. 1980) in differentiating definitive erythroid cells in the bone marrow (Nelson et al. 1980) and from red blood cells in the peripheral blood of developing chickens from approximately 20 days to 60 days post-hatch (Dietert et al. 1980). Sequential loss of CFA determinants may: (1) reflect the ability (avidity) of our antisera to detect different CFA determinants; (2) be due to post-translational modification of the CFA membrane glycoprotein by specific enzyme cleavage of sugars, or (3) represent the expression of specific gene families of CFA at different stages of cellular differentiation.

### *CFA Expression on Lymphoid Cells*

CFA is not an exclusive erythroid membrane antigen. Our understanding of CFA expression on lymphoid cells is not as extensive as our understanding of erythroid cell expression; however, we do know that CFA is present on lymphoid cells in the peripheral blood, bone marrow, bursa, thymus and on several virally transformed lymphoid cell lines in culture (Murthy et al. 1979; Kline et al. 1980). Not all of the CFA determinants are present on lymphoid cells since anti-CFA adsorbed with bursa or thymus cells contain antibodies that agglutinate CFA positive one-day-old chick red blood cells. Analyses of bursa cells and thymus cells (taken from individual thymus lobes) for differential CFA expression did not establish CFA as a marker for identifying subpopulations of chicken lymphocytes. However, the differential expression of CFA on splenic T and B-lymphocytes has not been performed.

## CFA as a Model for Investigation of the Cellular Differentiation Blockage Hypothesis

Studies of CFA expression on normal erythroid cells indicate that CFA is found on immature cells and suggests that CFA expression is controlled by cellular differentiation processes. Since cloned-REV-transformed lymphoid cells express different combinations of CFA (Table 2), we feel that CFA on lymphoid and erythroid cells serves as a good model for testing the cellular differentiation blockage hypothesis of cancer (Sanders 1980). The cellular differentiation blockage hypothesis of cancer is illustrated in Figure 6. The model shows (1) normal cellular differentiation in which stem cells give rise to progenitor cells that undergo normal

**Table 2.** CFA Expression on Cloned REV-Transformed Lymphoid Cell Lines.

| Cell line designation | CFA determinant expression |
|---|---|
| 1 | 1, 3, 5, 6 |
| 2 | 1 5 |
| 3 | 1 |

differentiation, giving rise to mature cells, (2) abnormal cellular differentiation in which cells are blocked in a cell cycle and are unable to complete cell division, and (3) abnormal cellular differentiation in which cells complete cell division but are unable to proceed forward in the cellular differentiation process. Cell cycle blockage would result in the accumulation of immature cells. Cell cycle blocked cells would not be able to be maintained in *in vitro* cell culture since they cannot complete cell division, and would depend on progenitor stem cells for increase in cell numbers. Cells blocked in a specific stage of cellular differentiation would accumulate more rapidly, depending on the cell growth properties of cells at a particular differentiation stage, and would grow in cell culture.

The cellular differentiation blockage hypothesis of cancer has several features that could account for several observed aspects of cancer: (1) Slow growing versus fast growing cancers (cell cycle blockage versus cellular differentiation stage blockage); (2) the ability or inability of cancer cells to be grown *in vitro* (cellular differentiation stage blockage versus cell cycle blockage); (3) the great individual diversity among cancers of a "single" cancer type (numerous cell cycle blockages and cell differentiation stage blockages could be postulated for every cell cycle and differentiation stage of a particular differentiation pathway, each blockage would give rise to a unique cell type, yet the end effect would be the same, i.e., no fully mature functioning cell type for this differentiation pathway); (4) the ability of some cancers within a "single" cancer type to respond to certain treatment forms while others of the same cancer type do not (differences between breaking cell cycle blockages in $G_1$,S,$G_2$, or M; and differences between breaking cell differentiation stage blockages in stages 1, 2, 3, 4, . . . . . M), (5) the great difficulty in finding cancer-specific markers, because all cells involved would represent some differentiation pathway stage or cell cycle phase of normal cellular processes.

Evidence supporting the cellular differentiation blockage hypothesis is accumulating. Alpha-fetoprotein studies by Becker et al. (1976) in two hepatoma cell lines, one producing AFP and the other not, indicate that AFP production occurs during a very brief period in the ontogeny of the liver cell. Hepatomas that synthesize AFP are considered to be "locked in" to a specific stage of development with respect to the gene for AFP, while hepatomas that do not produce AFP are "locked in" at a non-AFP-producing stage before or subsequent to the AFP-producing stage. In humans, well differentiated hepatomas do not produce AFP (Shikata and Sakakitara 1973). Sell et al. (1976) demonstrated AFP production to be associated with normal hepatocyte division in both fetal and adult rats.

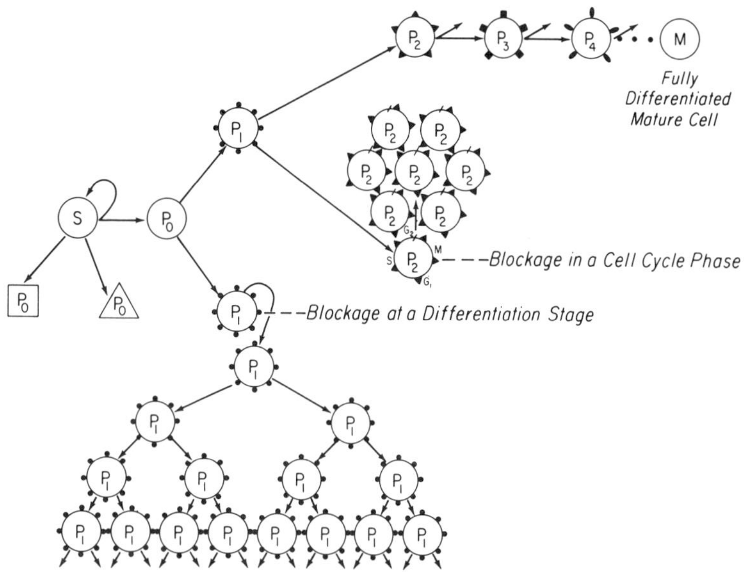


**Figure 6.** A model for the cellular differentiation blockage theory of cancer is depicted. Pluripotential stem cells (S) differentiate into $P_0$ cells that undergo further differentiation into (1) fully differentiated mature cells (top), (2) cells ($P_2$) that are blocked at the $G_2$ cell cycle phase (such blocked cells are dependent on $P_0$ cells for increasing in numbers since they cannot complete mitosis), and (3) $P_1$ cells that are capable of completing cell division, but are blocked in their ability to advance from the $P_1$ to the $P_2$ stage of cellular differentiation. Expression of different membrane antigens specific for different cellular differentiation stages are depicted as projections coming from the membranes of $P_1$, $P_2$, $P_3$ and $P_4$ cells.

Teratocarcinomas, a malignant tumor in mice, are composed of pluripotential stem cells (embryonal) as well as several different fully differentiated mature cells (Braun 1975). Injections of single embryonal-carcinoma cells, cells thought to be blocked in cellular differentiation, into mice results in teratocarcinomas in the recipient mice that have the same cell characteristics as the teratocarcinoma of the donor (Kleinsmith and Pierce 1964). The interpretation of these data is that the embryonal-carcinoma cell is a highly malignant pluripotential cell in the undifferentiated state, but is capable of differentiating into several distinct non-malignant differentiated cell types.

Another possible example of a cancer which may result from cellular differentiation blockage is neuroblastomas in humans (Braun 1975). Spontaneous regression of malignant neuroblastomas occurs in humans (Everson and Cole 1966). It is thought that some neuroblastoma cells differentiate into ganglion cells that have lost their malignant properties (Braum 1975). Nerve growth factor induces neuroblastoma cells to develop into ganglion cells (Everson and Cole 1966; Dyke and Mulkey 1967). Furthermore, neuroblastomas in humans can be classified into class 1 and class 2 neuroblastomas. Patients with class 1 neuroblastomas survive longer and their neuroblastoma cells will not grow in culture (suggestive of a cell cycle blockage); whereas, patients with class 2 neuroblastomas do not survive long and their neuroblastoma cells will grow in culture (suggestive of a cellular differentiation stage blockage).

CFA is currently serving as a model system for testing the differentiation blockage hypothesis. It has been known for several years that certain chemicals such as dimethyl sulfoxide (DMSO), and butyric acid can induce Friend leukemia cells (murine erythroid cells) to undergo cellular differentiation (Friend et al. 1971; Leder and Leder 1975; Graf et al. 1978). Experiments involving treatment of cloned REV and AEV-tranformed cells with cellular differentiation inducing agents (DMSO, butyric acid, and HMBA, 1,6 N-N diacetylhexane diamine hexamethylbisacetylamide) and testing for changes in CFA expression are currently in progress.

In the next two sections, two possible functions of CFA besides that of cellular differentiation stage markers will be examined: CFA as a possible cell-cell communication marker and CFA determinants as viral binding sites.

## CFA as Possible Cell-Cell Communication Molecules

The specific co-capping of non-identical markers on a membrane has been proposed as a prerequisite for membrane molecules serving as cell communication molecules for cell-cell interactions such as cellular migration (Bourguignon et al. 1978). The possibility that CFA is a cell-cell communication molecule is derived from co-capping studies that demonstrate CFA to co-cap with the B histocompatibility antigens (Table 3). The co-capping data is presented in the top line of Table 3. A total of 120 fluorescent cells, from the 22°C incubation, were examined. 43% of the cells formed caps with 30% of the capped cells being co-capped. Capping was not observed at 4°C.

**Table 3.** Co-Capping of CFA and B Locus Membrane Antigens.

| | Number of cells examined | | Percent of fluorescent cells with | | | |
|---|---|---|---|---|---|---|
| **Co-capping experimental design** | **Non-fluorescent** | **Fluorescent** | **No-caps** | **Co-caps** | **F*-caps only** | **R*-caps only** |
| R-anti-CFA + R*-G-anti-R-Ig (4°C) + C-anti-B2 + F*-R-anti-C-Ig (22°C) | | 120 | 57 | 30 | 0 | 13 |
| Controls | | | | | | |
| NRS + R*-G-anti-R-Ig (4°C) + NCS + F*-R-anti-C-Ig (22°C) | 200 | 0 | | | | |
| R-anti-CFA + R*-G-anti-R-Ig (4°C) | | 100 | 100 | 0 | 0 | 0 |
| R-anti-CFA + R*-G-anti-R-Ig (22°C) | | 100 | 70 | 0 | 0 | 30 |
| C-anti-B2 + F*-R-anti-C-Ig (4°C) | | 100 | 100 | 0 | 0 | 0 |
| C-anti-B2 + F*-R-anti-C-Ig (22°C) | | 100 | 72 | 0 | 28 | 0 |
| NRS + R*-G-anti-R-Ig (4°C) | 200 | 0 | | | | |
| NCS + F*-R-anti-C-Ig (4°C) | 200 | 0 | | | | |
| 0.75% NaCl + R*-G-anti-R-Ig (4°C) | 200 | 0 | | | | |
| 0.75% NaCl + F*-R-anti-C-Ig (4°C) | 100 | 0 | | | | |

Abbreviations used:
R* = Rhodamine labeled antibody.
F* = Fluorescein labeled antibody.
R-anti-CFA = Rabbit antisera specific for CFA.
G-anti-R-Ig = Goat antisera to rabbit Ig.
R-anti-C-Ig = Rabbit antisera to chicken Ig.
C-anti-$B_2$ = Chicken antisera to chicken $B_2$ histocompatibility antigen.
NRS = Normal rabbit serum.
NCS = Normal chicken serum.

Although CFA co-caps with histocompatibility membrane antigens on splenic lymphocytes, CFA is not a B antigen. Studies by Krsmanovic et al. (1979) show embryonic antigens on red blood cells to have a molecular weight of 48,000 daltons. SDS gel electrophoretic studies of radiolabeled immunoprecipitated proteins from one-day hatched chick red blood cells and from thymus and bursa lymphocytes show CFA to have a molecular weight of 48,000; it is not associated with beta-2-microglobulin (manuscript in preparation).

## CFA #9 as a Viral Binding Site

It has been known for many years that it is much easier to infect and trasform cells from embryos and young animals than from adults (Burmester et al. 1960; Baluda 1962; Bela et al. 1963). Several hypotheses have been proposed to account for what appears to be windows of specific periods of infectivity, most based on the immaturity of the immune response system. Here we propose that fetal antigens may be serving as viral binding sites for viral infectivity.

Proof that CFA #9 is a site for virus binding is derived from studies with Sindbis virus (Figure 7). The ability of Sindbis virus to bind and agglutinate red blood cells from different avian species is dependent upon whether or not the red blood cells express CFA determinant #9. Furthermore, reacting test red blood cells with Sindbis virus prior to testing for CFA#9 demonstrated that Sindbis binding to avian erythrocytes inhibited anti-9-antibodies from reacting with the CFA#9 erythrocyte antigens (Sanders et al. 1980). Anti-CFA is capable of preventing isotope labeled Sindbis virus from binding to one day hatched chicken red blood cells (Table 4). The ability of anti-CFA to prevent Sindbis binding decreases with serial dilution from 40% to 0%. Anti-CFA adsorbed with turkey red blood cells, which results in the removal of antibodies to CFA determinants #1 and #9, no longer inhibits Sindbis binding. Hemagglutination data and viral inhibition of antigen-antibody reactions clearly implicate CFA determinant #9 as a hemagglutination binding site for Sindbis. Whether CFA #9 not only binds virus but is essential for infectivity as a virus receptor is currently under investigation. The possible role of fetal membrane antigens as virus receptors is one intriguing possibility for explaining the distinct windows of viral infectivity observed in embryonic and young animals.

## Summary

Chicken fetal antigen is a complex of a minimum of thirteen serologically distinct membrane antigens that are found on immature hematopoietic-lymphoid cells. CFA determinants are differentially expressed on erythroid cells undergoing cellular differentiation. CFA's are useful membrane markers for studying normal cellular differentiation in hematopoietic-lymphoid cells and for testing the cellular differentiation blockage hypothesis of cancer. Studies implicate CFA as a possible cell-cell communication molecule and show CFA determinant #9 to be a viral binding site.

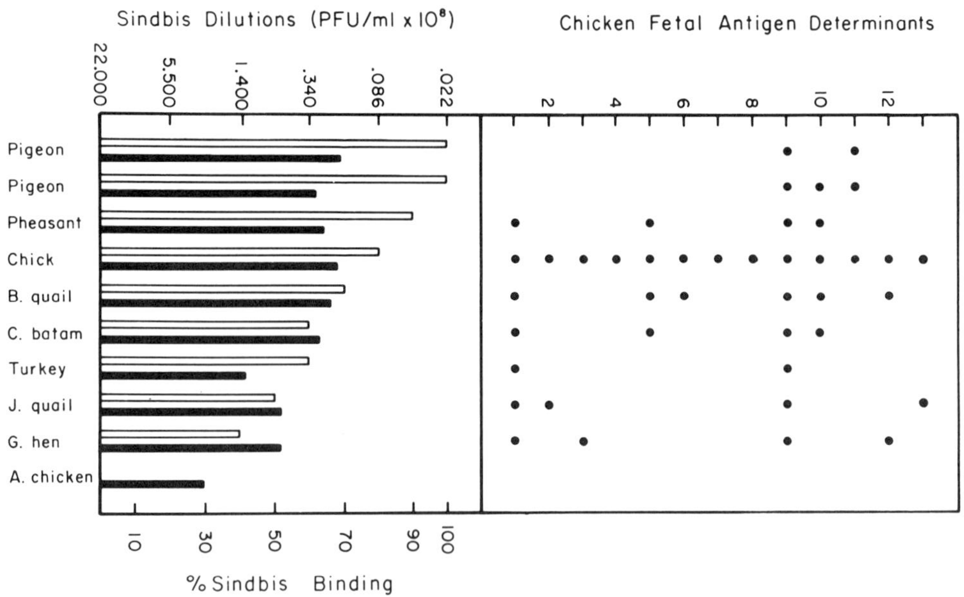


**Figure 7.** CFA determinants expressed on the erythrocytes from several avians are shown by the black circles in the top part of the figure. Absence of black circle(s) indicates that the CFA determinant is not expressed. The ability of serially diluted Sindbis virus ($22 \times 10^8$ to $0.22 \times 10^8$) to agglutinate red blood cells from several avians is depicted by open bars in the lower part of the figure. The percent isotope labeled virus bound to the different red blood cells is depicted by closed bars.

**Table 4.** Ability of Anti-CFA-Sera to Inhibit Sindbis Binding to Chicken Red Blood Cells.

| Source of chicken red blood cells | Percent isotope labeled Sindbis bound to red blood cells | | | | | | | |
|---|---|---|---|---|---|---|---|---|
| | | Anti-CFA | | | | | | Anti-CFA (−1,9) |
| | Controls | Undil | 1:4 | 1:8 | 1:16 | 1:32 | 1:64 | Undil |
| 1-Day-Hatch | 63 +/−4.8 | 38 +/−2.8 (40%)[a] | 48 +/−4.2 (24%) | 54 +/−3.6 (14%) | 57 +/−5.6 (10%) | 60 +/−7.2 (5%) | 61 +/−3.6 (3%) | 63 +/−4.6 (0%) |
| Adult | 33 +/−1.3 | 32 +/−2.2 (3%) | 34 +/−1.4 (0%) | 36 +/−1.4 (0%) | 35 +/−2.2 (0%) | 34 +/−2.8 (0%) | 33 +/−1.4 (0%) | 36 +/−2.8 (0%) |

[a]( ) = % inhibition of isotope binding by anti-CFA.

ACKNOWLEDGMENT
I would like to thank Kimberly Kline for her invaluable advice and help. This research is supported by the National Institutes of Health Grant CA12851.

## References

Abelev, G.I., Perova, S.D., Khramkova, N.I., Postnikova, Z.A., and Irlin, I.S. 1963. Production of embryonal alpha-globulin by transplantable mouse hepatomas. Transplantation 1:174.

Baluda, M. 1962. Properties of cells infected with avian myeloblastosis virus. Cold Spring Harbor Symp. Quant. Biol. 27:415.

Becker, J., de Neuchaud, B., and Potter, V.R. 1976. Two new rat hepatoma cell cultures for studying the unbalanced blocked ontogeny hypothesis. In Onco-Developmental Gene Expression. W.H. Fishman and S. Sell, eds. New York: Academic Press, p. 259.

Bela, R., Rappaport, H., and Shubik, P. 1963. Influence of dose and age on the induction of malignant lymphomas and other tumors by 7,12-dimethylbenz (a)-anthracene in Swiss mice. J. Natl. Cancer Inst. 30:723.

Blanchet, J.P. 1976a. Developmental changes of chick erythrocyte membrane antigens. Study by immunofluorescence. Exp. Cell Res. 102:1.

Blanchet, J.P. 1976b. The chick erythrocyte membrane antigens: Characterization and variation during embryonic and post-embryonic development. Dev. Biol. 48:411.

Blanchet, J.P., Samarut, J., and Nigon, V. 1976. Chick erythrocyte membrane antigens. Their expression in irradiated chickens grafted with hematopoietic tissue from different origins. Exp. Cell Res. 102:9.

Booth, S.N., King, J.P., Leonard, J.C., and Dykes, P.W. 1974. The significance of elevation of serum carcinoembryonic antigen (CEA) levels in inflammatory diseases of the intestine. Scand. J. Gastroenterol. 9:651.

Bourguignon, L.Y., Hyman, R., Trowbridge, I., and Singer, S.J. 1978. Participation of histocompatibility antigens in capping of molecularly independent cell surface components by their specific antibodies. Proc. Natl. Acad. Sci. U.S.A. 75:2406.

Braun, A.C. 1975. Differentiation and dedifferentiation. In Cancer: A Comprehensive Treatise. Biology of Tumors: Cellular Biology and Growth. F.F. Beck, ed. New York: Plenum Press, p 3.

Burmester, B.R., Fontes, A.K., and Walter, W.G. 1960. Pathogenicity of a viral strain (RPL 12) causing avian visceral lymphomatosis and related neoplasms. III. Influence of host age and route of inoculation. J. Natl. Cancer Inst. 24:1423.

Dietert, R.R. and Sanders, B.G. 1978. Expression of an onco-developmental antigen among avian species. J. Exp. Zool. 206:17.

Dietert, R.R. and Sanders, B.G. 1979. Genetic segregation and developmental phasing involving chicken fetal-leukemic antigen. J. Hered. 70:235.

Dietert, R.R., Ciratest, J., and Juran, M. 1980. Developmental changes in the presence of specific chicken-fetal-leukemic antigen determinants in the chicken, Japanese quail and the interspecific hybrid. Poult. Sci., in press.

Dyke, P.C. and Mulkey, D.A. 1967. Maturation of ganglioneuroblastoma to ganglioneuroma. Cancer 20:1343.

Everson, T.C. and Cole, W.H. 1966. Spontaneous Regression of Cancer. Philadelphia: Saunders, p. 560.

Friend, C., Scher, W., Holland, J.G., and Sato, T. 1971. Hemoglobin synthesis in murine virus-induced leukemic cells *in vitro:* Stimulation of erythroid differentiation by dimethyl sulfoxide. Proc. Natl. Acad. Sci. U.S.A. 68:378.

Gold, P. and Freedman, S.O. 1965. Demonstration of tumor-specific antigens in human colonia carcinomata by immunological tolerance and adsorption techniques. J. Exp. Med. 121:439.

Gold, P. and Freedman, S.O. 1966. Specific carcinoembryonic antigens of the human digestive system. J. Exp. Med. 122:467.

Graf, T., Beug, H., Royer-Pokora, B., and Meyer-Glauner, W. 1978. *In vitro* transformation of hematopoietic cells by avian erythroid and myeloid leukemia viruses: A model system for the differentiation of normal and neoplastic cells. In Differentiation of Normal and Neoplastic Hematopoietic Cells. B. Clarkson, P.A. Marks, and U.E. Till, eds. Cold Spring Harbor Conferences on Cell Proliferation Vol. 5, p. 625.

Kleinsmith, L.J. and Pierce, G.B., Jr. 1964. Multipotentiality of single embryonal carcinoma cells. Cancer Res. 24:1544.

Kline, K., Bose, H.R., Jr., and Sanders, B.G. 1980. CFA expression on peripheral erythroid cells of erythroleukemic adult chickens and on *in vitro* derived virally transformed tumor cell lines. (Submitted for publication).

Krsmanovic, V., Blanchet, J.P., Greenland, T.B., and Aupoix. M. 1979. Immunochemical properties of embryonic and adult specific antigens of chicken erythrocytes. Exp. Cell Res. 120:409.

Leder, A. and Leder, P. 1975. Butyric acid, a potent inducer of erythroid differentiation in cultured erythroleukemic cells. Cell 5:319.

Lucas, A.M. and Jamroz, C. 1961. Atlas of Avian Hematology. Agriculture Monograph 25. U.S. Department of Agriculture, Washington, D.C., p. 271.

Mahoney, K.A., Hyer, B.J., and Chan, L.N.L. 1977. Separation of primitive and definitive erythroid cells of the chick embryo. Dev. Biol. 564:12.

Marks, P.A. 1978. Introduction to the symposium on erythrocyte differentiation and regulation. In Differentiation of Normal and Neoplastic Hematopoietic Cells. Cold Spring Harbor Conference on Cell Proliferation, Vol. 5, p. 147.

Murthy, K.K., Dietert, R.R., and Calnek, B.W. 1979. Demonstration of chicken fetal antigen (CFA) on normal splenic lymphocytes, Marek's disease lymphoblastoid cell lines and other neoplasms. Int. J. Can. 24:349.

Nelson, C.H., Patel, N.H., and Sanders, B.G. 1980. Chicken fetal antigen expression on the definitive erythroid maturation series in the bone marrow of the adult chicken. J. Exp. Zool. 212:101–108.

Owen, R.D. and Mallek, P. 1954. Red blood cell antigens in chickens. In Biology Annual Report. Pasadena: California Institute of Technology.

Patel, N.H., Nelson, C.H., Ellison, J., and Sanders, B.G. 1980. Chicken fetal antigen (CFA) expression on the primitive erythroid maturation series. (Submitted for publication).

Quesenberry, Pl. and Levitt, L. 1979. Hematopoietic stem cells. N. Engl. J. Med. 301:755.

Sanders, B.G. and Wiley, K. L. 1971. Expression of embryonic and adult erythrocyte antigens in hematopoietic repopulated X-irradiated chickens. J. Exp. Zool. 178:393.

Sanders, B.G. and Kline, K. 1975. Fetal-tumor membrane associated antigens: Genetic and immunological implications. Trans. Am. Microsc. Soc. 94:470.

Sanders, B.G., Teplitz, R.L., Brodetsky, A.M., Fung, H., and Wiley, K.L. 1975. Investigation of fetal antigen in chickens with AMV-induced leukemia. In Proc. 13th Hanford Biol. Sump., The Cell Cycle in Malignancy and Immunity. Oak Ridge, Tennessee, USERDA, p. 348.

Sanders, B.G., Wan, K.M., Kline, K., Garry, R.F., and Bose, H.R., Jr. 1980. Chicken fetal antigens (CFA): Role as cell surface receptors for Sindbis virus hemagglutinin. J. Virol. 106:183–186.

Sanders, B.G., Dietert, R.R., Kline, K., and Dietert, M. 1980. Chicken fetal antigen: Example of an antigenically complex onco-developmental membrane glycoprotein. Onco-Dev. Biol. Med., in press.

Sell, S., Becker, F.F., Leffert, H.L., and Watabe, H. 1976. Expression of an onco-developmental gene product (alpha-fetoprotein) during fetal development and adult oncogenesis. Cancer Res. 36:107.

Shikata, T. and Sakakitara, K. 1973. Relationship between alpha-fetoprotein and histological patterns of hepatoma and localization of alpha-fetoprotein hepatoma cells using the peroxidase antibody technique. Gann. Monogr. Can. Res. 14:269.

Sung, M.T. 1977. Phosphorylation and dephosphorylation of histone V (H5): Controlled condensation of avian erythrocyte chromatin. Biochemistry 16:286.

Sung, M.T. and Freedlender, E.F. 1978. Sites of *in vivo* phosphorylation of histone H5. Biochemistry 17:1884.

Tatarinov, Y.S. 1964. Detection of embryo-specific alpha-globulin in the blood sera of patients with primary liver tumors. Vop. Med. Khim. 10:90.

Teplitz, R.K., Sanders, B.G., Broadetsky, A.M., Fung, H., and Wiley, K.L. 1974. Fetal-leukemia antigen of chicken blood cells. Cancer Res. 34:1049.

Von Kleist, S. 1976. The use of CEA (carcinoembryonic antigen) and other carcinofoetal antigens in human cancer. In Clinical Tumor Immunology. J. Wybran and M.J. Staquet, eds. London: Pergamon Press, p. 89.

Williams, A.F. 1972. DNA synthesis in purified populations of avian erythroid cells. J. Cell Sci. 10:27.

Hildemann, ed. Frontiers in Immunogenetics

# Homologous T-Cell Differentiation Antigens of Mouse and Man

Leonard A. Herzenberg and Jeffrey A. Ledbetter

*Department of Genetics, Stanford University School of Medicine, Stanford, California*

## Introduction

Delighted as I am to participate in this symposium honoring Ray Owen, I must confess that I am an illegitimate participant. I never was formally a student or postdoctoral fellow of Ray's. However, he has played such an important role in my personal and professional development and that I greatly appreciate this opportunity to join with his legitimate "offspring" on this wonderful occasion.

In many ways I do consider myself a student of Ray's. In my graduate student days at Caltech, each of us was required to have a minor thesis and minor subject area and I took Ray's course in immunology. He introduced me to the concepts and facts of immunology and immunogenetics in a marvelous, stimulating and eventually compelling fashion. Most people now consider me more of an immunologist or immunogeneticist than a practitioner in the areas of my pre- and postdoctoral work: biochemical genetics and what has now become known as molecular biology.

Much of the work in our lab and increasingly in cellular immunology generally makes extensive use of the fluorescence-activated cell sorter (FACS) (Bonner et al., 1972; Boyse et al., 1971; Cantor and Boyse, 1975). With hybridoma-produced monoclonal antibodies to cell surface antigens (Cantor et al., 1975; Cantor et al., 1976; Cantor and Boyse, 1977a). providing the opportunity of overcoming the remaining major technical problem for analyzing and sorting distinct lymphoid cells viably, we have focused our efforts on characterization of subpopulations of T and B-cells. Here we present our recent work on T-cells of mice and men (Cantor and Boyse, 1977b; Evans et al., 1977).

The mouse Lyt-1, Lyt-2 and Lyt-3 lymphocyte surface antigens have been used for some years now as immunogenetic markers whose selective expression distinguishes maturational and functional T-cell subpopulations (Evans et al., 1978; Fatham et al., 1975). Lyt-2 and Lyt-3, for example, are selectively expressed on cytotoxic and suppressor T-cells but are not found on helper T-cells (Herzenberg et al., 1976; Herzenberg and Herzenberg, 1978). Similarly, cytotoxic depletion studies originally indicated that Lyt-1 is selectively expressed on helper T-cells but not on suppressor or cytotoxic T-cells (Jandinski et al., 1976; Köhler and Milstein, 1975). More sensitive immunofluorescence techniques, however, have now shown that Lyt-1 is found on all T-cells (Cantor and Boyse, 1977a; Cantor and Boyse, 1977b; Ledbetter and Herzenberg, 1979; Ledbetter et al., 1980) but is present in higher levels on helper T-cells than on suppressor or cytotoxic T-cells (Cantor and Boyse, 1977b). In addition, each of the Lyt-1, Lyt-2 and Lyt-3 antigens undergoes characteristic changes in surface density expression as T-cells mature in the thymus and peripheral lymphoid tissues (Cantor and Boyse, 1977b; Ledbetter et al., 1980) as shown in the following sections.

## *Lyt-1 is on All T-Cells and Increases During Maturation*

All thymocytes and splenic (Thy-1-bearing) T-cells express Lyt-1 antigen; however, there is a clear bimodal distribution of antigen densities that correlates with maturation (Figure 1a). In thymus, approximately 15-20% of the cells stain brightly for Lyt-1. These form a "shoulder" on the brighter side of the main population. The splenic or lymph node Lyt-1$^+$ cells are about four times brighter than the main thymocyte population and correspond in brightness to the smaller number of bright thymus cells. Since this latter is the cortisone-resistant thymocyte population (Cantor and Boyse, 1977a), these data indicate that levels of Lyt-1 antigen increase during T-cell maturation (Table 1).

**Table 1.** Quantitative Cellular Expression and Density of T-Cell Antigens by FACS Analysis.[a]

| | Thymus | | Spleen | | Lymph node | |
|---|---|---|---|---|---|---|
| **Antibody** | **Positive cells (%)** | **Antigen density[b]** | **Positive cells (%)** | **Antigen density[b]** | **Positive cells (%)** | **Antigen density[b]** |
| α-Thy-1.2 (53-2.1) | 100 | 85 | 30 | 37 | 57 | 39 |
| α-Lyt-1 (53-7.3) | >95 | 1.5 | 34 | 3.8 | 59 | 4.4 |
| α-Lyt-2 (53-6.7) | 82 | 5.7 | 13 | 6.5 | 21 | 6.7 |
| α-Lyt-3 (53-5.1) | 82 | 6.0 | 11 | 6.8 | 20 | 7.2 |

[a]C57BL/6.Lyt-2.1 cells were stained with directly fluorescein-conjugated antibodies and analyzed on a FACS-II.

[b]Antigen densities of positive cells are expressed as mean number of antibody molecules bound/cell ($\times 10^4$), calculated as described in Materials and Methods section.

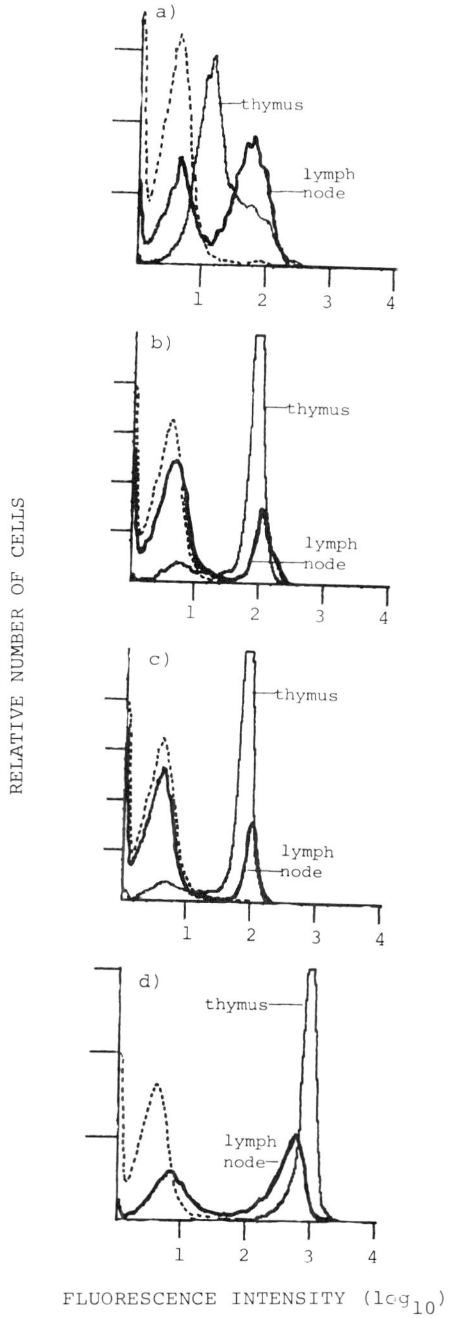


**Figure 1.** Immunofluorescence staining of C57BL/6J thymocytes and lymph node cells with (a) anti-Lyt-1 (53-7.3): (b) anti-Lyt-2 (53-6.7); (c) anti-Lyt-3 (53-5.1); and (d) anti-Thy-1.2 (53-2.1). Cells were stained with directly fluorescein-conjugated antibodies and analyzed on a FACS-II with a logarithmic amplifier. The dotted line shows the autofluorescence of unstained lymph node cells.

### *Lyt-2 and Lyt-3 Are Lost From Most T-Cells as Thymocytes Mature and Migrate to the Periphery*

Lyt-2 and Lyt-3 bearing cells comprise between 80-90% of thymocytes. The fluorescence distribution patterns are identical for Lyt-2 and Lyt-3 (Figure 1). The antigen densities of Lyt-2 and Lyt-3 are almost identical (Table 1) and these two antigens are expressed on the same cells (Ledbetter et al., 1981 and our unpublished two-color immunofluorescence data). The variation in frequency of Lyt-$2^+3^+$ cells in thymus which is seen between individual mice is not due to estimation errors which are at most 1 or 2%.

The frequency of Lyt-$2^+3^+$ cells in spleen and lymph node of normal mice is usually only 27-40% of the Thy-1 cells. Again, the variation is between individual mice and not due to estimation problems. These data indicate the Lyt-2 and Lyt-3 are lost from the majority of T-cells during maturation, and that Lyt-$1^+2^-3^-$ cells already exist in the thymus. Other data (manuscript in preparation) indicate that these cells are all in the hydrocortisone-resistant subpopulation of thymocytes.

The average Lyt-2 and Lyt-3 antigen densities are slightly higher in spleen and lymph node than in thymus (Table 1). However, the peripheral (spleen or lymph node) Lyt-$2^+3^+$ cells correspond in brightness to the brightest thymocytes, indicating that these antigens do not change substantially in amounts on positive cells during maturation.

### *Thy-1.2 Decreases in Amount During Maturation*

For Thy-1.2, we found the immunofluorescence of thymocytes and peripheral T-cells closely agreed with previous reports using conventional reagents (Evans et al., 1978; Loken et al., 1977; Mathieson et al., 1979). Thy-1.2-stained thymocytes give a very bright peak with a duller shoulder (Figure 1-d). The latter corresponds to the hydrocortisone-resistant subpopulation (manuscript in preparation). In spleen and lymph node, the brighter Thy-1.2 bearing cells were equivalent in brightness to the dullest cells in the thymus.

In summary, the results of the quantitative staining analyses for Thy-1.2, Lyt-1, Lyt-2, and Lyt-3 antigens in thymus, lymph node, and spleen imply the following changes during T-cell maturation: (a) Lyt-1 increases substantially; (b) Thy-1 decreases substantially; and (c) Lyt-2 and Lyt-3 are lost from most cells.

Thus, by comparing thymus, spleen, and lymph node cells on a population basis, Lyt-1 and Thy-1 antigen densities appear to change in opposite directions during T-cell development but frequencies remain essentially the same. In contrast, Lyt-2 and Lyt-3 change in frequencies of positive T-cells but only slightly in density on positive cells.

### *Two-color Cell Suspension Immunofluorescence for Thy-1.2, Lyt-1, and Lyt-2*

The correlations of staining with the monoclonal T antibodies are readily examined by FACS simultaneous detection of fluorescein and rhodamine on individual cells (Micklem et al., 1980). Nylon-purified splenic T-cells were used. Figure 2 shows

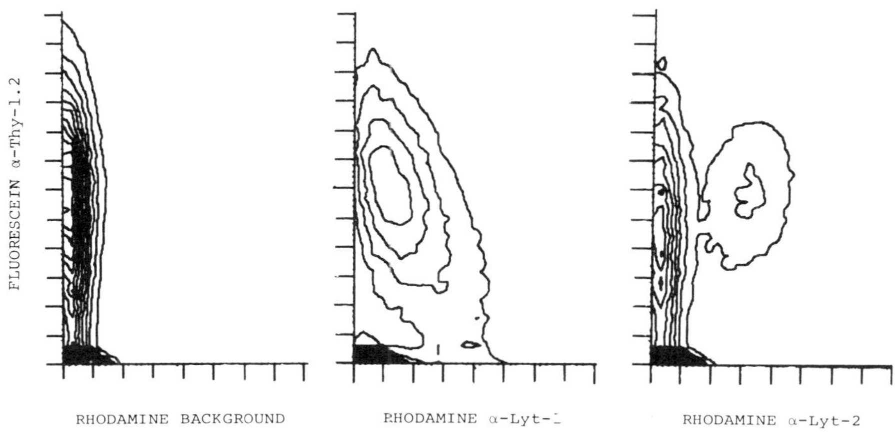


**Figure 2.** Two-color immunofluorescence analysis of BALB/cNHz nylon-enriched splenic T-cells on a FACS-II with standard linear amplifiers. Staining for Thy-1.2 in each panel was with directly fluorescein-conjugated anti-Thy-1.2 (30-H12). Staining for Lyt-1 or Lyt-2 was with biotin-conjugated antibodies (53-7.3 or 53-6.7) followed by rhodamine-conjugated avidin. The first panel shows the fluorescein anti-Thy-1.2 staining and the rhodamine background (rhodamine-avidin alone). The contour lines represent 75 cells/channel intervals.

the negative correlation between Thy-1 and Lyt-1 antigen densities using fluorescein-conjugated anti-Thy-1.2 in combination with biotin-anti-Lyt-1 followed by rhodamine-conjugated-avidin (panel B). In panel C, the Lyt-2 cells are seen as a discrete population with intermediate to bright levels of Thy-1. The contour plots from these data graphically illustrate the correlations of Thy-1 with the Lyt antigens and agree well with the cytotoxicity results presented above.

Similar two-color staining experiments for Lyt-1 and Lyt-2 depicted on contour plots (Figure 3) show that the brightest Lyt-1 cells are Lyt-2 negative. Conversely, Lyt-2 positive cells stain dully for Lyt-1. Again, quantitative staining analysis rationalizes how selective cytotoxic depletion of the "Lyt-1 subset" or of the "Lyt-2 subset" can occur at certain antibody concentrations. These data also rationalize the failures to get total depletion of the Lyt-2 cells using anti-Lyt-1 and complement, since most of the Lyt-2 cells express low density Lyt-1.

Functional subpopulations of human T-cells selectively express surface antigens analogous to the mouse Lyt-1, Lyt-2 and Lyt-3. Two subpopulations of human T-cells were originally defined by a xenogeneic antiserum termed :ga$TH_2$ (Oi et al., 1978). TH:i2$^+$ cells were shown to mediate suppressor effects *in vitro* and to be responsible for most of the killing in cell-mediated lympholysis (CML) (Reinherz et al., 1979a). In contrast, $TH_2^-$ cells had markedly less cytotoxic activity in CML but were found to amplify the functions of other cells and to proliferate in response to specific antigens (mumps, tetanus toxoid) (Reinherz et al., 1979a).

Recently, both of these subsets have been redefined by monoclonal antibodies

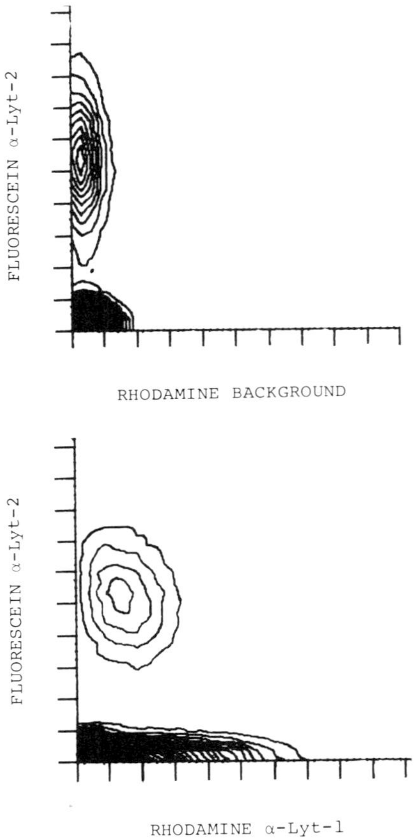


**Figure 3.** Two-color immunofluorescence analysis of BALB/cNHz nylon-enriched splenic T-cells on a FACS-II with standard linear amplifiers. Directly fluorescein-conjugated anti-Lyt-2 (53-6.7) and biotin-conjugated anti-Lyt-1 (53-7.3) followed by rhodamine-conjugated avidin were used. The first panel shows the fluorescein anti-Lyt-2 staining and the rhodamine background (rhodamine-avidin alone). The contour lines represent 75 cells/channel intervals.

(Reinherz et al., 1979b; Reinherz et al., 1980; Shiku et al., 1975).[1] Two antibodies, SK1 and SK2, defining Leu-2a and Leu-2b antigenic determinants, respectively, appear to react with the same surface antigen identified by the original $\alpha TH_2$ serum since both of these monoclonal antibodies block the binding of $TH_2$ antiserum.[1] Two other antibodies, SK3 and SK4 defining Leu-3a and Leu-3b determinants, respectively, react with $TH_2^-$ subsets.[1] These two subsets (Leu-$2^+$ and Leu-$3^+$ T-cells) were shown not to overlap and to comprise subpopulations of ERF-C, pre-

[1]Evans, R.L., Wall, D.C., Platsoucas, C.D., Siegal, F.P., Fikrig, S.M., Testa, C.M., and Good, R.A. Thymus-dependent membrane antigens in man: Inhibition of cell-mediated lympholysis by monoclonal antibodies to the $T_{H2}$ antigen, manuscript in preparation.

viously defined by a T-cell membrane component (Leu-1) (Wang et al., 1980). The Leu-1 antigen, unlike other human T-cell membrane antigens thus far defined by monoclonal antibodies, is found on Ig$^+$ leukemic cells from the majority of patients with chronic lymphocytic leukemia (CLL) (Wang et al., 1980), but is not detected on normal B-cells.

We have recently completed a series of comparative studies showing that the human T-cell antigens, Leu-1, Leu-2a, and Leu-2b, have strong analogies to the mouse Lyt-1, Lyt-2, and Lyt-3 antigens, respectively. Similar studies to those shown above (Ledbetter et al. 1981) indicate that molecules carrying the human Leu antigens approximate the size, charge, and subunit composition of the corresponding molecules carrying the mouse Lyt antigens (data not shown). Moreover, each of these structurally homologous antigen systems have similar sensitivities to trypsin and similar fluorescence distributions on thymocytes and T-cells (see Figure 4).

Analogies between the human and mouse T-cell differentiation antigens are formalized below:

Analogies between Leu-1 on human T-cells and Lyt-1 on mouse cells:

1. Present on all peripheral T cells and thymocytes.
2. Amount per cell varies widely (14-fold range in peripheral T).
3. FACS profiles have similar features. Thymocyte profile has a bright shoulder that derives from the mid-size (C-R) population and coincides with the peak of the peripheral T-cell profile. Peripheral T-cell profile has a dull shoulder that derives from Lyt-2,3$^+$/Leu-2a,2b$^+$ cells.
4. Single chain molecule.

**Figure 4.** Immunofluorescence staining of human thymocytes with anti-Leu-1 and anti-Leu-2a antibodies. The anti-Leu-1 staining was with monoclonal antibody SK5 followed by a fluorescein-conjugated goat anti-mouse IgG2 second step antibody. The anti-Leu-2a staining was with monoclonal antibody SK1 followed by a fluorescein-conjugated goat anti-mouse IgG1 second step antibody. The background staining with second step alone is shown by a dotted line in each panel.

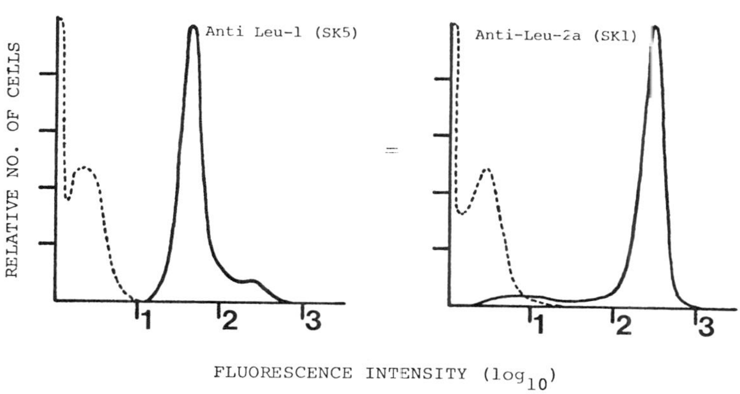

5. Mr 65-71 K.
6. Found on malignant B-cells from some individuals.

Analogies between Leu-2a,2b molecule on human T-cells and Lyt-2,3 molecule on mouse T-cells:
1. Present on 25-35% of peripheral T-cells and 80-90% of thymocytes.
2. Present on suppressor and cytotoxic T-cells but not on helper T-cells.
3. Amount per cell is relatively constant (4-fold range).
4. Positive cells carry less Lyt-1/Leu-1 than negative cells.
5. Composed of at least two non-identical subunits (30-45 K Mr).
6. Subunits are disulfide-bonded into multimeric forms.
7. More basic than most cell surface molecules.
8. Leu-2a and Lyt-2 relatively stable to trypsin.
9. Leu-2b and Lyt-3 easily destroyed by trypsin.

The molecules carrying the Leu and Lyt antigens have undergone evolutionary change since no cross-reactivity was observed between murine and human T-lymphocyte antigens when staining with either anti-Lyt or anti-Leu antibodies. Nevertheless, these molecules appear to have conserved their basic properties such as surface expression patterns and molecular configuration.

This apparent conservation of the molecular structure and subpopulation density distributions for the Leu and Lyt antigens suggests that these surface structures are not simply convenient markers that allow the distinction of T-cell populations at various stages of maturity or with different functional capabilities. Rather, the maintenance of these structures through evolution seems more likely to have occurred because these molecules perform essential functions for the cells on which they are found. Such functions are probably reflected in the absolute changes that occur during differentiation (i.e., Lyt-$2^+$Leu-$2a^+$ to Lyt-$2^-$/Leu-$2a^-$), the quantitative changes that occur (e.g., Lyt-1/Leu-1 dull to Lyt-1/Leu-1 bright) and the maintenance of selective quantitative expression patterns in different subpopulations (e.g., less Lyt-1/Leu-1 on Lyt-$2^+$/Leu-$2a^+$ cells than on Lyt-$2^-$/Leu-$2a^-$ cells); which, if any, of these changes are directly related to effector functions and which are involved in the ability to send or receive differentiation signals is not clear.

## References


Bonner, W.A., Hulett, H.R., Sweet, R.G., and Herzenberg, L.A. 1972. Fluorescence activated cell sorting. Rev. Sci. Instru. 43:404–409.

Boyse, E.A., Itakura, K., Stockert, E., Iritani, C.A., and Miura, M. 1971. Lyc: A third locus specifying alloantigens expressed only on thymocytes and lymphocytes. Transplantation 11:351.

Cantor, H. and Boyse, E.A. 1975. Functional subclasses of T-lymphocytes bearing different Ly antigens. I. The generation of functionally distinct T-cell subclasses in a differentiative process independent of antigen. J. Exp. Med. 141:1376.

Cantor, H., Simpson, E., Sato, V., Fathman, C.G., and Herzenberg, L.A. 1975. Characterization of subpopulations of T-lymphocytes. I. Separation and functional studies of peripheral T-cells bearing different amounts of fluorescent anti-Thy-1.2 (theta) antibody using a fluorescence-activated cell sorter (FACS). Cell. Immunol. 15:180–196.

Cantor, H., Shen, F.W., and Boyse, E.W. 1976. Separation of helper from suppressor T-cells expressing Ly components. II. Activation by antigen: After immunization, antigen specific suppressor and helper activities are mediated by distinct T-cell subclasses. J. Exp. Med. 143:1391.

Cantor, H. and Boyse, E.A. 1977a Lymphocytes as models for the study of mammalian cellular differentiation. Immunol. Rev. 33:105.

Cantor, H. and Boyse, E.A. 1977b. Regulation of cellular and humoral immune responses by T-cell sub classes. Cold Spring Harbor Symp. Quant. Biol. 41:23.

Evans, R.L., Breard, J.M., Lazarus, H., Schlossman, S.F., and Chess, L. 1977. Detection, isolation and functional characterization of two human T-cell subclasses bearing unique differentiation antigens. J. Exp. Med. 145:221.

Evans, R.L., Lazarus, H., Penta, A.C., and Schlossman, S.F. 1978. Two functionally distinct subpopulations of human T-cells that collaborate in the generation of cytotoxic cells responsible for cell-mediated lympholysis. J. Immunol. 129:1423.

Fathman, C.G., Small, M., Herzenberg, L.A., and Weissman, I.L. 1975. Thymus cell maturation. II. Differentiation of three "mature" subclasses *in vivo*. Cell. Immunol. 15:109–128.

Herzenberg, L.A., Sweet, R.G., and Herzenberg, L.A. 1976. Fluorescence activated cell sorting: A new tool for isolating functional cell types. Sci. Am. 234:108–117.

Herzenberg, L.A. and Herzenberg, L.A. 1978. Analysis and separation using the fluorescence activated cell sorter (FACS). In Handbook of Experimental Immunology, third edition. D.M. Weir, ed. Oxford, England: Blackwell Scientific Publications, chap. 22, pp. 22 1–22.21.

Jandinski, J.H., Cantor, H., Tadakuma, T., Peavy, D.L., and Pierce, C.W. 1976. Separation of helper T-cells from suppressor T-cells expressing different Ly components. I. Polyclonal activation: Suppressor and helper activities are inherent properties of distinct T-cell subclasses. J. Exp. Med. 143:1382.

Köhler, G. and Milstein, C. 1975. Continuous cultures of fused cells secreting antibody of predefined specificity. Nature 256:495–497.

Ledbetter, J.A. and Herzenberg, L.A. 1979. Xenogeneic monoclonal antibodies to mouse lymphoid differentiation antigens. Immunol. Rev. 47:63–90.

Ledbetter, J.A., Rouse, R.V., Micklem, H.S., and Herzenberg, L.A. 1980. T-cell subsets defined by expression of Lyt-1,2,3, and Thy-1 antigens. Two parameter immunofluorescence and cytotoxicity analysis with monoclonal antibodies modifies current views. J. Exp. Med. 152:280–295.

Ledbetter, J.A., Evans, R.L., Lipinski, M., Cunningham-Ruddles, C., Good, R.A., and Herzenberg, L.A. 1981. Evolutionary conservation of surface molecules that distinguish T-lymphocyte helper-inducer and T cytotoxic/suppressor subpopulations in mouse and man. J. Exp. Med., in press.

Loken, M.R., Parks, D.R., and Herzenberg, L.A. 1977. Two-color immunofluorescence using a fluorescence-activated cell sorter (FACS). J. Histochem. Cytochem. 25:899–907.

Mathieson, B.J., Sharrow, S.O., Campbell, P.S., and Asofsky, R. 1979. An Lyt differentiated subpopulation of thymocytes detected by flow microfluormetry. Nature 277:478.

Micklem, H.S., Ledbetter, J.A., Eckhardt, L.A., and Herzenberg, L.A. 1980. Analysis of lymphocyte subpopulations with monoclonal antibodies to Thy-1, Lyt-1, Lyt-2 and ThB antigens. In Regulatory T-Lymphocytes. B. Pernis and H.J. Vogel, eds. New York: Academic Press, pp. 119–132.

Oi, V.T., Jones, P.P., Goding, J.W., Herzenberg, L.A., and Herzenberg, L.A. 1978. Properties of monoclonal antibodies to mouse Ig allotypes, *H-2* and *Ia* antigens. Curr. Top. Microbiol. Immunol. 81:115–129.

Reinherz, E..L., King, P.C., Goldstein, G., and Schlossman, S.F. 1979a Separation of functional subsets of human T-cells by a monoclonal antibody. Proc. Natl. Acad. Sci. U.S.A. 76:4061.

Reinherz, E.L., King, P.C., Goldstein, G., and Schlossman, S.F. 1979b. Further characterization of the human inducer T-cell subset defined by monoclonal antibody. J. Immunol. 123:2894.

Reinherz, E.L., King, P.C., Goldstein, G., Levey, R.H., and Schlossman, S.F. 1980. Discrete stages of intrathymic differentiation: Analysis of normal thymocytes and leukemic lymphoblasts of T lineage. Proc. Natl. Acad. Sci. U.S.A., in press.

Shiku, H., Kiseielow, P., Bean, M.A., Takahashi, T., Boyse, E.A., Oettgen, H.T., and Old, L.J. 1975. Expression of T-cell differentiation antigens on effector cells in cell-mediated cytotoxicity *in vitro*. J. Exp. Med. 141:227.

Wang, C.Y., Good, R.A., Ammirati, P., Dymbort, G., and Evans, R.L. 1980. Identification of a p69,71 complex expressed on human T-cells sharing determinants with B-type chronic lymphatic leukemia cells. J. Exp. Med. 151:1539.

# SECTION IV:

# Immunogenes and Disease

Hildemann, ed. Frontiers in Immunogenetics

# Genetics of Retrovirus–Host Interactions

Raymond V. Gilden, Stephen Oroszlan, Howard A. Young, Nancy R. Rice, Matthew A. Gonda, Maurice Cohen, and Alan R. Rein

*Biological Carcinogenesis Program, Frederick Cancer Research Center, Frederick, Maryland*

## Introduction

Retroviruses constitute a large family of RNA viruses united by the common property of multiplication via a DNA intermediate which then integrates into the host cell genome. Members of the family exist as conventional horizontally transmitted viruses and as inherited genetic elements, generally present in relatively high copy numbers. These viruses are evidently capable of multiple random integration events. The pathogenic members are associated with a variety of diseases including malignancies, neurologic disorders, and arthritis in several infra-human species but, to date, no convincing isolates have been made from man. The oncornavirus subfamily (*onco*genic *RNA*) of retroviruses has received the greater attention in recent years and current evidence indicates that acute acting members of this subfamily acquire malignant potential by acquisition of cellular transforming genes. Subacute acting members, classified in this way because of the long latent period of disease induction, may not carry a specific transforming gene and, thus, may mediate their activity through indirect means. It is not surprising that the retrovirus family has attracted a great deal of interest from various disciplines and that much speculation has centered on the possible roles of inherited viral or viral-related genes in normal development. An alternate view is that these genetic elements represent one stage in the life cycle of a highly successful parasite—a viewpoint easily understood based on recent information (Dhar et al. 1980) that integrated provirus has a structure remarkably similar to bacterial transposons (Figure 1). This provides for considerable mobility and potential independence from host responses successful in dealing with conventional viruses. The current paper summarizes ongoing studies involving (1) the interrelationships among retroviruses based on primary structure analyses

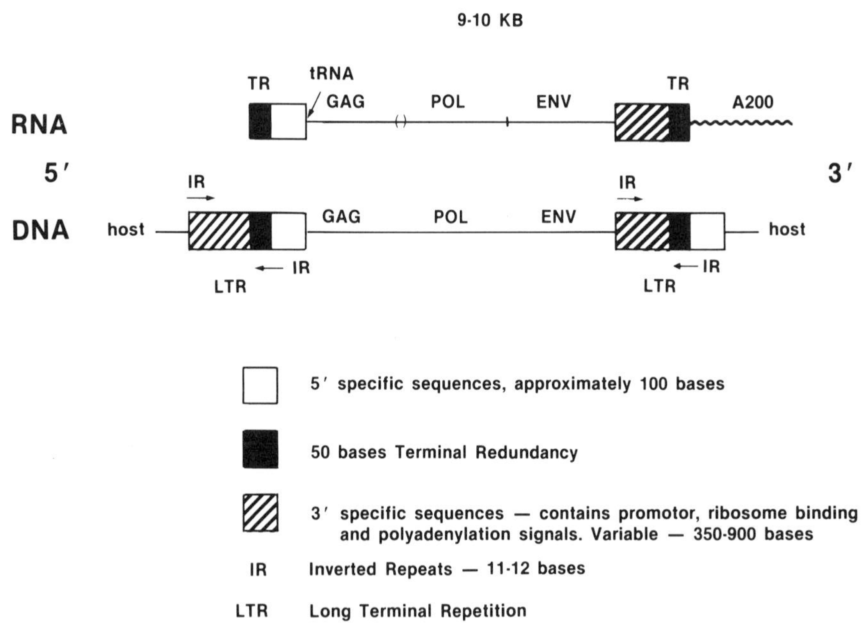


**Figure 1.** Structure of viral RNA and integrated proviral DNA.

of their proteins; (2) the origin and biology of sarcoma viruses with emphasis on the rat-derived sarcoma virus—a complex system involving three genetic elements, a rat type C virus, a viral-like RNA sequence designated 30S (based on sedimentation rate), and a normal cell-transforming gene; (3) the origin and biology of acute acting leukemia viruses with emphasis on the avian reticuloendotheliosis virus—an avian virus most unusual in that its structural genes are highly related to those of primate viruses and its transforming gene appears to be of avian origin; (4) the sequence organization of the multiple integrated genomes of a primate type C virus, the endogenous virus of baboons—the presence of multiple copies (~100) makes this an interesting system for understanding the functional significance of endogenous genomes; and (5) the complexity of viral isolates in mice with emphasis on a new replication-defective virus isolated from leukemic cells.

Collectively, these topics give a glimpse of the complex biology of a most intriguing virus family.

## Primary Structural Relationships of Retroviral Proteins

Primary structure analysis provides the essential information for evaluation of the precise degree of genetic relationship between structural and functional protein homologs of retroviruses. The immunologic methods most commonly used for establishing this relatedness have been of great value, but have inherent sensitivity limitations and may give variable results depending on the antiserum used. The *gag* and *env* gene products of retroviruses are synthesized in the form of large precursor polyproteins which are post-translationally cleaved to yield the viral structural proteins. Amino acid sequence analysis of the natural cleavage products provides the best approach for determining the structure of a primary translational unit. Such analyses have identified the pertinent coding regions of the viral genome and have revealed previously undescribed relationships between retroviruses and between retroviruses and cellular proteins.

### *Classification of Mammalian Type C Viruses Based on Amino Acid Sequences of p30s*

#### Subgroups I–IV

The mammalian p30s (protein molecules of 30,000 daltons) have shown cross-reactive (interspecies) determinants (Oroszlan and Gilden 1978), as established by both immunodiffusion and radioimmunoassays, and they have been found to be compositionally similar (Oroszlan et al. 1975). Sequence analysis provided support for the immunological findings and showed that the $NH_2$-terminal regions of p30s of mammalian type C viruses are highly conserved (Oroszlan et al. 1975). We have identified four major subgroups based on alignments of amino acid terminal sequences of p30s. This classification is shown in Figure 2. All p30s initiate with a common tripeptide, viz., prolylleucylarginine, and contain a highly homologous (conserved) region beginning with glutamine at position 11 in the Subgroup I

```
Subgroup I        1       5         10        15        20        25        30
  Mouse
    R-MuLVa       P L R L G G N G Q L Q Y W P F S S S D L Y N W K X D N P A F

  Rat
    MSV (RaLV)    P L R Q G A X G X M Q Y W X F

  Cat
    FeLV          P L R E G P N N R P Q Y W P F S A S D L Y N W K S H N P P F

Subgroup II
  Baboon
    BaEV          P L R T * V N R T I Q Y W P F S A S D L Y N W K T H N P X F

  Cat
    RD-114        P L R T * V N R T V Q Y W P F S A S D L Y N W K T H N P X F

Subgroup III
  Gibbon ape
    GaLVb         P L R A I G N G P L Q Y W P F S X A D L Y
                             ↑   ↑
                             |  (L V)
                             |
                        (P P A E P)

Subgroup IV
  Rhesus
    MAC-1c        P L R E I G T G R L M Y W P F S T S D L Y N W K
                             ↑   ↑
                             |  (L S)
                             |
                        (S L D D)
```

**Figure 2.** Classification of mammalian type C viruses based on alignment of $NH_2$-terminal sequences of p30s*.

[a]All mouse p30s have identical sequences except position 4 where L may be exchanged for S and A.

[b]Sequence of SSV-1 p30 is identical.

[c]Sequence of MMC-1 p30 is identical with the possible exception of residue 14, serine, in second insert. REV belongs to this subgroup.

*Note:* The one letter code used for amino acids is: A, alanine; D, aspartic acid; E, glutamic acid; F, phenylalanine; G, glycine; H, histidine; I, isoleucine; K, lysine; L, leucine; M, methionine; N, asapragine; P, proline; Q, glutamine; R, arginine; S, serine; T, threonine; V, valine; W, tryptophan; X, unidentified; Y, tryosine.

sequences (a few additional substitutions also occur in this region). While in the first subgroup (mouse, rat, and cat leukemia viruses) residues 4–10 are variable and essentially species-specific, the p30s in Subgroup II, baboon endogenous virus (BaEV) and cat endogenous virus (RD-114), differ only in position 9 and both have a deletion in position 5. Gibbon ape leukemia virus (GaLV) and simian sarcoma-associated virus (SSAV) in Subgroup III have identical sequences throughout the known first 28 residues and both have two inserts involving a total of seven residues in the variable region of the mammalian p30s. In Subgroup IV, the p30s of the recently isolated endogenous rhesus monkey *(Macaca mulatta)* virus MMC-1 (Rabin et al. 1979) and that of *Macaca arctoides* MAC-1 (Todaro et al. 1978) are also identical, but have a six-residue insert which is divided in the alignment into two inserts, one involving four and the other two residues. These sequences have the first residue glutamine in the conserved region substituted with methionine.

## *Relationship of Avian Reticuloendotheliosis Virus (REV) to Mammalian Type C Viruses*

Comparing the avian reticuloendotheliosis virus (REV) p30 sequence with the previously published sequences of mammalian type C virus (Oroszlan et al. 1975), Hunter et al. (1978) surprisingly found that these showed an extensive homology. They aligned the sequences of REV p30 and Rauscher murine leukemia virus (R-MuLV) and feline leukemia virus (FeLV) p30s by introducing a six-residue gap between proline and phenylalanine, positions 14 and 15, in the conserved region of R-MuLV and FeLV p30s and found approximately 40% identity with the sequence of REV p30.

In a recent analysis, we also determined the $NH_2$-terminal sequence of REV p30 (strain T) (Oroszlan et al., unpublished data) and confirmed the majority of the sequence assigned by Hunter et al. (1978). However, in position 6 we found glycine instead of threonine and in position 26 leucine instead of isoleucine. In addition, we were able to assign aspartic acid in the previously unidentified position 25. The alignment of this REV p30 sequence, as determined in our laboratory, with R-MuLV and FeLV p30 sequences is shown in Figure 3. In this alignment, we do not put the six-residue insert of REV p30s into the conserved region of mammalian p30s, but instead, divide it into two inserts (one of four residues, the other of two residues) and introduce them between residues 6 and 7 and 8 and 9, respectively, in the R-MuLV/FeLV p30 sequences in exactly the same manner as used in the alignment of all mammalian p30s (Figure 2). Such an analysis results in a higher degree of homology between REV and R-MuLV/FeLV p30s. The amino acid sequence data thus indicate that REV is more closely related to mammalian type C viruses than to the viruses of the avian leukemia-sarcoma virus (ALSV) group. Since REV is not represented in normal avian DNA (Kang and Temin 1974), it

**Figure 3.** Alignment of $NH_2$-terminal sequence of REV p30 with the sequences of R-MuLV and FeLV p30s.

```
R-MuLV     P L R L G G N G Q L Q Y W P F S S S D L Y N W K

FeLV       P L R E G P N N R P Q Y W P F S A S D L Y N W K

REV        P L R E G T G G R X T Y V A F D T T D L Y N W K
                      ↑   ↑
                      | (R P)
                      |
                  (E E D M)
```

```
               1       5         10        15        20        25
MMC-1 p27    P L R E I G S L D D T G L H R L M Y W P F X T X D L Y N
REV p30      P L R E T G E E D M G G R P R X T Y V A F T T T D L Y N
GaLV p29     P L R A I G P P A E P G L V P L Q Y W P F S X A D L Y N
                                 ↑
                                 N
```

**Figure 4.** $NH_2$-terminal sequences of MMC-1 type C virus p30 aligned with sequences of REV and GaLV p30s. REV p30 aligns with MMC-1 p27 without any gaps. Fifteen of 28 residues are positionally identical. This corresponds to an ~54% homology. GaLV p29 aligns with MMC-1 p27 by introducing a gap between positions 11 and 12 in the MMC-1 sequence (an insert of N in GaLV sequence). Alignment of REV p30 to GaLV p29 gives 11 identities.

may well be a mammalian type C virus reintroduced in aves, or it is equally plausible to speculate that mammalian type C viruses originated from REV.

REV p30, however, aligns best with MMC-1/MAC-1 and GaLV/SSAV p30 sequences (Figure 4). Such an alignment with MMC-1 p30 does not require the introduction of any gap and results in a higher number of identities between REV and MMC-1 p30s than that obtainable between sequences of REV and other mammalian p30s, including GaLV and SSAV p30s. Therefore, on the basis of the sequence homology of p30s, REV is tentatively best classified as belonging to Subgroup IV (Figure 2) of mammalian type C viruses since it appears to be most closely related to the endogenous viruses of macaques. It should be noted that recently the immunological relatedness of REV and mammalian type C viruses has also been detected. Not only the p30s show cross-reaction (Charman et al. 1979; Barbacid et al. 1979), but cross-reactivity between spleen necrosis virus (SNV, a member of the REV group) reverse transcriptase and the Moloney murine sarcoma virus (MSV) enzyme has also been documented (Bauer and Temin 1979). Moreover, in collaboration with Drs. Barbacid and Aaronson, we have found that REV p30 is also more highly related immunologically to MMC-1 p30 than to p30s of other subgroups.

## *Homology between Nucleoproteins of Avian and Mouse Viruses*

The $NH_2$-terminal amino acid sequences of mammalian p30s and the structural homolog p27 of endogenous avian type C viruses show no obvious sequence homology (Niall et al. 1970; Oroszlan et al. 1975; Hunter et al. 1978). Reliable serological analyses, including highly sensitive radioimmunoassays, have not revealed antigenic cross-reactions between *gag* gene products of endogenous viruses of the avian leukosis-sarcoma group and of mammalian type C viruses (Barbacid et al. 1980).

Due to the inherent limitations of immunoassays, the lack of immunological cross-reactivity does not mean that avian and mouse type C viruses are not genetically related. Indeed, we have predicted that homology in primary structure should exist between the *gag* gene products of avian and mammalian oncornaviruses. The underlying assumption is that contemporary viral genes are descendants of a common ancestral gene that has undergone divergence in the various viral species (Oroszlan and Gilden 1978). Since mouse p10 is highly conserved (based on the sequence analysis of several mouse p10s) and avian p12 is considered to be a functional homolog, a comparison of the sequences of these proteins should provide a sensitive measure of the potential interviral relationship. This is now possible since the complete structures of both avian p12 (Misono et al. 1980) and R-MuLV p10 have been determined (Henderson et al. 1981). The alignment of the two sequences is shown in Figure 5. The statistical analysis, according to Dayhoff (1976), indicates an alignment score of 4.31 which suggests a definite evolutionary relationship between these avian and mouse type C virus *gag* gene encoded proteins.

### *Sequence Homology with Cellular Histones*

We have recently found (Henderson et al. 1979) that the $NH_2$-terminal amino acid sequences of mouse leukemia virus phosphoproteins show definite homology with the $NH_2$-terminal conserved region of H5 histones, the phosphorylated nuclear proteins of nucleated erythrocytes.

When the $NH_2$-terminal amino acid sequences of H5 histones of goose and chicken are aligned with the $NH_2$-terminal sequences of various leukemia virus (R-MuLV, AKR-MuLV, M-MuLV) p12 proteins by introducing gaps, the maximum number of identities are obtained (Figure 6). In addition to the positionally identical amino acids (underlined with solid line), functionally homologous residues appear in several positions. Based on the comparison, the degree of relatedness of M-MuLV p12 to goose or chicken H5 is as high or higher than that of chicken H5 to goose H5 or that of AKR-MuLV p12 to R-MuLV p12.

As described by Henderson et al. (1979), differences in the amino acid composition of the two groups of proteins rule out the possibility that H5 histones and viral p12s evolved from a single ancestral gene by divergent evolution. However, our statistical analysis indicated that the observed sequence homology is not a result of random chance and that the posibility that viral p12s evolved from H5 histones or related cellular proteins through genetic recombination should be considered. Alternately, the sequence homology may be a result of convergent evolution. Whatever the case may be, the conserved structural feature may indicate a common function. Both sets of proteins bind specifically to nucleic acids through interactions modulated by phosphorylation. The homologous $NH_2$-terminal sequences may represent regions involved in nucleic acid binding or phosphorylation or both. It will be of interest to see whether phosphoproteins of other type C viruses, such as avian p19, also contain similar sequences. The sequence homology between type C virus phosphoproteins and H5 histones may represent the first example of usurpation of a normal cellular transcriptional unit for use in a retrovirus.

As we previously emphasized (Henderson et al. 1979), the findings of sequence homology between viral and cellular proteins is consistent with the emergence of

```
              1       5         10        15        20        25        30        35        40        45
RSV p12*      - A V V N R E R D G Z T G S G G R S R G L C Y T C G S P G H Y Q A Q C P K K R K S G N S R

R-MuLV p10    A T V V S G O R Q D R Q G - G E R - - - - - - - - - - - - - - - - - - - - - R R P Q L D R

Common            V V       R         G   G   R                                         R           R


                      50        55        60        65        70        75        80        85
RSV p12       E R C E L C N G M G H N A K Q C R K R D G N Q G Q R P G R G L S S W P G P E P P A V S

R-MuLV p10    D Q C A Y C K E K G H W A K D C P K K - - - - - - - - P - R G - - - - P R P E A S L L -
```

**Figure 5.** Alignment of RSV p12 and R-MuLV p10 sequences. 22 identities out of 54 possible identities. Alignment Score: 4.31, $P = 0.317 \times 10^{-4}$.

*K.S. Misono, F.S. Sharief and J. Leis, Fed. Proc. *39:* 1611, 1980.

| Source | Protein | Sequence |
|---|---|---|
| | | 1 2 3 4 5 6 7 8 9 10 11 12 13 14 15 |
| R-MuLV | p12 | Pro-Thr-Leu-Thr-Ser-Pro-Leu-Asn-Thr-Lys-Pro-Arg-Pro-Gln-Val |
| AKR-MuLV | p12 | Pro-Ala-Leu-Thr-Pro-Ser-Ile- * - * -Lys-Pro-Arg-Pro-Ser-Leu |
| Rad-MuLV | p12 | Pro-Ala-Leu-Thr-Pro-Ser-Ile- * - X -Lys-Pro-Arg-Pro-Ser-Lys |
| M-MuLV | p12 | Pro-Ala-Leu-Thr-Pro-Ser-Leu-Gly-Ala-Lys-Pro-Lys-Pro-Gln-Val |
| Goose | H5 | Thr-Asp-Ser-Pro-Ile-Pro-Ala-Pro-Ala-Pro-Ala-Ala-Lys-Pro-Lys- * -Arg-Ala |
| Chicken | H5 | Thr-Glu-Ser-Leu-Val-Leu-Ser-Pro-Ala-Pro- * -Ala-Lys-Pro-Lys- * -Gln-Val |

**Figure 6.** Alignment if amino terminal amino acid sequences of type C leukemia virus p12 proteins to avian histone H5 proteins. Taken from Henderson et al. (1979); p12 sequences are aligned with goose and chicken histone H5 sequences with the introduction of gaps (- * -). Residues underlined with solid line (——) are positionally identical when comparing at least one of the H5 histones to one of the p12s; residues underlined with dashed line (---) are considered to be functionally homologous in the two groups of proteins.

infectious entities by a process of differentiation from preexisting cellular genes. Vestiges of these primordial origins might be more readily detected in retroviruses because of their inheritance in the cellular genome. Given recent information on mRNA splicing (Darnell 1978; Crick 1979) and shifts in the physical location of specific DNA segments during maturation of the immune system (Hozumi and Tonegawa 1976), it is not unreasonable to suggest that similar mechanisms might have contributed to the origin of viral structural proteins. Thus, several cellular genes or coding domains of diverse function (Gilbert 1978) could have contributed to the origin of individual virion polypeptides. Further analyses of complete sequences of retrovirus polypeptides will be necessary to fully evaluate these speculations; however, this could provide a most vigorous evaluation of current theories of retrovirus origin.

### *Homologies of Bovine Leukemia Virus (BLV) p24 and Equine Infectious Anemia Virus (EIAV) p30 with Mammalian Type C Virus p30s*

In spite of the differences in primary structure (Oroszlan et al. 1980), statistical analysis using Dayhoff's computer program ALIGN (Dayhoff 1976) revealed a significant homology between bovine leukemia virus (BLV) p24 and mammalian p30s. The alignment of the first 35-residue sequence of p24 with the sequences of FeLV, wild-mouse murine leukemia virus (W-MuLV) and baboon leukemia virus (BaLV) p30s is shown in Figure 7. In the alignment there are 10 amino acid residues that are common to BLV p24 and FeLV p27 sequences. For these two proteins, an alignment score of 3.76 was obtained, which indicates that the probability is only $8.5 \times 10^{-5}$ that the similarity between these sequences is the result of chance alone. This statistically significant value suggests that BLV p24 and FeLV p24 are evolutionarily related viral proteins. While the values for the pair of BLV p24 and W-MuLV p31 and for the pair of BLV p24 and BaLV p28 alone are not considered to be statistically significant, the fact that the p30s of FeLV, W-MuLV, and BaLV are very highly related permitted us to group BLV p24 with the mammalian p30s in an evolutionarily related super-family of proteins.

The finding of a definite distant relationship between the $NH_2$-terminal regions of a single protein in BLV and mammalian type C viruses establishes the origin of the contemporary viruses from common progenitor genes. Examples from other viruses, notably influenza (Webster and Laver 1971), indicate that such relationships

**Figure 7.** Alignment of $NH_2$-terminal sequence of BLV p24 with that of mammalian type C virus p30 homologs. Positionally identical-amino acids are underlined. Hyphen (-) indicates a break.

```
BLV      P I I S E G N R N R H R A W A L R E L Q D I K K E I E N K A P G S Q
FeLV     P L - R E G P N N R P Q Y W P F S A - S D L Y N W K S H N P P F S Q
W-MuLV   P L R S G G N - G Q L Q Y W P F S S S D L Y N W K X D N P A F S Q D
BaLV     P L - R T V N R T V Q - Y W P F S A S D L Y N W K T H N P X F S Q D
```

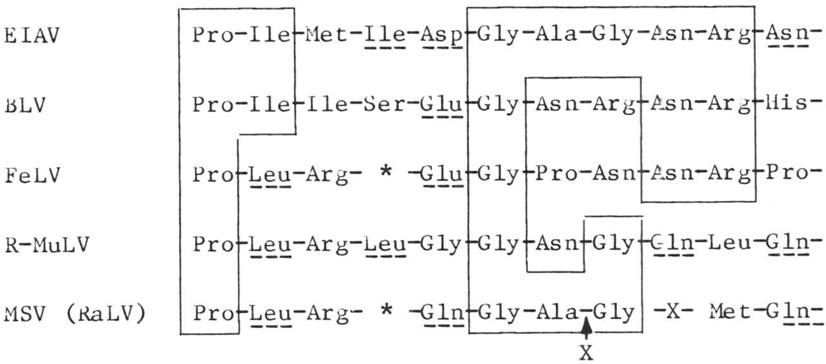


**Figure 8.** Alignment of the $NH_2$-terminal sequence of EIAV p30 with sequences of other retrovirus major structural proteins.

between viruses need not be constant for each gene product. For example, the analysis of the envelope glycoprotein of BLV may indicate a closer relationship to mouse mammary tumor virus (MMTV) than to the gp70s of type C viruses.

A short $NH_2$-terminal sequence of the p30 of another unclassified retrovirus, equine infectious anemia virus (EIAV), was determined. In Figure 8, EIAV is compared with sequences of type C virus p30s and with the structural homolog of BLV. Substantial homology at the $NH_2$-terminal region of these proteins is apparent and may indicate conservation of progenitor cleavage sites.

### *Amino Acid Sequences of env Gene Products*

The $NH_2$-terminal sequences of envelope glycoproteins of R-MuLV, Moloney murine leukemia virus (M-MuLV), and FeLV have been determined. The alignment is shown in Figure 9. The gp70s of mouse viruses show only three differences out of 26 residues and the sequence of FeLv gp70 also shows substantial homology with both R-MuLV and M-MuLV gp70s. The sequence also shows the position of a glycosylated asparagine residue (residue 12 in the alignment). In this alignment, 11 residues out of 23 possible comparisons are found positionally identical. In general, those amino acids which are positionally different require only a single base change in the codon (except Leu → Gly which requires two base changes).

## Origin of Transforming Sequences in Rat-Derived Sarcoma Viruses

Mammalian sarcoma viruses are type C retroviruses which are capable of transforming either fibroblasts or epithelial cells in tissue culture and causing the production of sarcomas in animals. These transforming viruses have been isolated from a number of different mammals, including mice, rats, cats, and a single woolly monkey (Hanafusa 1978; Van Zaane and Bloemers 1978; Shih and Scolnick 1980). All such mammalian viruses thus far reported are defective, i.e., they require the

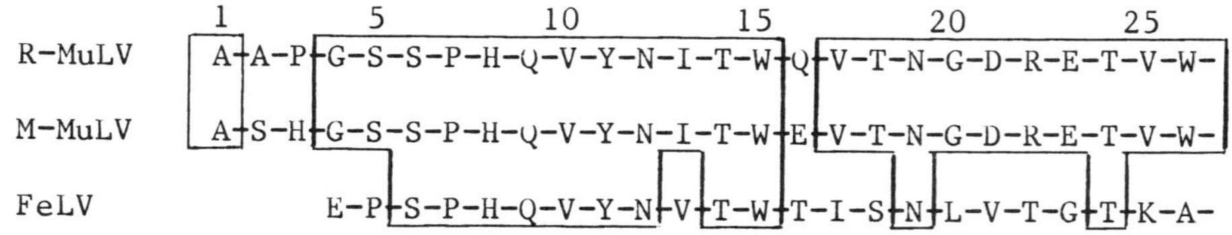


**Figure 9.** Alignment of mammalian type C virus gp70 $NH_2$-terminal sequences. N in position 12 is a carbohydrate attachment site. Alignment score: R-M 10.5; R-Fe 4.6; M-Fe 4.9.

presence of competent helper viruses for replication and infection of new host cells. The RNA of these transforming viruses consists predominantly of helper virus RNA with the insertion of a new gene *(src)* whose presence in the viral genome is required for transformation to occur. It is thought that this viral *src* gene represents a cellular transforming gene *(sarc)* whose expression is normally under strict cellular control, but when inserted into a viral genome becomes free of cellular control elements and is then expressed at much higher levels. This hypothesis has received strong support from recent experiments which have demonstrated that the gene responsible for transformation by Moloney sarcoma virus resides independently in the mouse genome from retroviral sequences and, by itself, cannot cause transformation in tissue culture. However, when this gene is spliced to specific retroviral sequences, transformation does occur (Oskarsson et al. 1980).

Within the past two years, there have been numerous reports of specific gene products associated with transformation by mammalian sarcoma viruses. The size of these gene products varies widely, ranging from 21,000 Mr in the Harvey and Kirsten sarcoma viruses to over 10,000 Mr in the Abelson leukemia virus. Many of these gene products appear to be similar in a number of respects—there appears to be a portion of the helper virus *gag* gene product synthesized as part of the viral *src* gene product, the proteins are phosphorylated, and many of the *src* proteins have been reported to have kinase activity. Thus, for the majority of the mammalian sarcoma viruses studied, there seems to be a preferential site for *sarc* gene recombination toward the 5′ end of the helper virus genome. This is true for some, but not all, isolates of Moloney sarcoma virus, Abelson leukemia virus, rat sarcoma virus, the three isolates of feline sarcoma virus, and woolly sarcoma virus. It should be pointed out that the non-*gag* portions of the *src* gene product of these different viruses do not cross-react, thus indicating that the individual viral *src* genes appear to be restricted (i.e., with respect to incorporation into a viral genome) to the species of origin.

Transforming viruses of rat origin, however, appear to be somewhat unique among mammalian sarcoma viruses. Three separate isolates have been reported (Harvey 1964; Kirsten and Mayer 1967; Rasheed et al. 1978), two resulting from animal experiments (Harvey and Kirsten) and one derived from tissue culture studies (rat sarcoma virus). What makes these viruses unique is that even though they were derived from different strains of rats, they all appear to code for an immunologically related *src* protein. A demonstration of this can be seen in Figure 10. Antisera used in this experiment were derived by injection of viral transformed nonproducer cells into syngeneic rats and collection of sera obtained 6 to 10 weeks after tumor appearance. As seen in this figure, when sera produced against either Harvey sarcoma virus nonproducer normal rat kidney (NRK) cells (lanes 5–8) or rat sarcoma virus transformed nonproducer Fischer rat embryo (FRE) cells (lanes 9–12) was used, a viral-specific protein was immunoprecipitated. In the case of Harvey and Kirsten sarcoma virus (lanes 6, 7, 10, 11), a protein of 21,000 Mr is observed, while rat sarcoma virus produces a protein of approximately 29,000 Mr (lanes 8, 12). A number of interesting features can be observed in this experiment. First, the

**Figure 10.** Immunoprecipitation of rat-derived retrovirus transformation-specific proteins. Procedures for labeling cells with 35-methionine, immunoprecipitation of cellular extracts, SDS-polyacrylamide gel electrophoresis, and autoradiography have been described in detail elsewhere (Young et al. 1979). Cells utilized in this experiment are NRK (normal rat kidney), lanes 1, 5, and 9; Kirsten sarcoma virus transformed NRK, lanes 2, 6, and 10; Harvey sarcoma virus transformed NRK, lanes 3, 7, and 11; and rat sarcoma virus transformed Fischer rat embryo cells (FRE), lanes 4, 8, and 12.

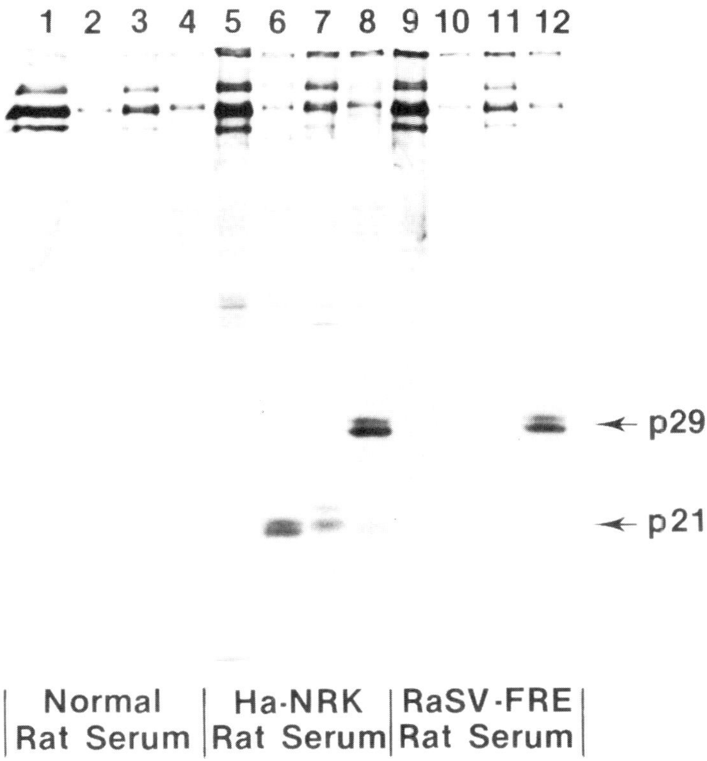

*src* proteins appear as doublets in the immunoprecipitate. While no explanation is currently available for this observation, possibilities such as acetylation or glycosylation of the *src* protein have not been ruled out. Also, additional bands of 25,000 and 21,000 Mr can be seen in immunoprecipitates of rat sarcoma virus transformed cellular extracts (lanes 8, 12). These appear to result from cleavage of the *src* protein, probably in the extra 8000 Mr region of the protein, during the extraction and immunoprecipitation. These bands do not appear to be the result of processing of the 29,000 Mr protein since pulse-chase experiments do not result in an increased level of the 21,000 Mr species (unpublished observations). Additionally, it appears that antisera produced against rat sarcoma virus nonproducer cells does not precipitate the Kirsten or Harvey *src* protein as well as antisera produced against Harvey nonproducer cells (lanes 6, 7 versus 10, 11). Thus, some type-specificity does appear to exist among these antisera. The *src* proteins common to these three viruses have a number of similar properties (Shih et al. 1979a; Young et al. 1979; Scolnick et al. 1979): (1) they are expressed (as shown in Figure 10) when cells of other species are transformed by these viruses; (2) they can be translated (though as a single band) from the respective viral RNAs; (3) they are phosphorylated; (4) apparently have the ability to bind GTP and GDP; and (5) they are located just inside the cell membrane. In the case of a temperature sensitive mutant of Kirsten sarcoma virus, the ability to immunoprecipitate the p21 *src* protein and bind GDP is lost at the nonpermissive temperature (Shih et al. 1979b). In addition, the Harvey sarcoma virus p21 and rat sarcoma virus p29 share almost identical $^{35}S$-methionine tryptic peptide maps (unpublished observations).

The rat sarcoma virus p29 is unique, however, in that it contains a portion of a rat helper type C virus structural protein, probably p15. The origin of the extra portion of this protein was determined from experiments using antiserum derived against rat type C virus. This antiserum was able to precipitate the p29, but not the Harvey or Kirsten sarcoma virus p21. In addition, this antiserum could not precipitate the p21 seen in rat sarcoma virus transformed cells (Young et al. 1979).

Thus, the selection of transforming viruses in the rat seems to have arisen through the incorporation of a specific unique cellular gene into a retroviral genome. While these rat transforming viruses appear to contain the same *src* protein, the genetic structure of the viruses differs. Harvey and Kirsten viruses were both obtained by the passage of uncloned mouse leukemia viruses through mice, then through rats and, finally, back into mice. These transforming viruses are recombinants between a mouse type C virus and an endogenous replication-defective viral-like sequence found in rats (30S). These rat sequences have many of the typical properties of viral sequences: they are approximately 6000–7000 nucleotides in length (i.e., 30S); they contain poly A; they can be packaged into virus particles by helper virus proteins; and they are inducible by halogenated pyrimidines and protein synthesis inhibitors. However, these sequences have not been shown to code for any known proteins, viral or otherwise. Nevertheless, they are expressed in high levels in specific rat tissues, rat mammary tumors, and many transformed tissue culture rat

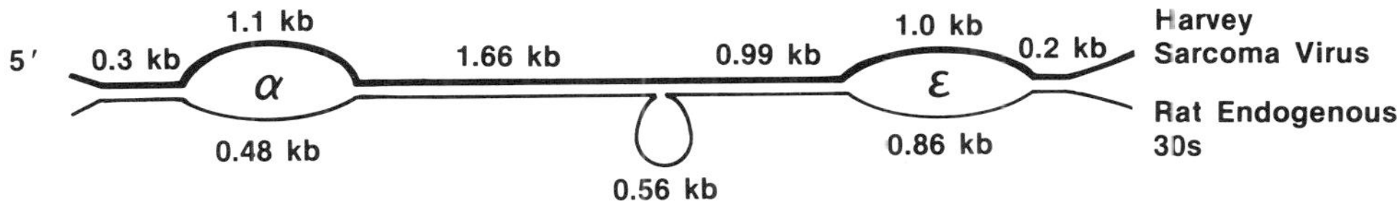


**Figure 11.** Heteroduplex analysis of endogenous rat virus and Harvey sarcoma virus. This Figure represents a simplified diagram of the heteroduplex obtained between cloned rat endogenous (30S) retrovirus DNA and cloned Harvey murine sarcoma virus DNA. Values are ± 0.04–0.13 kb.

cell lines. Harvey and Kirsten sarcoma viruses are composed mostly of these 30S sequences. The first 100–150 nucleotides at the 5′ and the last 1000 nucleotides at the 3′ end are of mouse virus origin with the remainder of the genomes being of rat origin (Shih et al. 1978). Thus, these viruses represent true interspecies recombinants. Through the use of recombinant DNA technology it has been possible to directly compare the relationship of the endogenous rat 30S sequence to Harvey sarcoma virus. Figure 11 shows a simplified schematic representation of the results of heteroduplex analysis of cloned rat 30S DNA and Harvey sarcoma virus DNA. The major features of this figure indicate that there are two major regions of nonhomology between 30S and Harvey (α and ε). The ε region, near the 3′ end of the genome, represents that portion of Harvey sarcoma virus which is mouse in origin. The α region lies precisely in the region of Harvey sarcoma virus that is required for transformation, based on restriction enzyme analysis, transfection of subgenomic fragments of Harvey sarcoma virus, generation of specific mutations of Harvey sarcoma virus, and qualitative RNA studies of cells transformed by Harvey sarcoma virus (Chang et al. 1980). Thus, it would appear that the cellular *sarc* gene was inserted into the 30S genome, although it is not clear whether this occurred before or after recombination with the mouse helper virus took place.

The α region of Harvey is approximately 1.1 kb in length. This region is larger than that required to code for a gene product of 21,000 Mr. Thus, it will be of interest to determine if the additional sequences represent controlling regions for *src* gene expression and if these same sequences are present in Kirsten sarcoma virus.

Rat sarcoma virus was derived in a manner entirely distinct from Harvey and Kirsten sarcoma virus and has an apparently different genetic structure. This virus was obtained by cocultivation of a Sprague-Dawley spontaneously transformed rat cell line (SD-1) producing high levels of rat type C virus with a chemically transformed Fischer rat cell line (4NQ) which had been passaged through a rat (Rasheed et al. 1978). Both of these cells express rat 30S sequences, but neither express rat sarcoma virus p29. Also, neither cell by itself is producing a transforming virus. The cocultivation, however, results in the formation of a stable transforming virus. Interestingly, the SD-1 cell is required in this cocultivation, whereas a number of other rat cells can be substituted for the 4NQ cells. These cells also express rat 30S

RNA. Regardless of the cell substituted for the 4NQ cell, the resulting sarcoma virus always codes for a protein of 29,000 Mr and it appears that a preferential site exists in the sarcoma virus genome for insertion of the cellular *sarc* gene.

While the Kirsten and Harvey sarcoma viruses are composed largely of the rat 30S genome, the rat sarcoma virus was not found to contain any 30S information. Instead, the genome was found to consist almost entirely of the rat helper virus genome and, in this respect, is similar to other mammalian transforming viruses (Young et al. 1979). Also, if the extra portion of the 29,000 Mr *src* protein is the viral p15, this would place the *src* gene near the 5′ end of the viral genome, similar to that seen in Harvey sarcoma virus (Figure 11).

The unique observation that three independently derived transforming viruses code for an immunologically related protein raises a number of interesting questions. Of prime importance is the relationship of the p21 gene to the viral genomes in the germ line of rats. It is currently not known whether this gene is normally associated with a viral genome in the rat DNA or if it exists independently of such sequences. Also, it is unclear as to what the relationship of p21 is to the 30S genome, especially in the generation of the rat sarcoma virus. Additionally, there is currently little information as to what cellular mechanisms act to control p21 expression. Low levels of p21 have been detected in cells of many mammalian species, but the relationship of this gene to the viral p21 and the function of these gene products remains unknown at this time.

In summary, the rat offers a unique and potentially highly rewarding model system in which to study the origin and function of mammalian sarcoma viruses and sarcoma virus gene products. Through the use of current genetic and biochemical technology, it should be possible to gain a much better understanding of the process by which mammalian retroviruses act to induce malignancy.

## The Transforming Sequences of Avian Acute Leukemia Viruses

Among the oncogenic retroviruses, some (e.g., avian acute leukemia virus, ALV, and MMTV) produce disease which typically arises only after a long latent period. In contrast, other retroviruses (including avian sarcoma virus, ASV, feline sarcoma virus, FeSV, the avian and murine defective leukemia viruses, and REV) act much more quickly; cell transformation in culture, as well as disease and death in the infected animal, occurs within only a few days to weeks after infection. Whereas a long latent period may imply the necessity of additional events subsequent to infection (e.g., hormonal stimulation, development of a sensitive cell type, generation of recombinant virus), the extreme virulence of this second group strongly suggests both that the sensitive cell type(s) is already present in the host and that the input virus itself is responsible for the resultant malignancy. For this reason, we shall consider these viruses in some detail, emphasizing the avian defective leukemia viruses and reticulendotheliosis virus (REV).

Of the four known reticuloendotheliosis viruses (spleen necrosis virus, Trager duck infectious anemia virus, chick syncytial virus, and REV-T), only REV-T has been shown to be oncogenic. REV-T is capable of transforming cultured avian fibroblasts, as well as bone marrow and spleen cells, both *in vivo* and *in vitro* (Franklin et al. 1974; Rup et al. 1979). In young chicks, the virus produces a rapidly fatal disease characterized by proliferation of reticuloendothelial cells in the liver, spleen, and other internal organs.

The other known avian defective leukemia viruses can be classified into several groups (Graf and Beng 1978). Avian erythroblastosis virus (AEV, strains ES4 and R) transforms cells which are erythroblast-like; clone-purified virus produces an acute erythroleukemia in the host, as well as sarcomas at the site of infection. Avian myeloblastosis virus (AMV, strains BAI/A and E26) transforms myeloblast-like cells both *in vivo* and *in vitro,* while the cells transformed by avian myelocytomatosis virus (strains MC29, CMII, OK10, and MH2) are predominantly macrophage-like, though carcinomas and sarcomas are also observed. As with AEV, clone-purified preparations of MC29 and CMII are able to transform cloned chick embryo fibroblasts, as well as the hematopoietic cell types mentioned.

These avian acute leukemia viruses share a number of significant properties. First, dilution experiments have shown that each of them consists of at least two biologically distinguishable elements; one is capable of replicating in a variety of cell types, but cannot transform them, while the other can transform the sensitive cell type, but is replication-defective (Graf and Beng 1978; Hoelzer et al. 1979). When both are present in the same cell, functions supplied by the helper virus permit replication and production of infectious particles containing the defective transforming virus. In the case of REV, we propagate the helper virus (REV-A) in a line of canine thymus cells (avian fibroblasts have also been used in other laboratories), while a mixture of the two viruses (REV-T) is produced in the transformed chicken bone marrow line established by Franklin et al. (1974).

In all of the avian acute leukemia viruses, the RNA genomes of the two entities differ in size (Hu et al. 1979; Lai et al. 1979; Gonda et al. 1980). In electron microscope spreads (Figure 12), RNA from the REV helper virus exhibited a typical retroviral dimeric structure with linkage close to the 5′ ends and with poly A tracts at both 3′ ends. The monomer length averaged 8.8 ± 0.7 kb. When REV-T RNA was treated in the same way, more than one population of molecules was seen. First, REV-T contains a large dimer very similar in size and conformation to that seen in REV-A. Second, REV-T contains an even larger number of molecules of smaller size, with average monomer length 5.3 ± 0.7 kb. Similar values have also been obtained for the helper and defective genomes of AEV (Lai et al. 1979) and of MC29 (Hu et al. 1979). We know from hybridization experiments that some of the sequences present in the helper genome are also present in the defective genome (Gonda et al. 1980), but based on these sizes alone, it is clear that the transforming genome is missing a significant fraction of the replication-competent genome.

Again, in all cases the transforming genome has been found to contain some sequences not present at all in the helper. In the case of REV, we have used reverse transcriptase to synthesize complementary DNA copies of REV-T viral RNA and we have found that, while most of this cDNA is subsequently able to hybridize

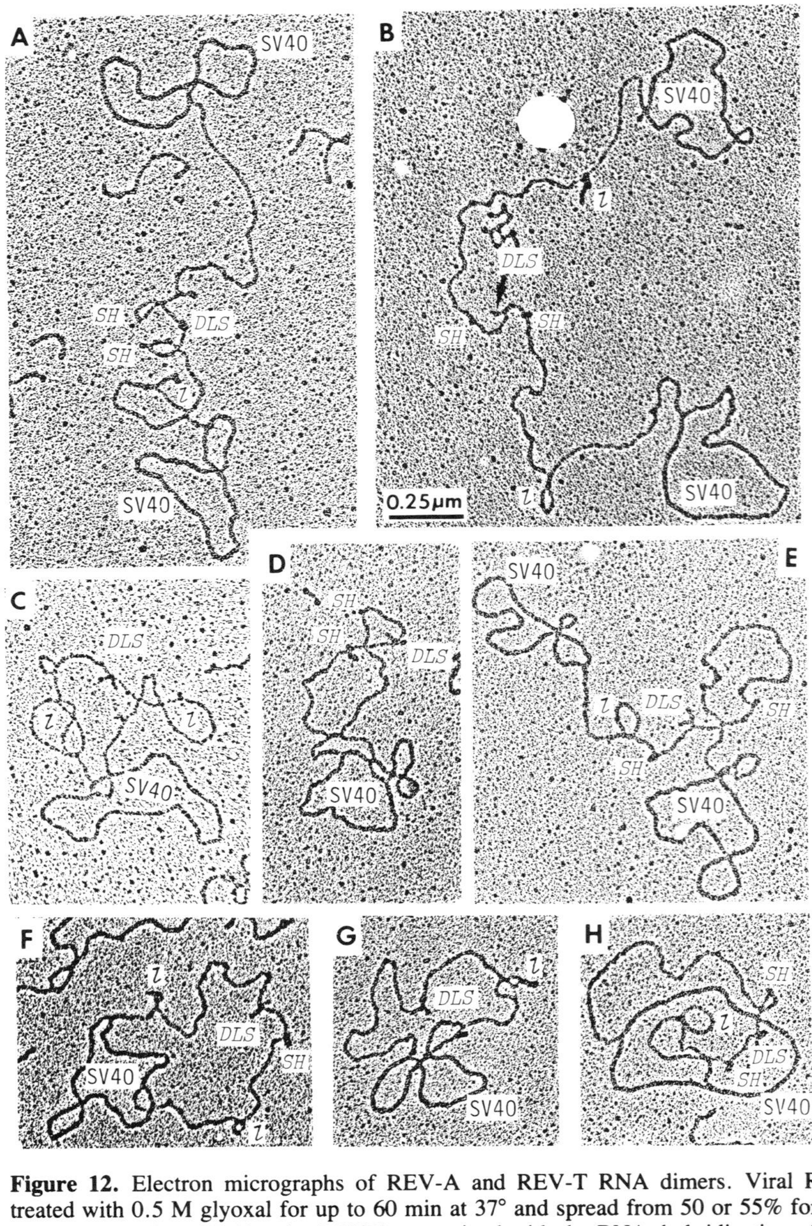


**Figure 12.** Electron micrographs of REV-A and REV-T RNA dimers. Viral RNA was treated with 0.5 M glyoxal for up to 60 min at 37° and spread from 50 or 55% formamide. Prior to spreading, SV40-poly (BUdR) was mixed with the RNA; hybridization of the poly BUdR to the poly A tracts typically found at the 3′ end of retroviral RNA results in the deposit of a circular SV40 DNA molecule at the RNA 3′ ends. These DNA circles were used as an internal length standard, taking a contour length of 1.76 μm to represent 5.45 kb. (A) REV-A dimer; (B) REV-T large RNA dimer; (C–H) REV-T small dimers. DLS, dimer linkage structure; l, loop; SH, short hairpin structure. All micrographs were printed at × 50,000 magnification.

with RNA of the purified helper virus, some (about 10% of the total) is not (Simek and Rice 1980). We then asked whether this REV-T-specific cDNA could hybridize with the small size RNA molecules seen in the electron microscope and it was found that it could (Gonda et al. 1980). Figure 13 shows REV-T RNA electrophoretically separated by size, transferred and immobilized on paper, and hybridized with cDNA. Lane B demonstrates that both the 9.3 and 5.7 kb RNAs can hybridize with cDNA of purified helper virus, while lane C shows that only the 5.7 kb RNA can hybridize with REV-T-specific cDNA. Thus, this 5.7 kb defective genome is a recombinant form which contains both helper-related and helper-unrelated sequences. Heteroduplex experiments with AEV and with MC29 have demonstrated

**Figure 13.** Hybridization of REV-T RNA transferred from a denaturing agarose gel. After electrophoresis in a 0.8% agarose gel containing 10 mM $CH_3H_gOH$, REV-T RNA was transferred to diazobenzyloxymethyl paper and hybridized with $^{32}$P-cDNA. Filters were washed, dried, and analyzed by autoradiography at −70° using Kodak No Screen film. Lane A, molecular weight standards stained with ethidium bromide and printed as a negative: RD-114 RNA (10 kb), chicken 28S rRNA (4.7 kb), *E. coli* 23S rRNA (3.1 kb), chicken 18S rRNA (2.0 kb), and *E. coli* 16S rRNA (1.7 kb). Lane B, REV-T RNA hybridized with REV-A $^{32}$-P cDNA. Lane C, REV-T RNA hybridized with $^{32}$-cDNA specific to REV-T.

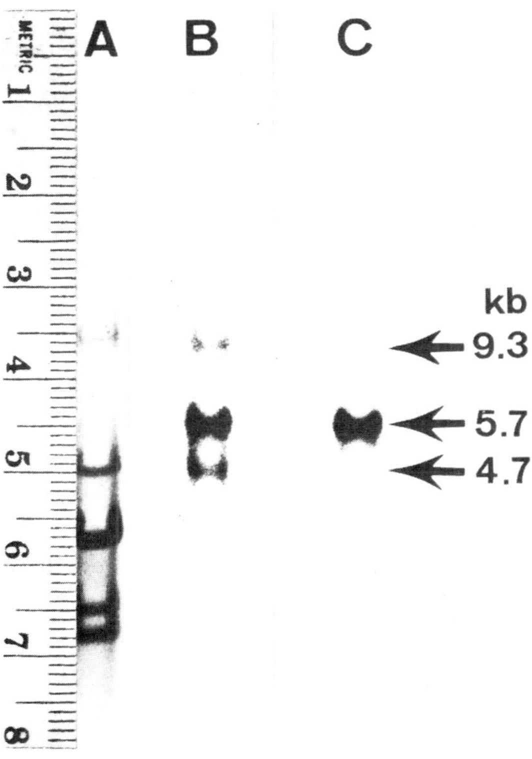

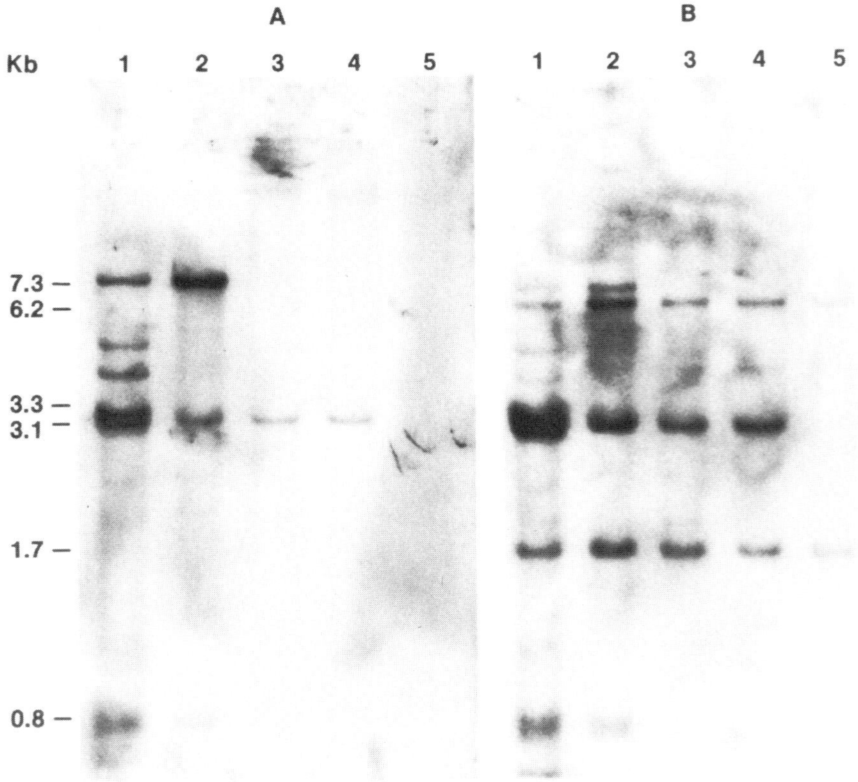


**Figure 14.** Hybridization of DNA from REV-producing and nonproducer chicken transformed cell lines. DNAs were digested with Sac-1, electrophoresed in a 1% agarose gel, blotted onto nitrocellulose paper, and hybridized with (A) REV-$^{32}$-P cDNA or (B) $^{32}$-P cDNA specific to REV-T. Filters were washed, dried, and analyzed by autoradiography. Lanes 1 and 2, DNA from transformed virus-producing cell lines; Lanes 3 and 4, DNA from transformed nonproducer cell lines; and Lane 5, DNA from uninfected chicken.

that the sequences specific to the defective genome amount to 2–3 kb located in the middle of the RNA, and that helper and defective genomes are related at their 5′ and 3′ ends (Lai et al. 1979; Hu et al. 1979).

If this defective genome is indeed the cause of cell transformation, then these REV-T–specific sequences should be found in all cells transformed by REV-T, including those which were not infected by the helper virus and which, therefore, are not producing virus. Figure 14 shows this to be the case. In this experiment, DNA from various REV-T transformed chicken cell lines has been digested with the restriction endonuclease Sac-1, electrophoresed in an agarose gel, blotted onto nitrocellulose paper, and hybridized either with helper virus cDNA or REV-T-specific cDNA. DNA from the transformed virus-producing bone marrow cell line is shown in Lane A-1. We see that helper virus cDNA hybridizes predominantly with a 7.3 kb DNA fragment, which we know from other experiments to be part of the helper virus genome, and with a 3 kb fragment, which we know to be part of the defective genome. Indeed, Lane B-1 shows that only the 3 kb DNA and not the 7.3 kb DNA can hybridize with REV-T-specific cDNA. DNA from a second transformed virus-producing line, shown in Lanes A-2 and B-2, also contains both of these fragments. Lanes A-3, B-3, A-4, and B-4 have DNA from two transformed lines which are not producing virus; we find that they contain the 3 kb fragment, but not the 7.3 kb fragment. Thus as expected, the helper virus genome is not necessary for transformation, whereas the 5.7 kb genome is consistently associated with the transformed state. Our goal in these ongoing studies is to define the specific region of the defective genome which is responsible for transformation and to characterize the product for which it codes.

Another feature common to all of the defective acute transforming viruses is the origin of these transformation-specific sequences. For each virus examined to date, it has been demonstrated that the nonhelper sequences in the defective genome are highly related to sequences in normal DNA of the natural host. Thus, the 3.25 kb specific to AEV and the 1.8 kb specific to MC29, though unrelated to each other, are each very similar to normal genes of the chicken (Sheiness and Bishop 1979, Roussel et al. 1979). The same is also true of the Abelson acute leukemia virus of the mouse (Shields et al. 1979) and of the murine sarcoma viruses (Frankel et al. 1976), and appears to be true of REV as well (Simek and Rice 1980). Each virus has a sequence in its defective component which is unrelated to either its helper or to the specific sequences in any of the other acute oncogenic viruses, which appear to be the cause of cell transformation, and which is highly related to sequences present at the level of one or a few copies per haploid genome in normal host DNA. This finding has lead to the hypothesis that these transforming viruses have arisen through a recombinational event between the nontransforming helper virus and host DNA and that it is this excised segment of host DNA which, when exogenously introduced into an appropriate cell, results in transformation. Indeed, Oskarsson et al. (1980) have found that the normal sequence in mouse DNA which is related to the *src* region of MSV can be isolated and that it carries transforming potential. This brings us to the hope that we might be able to identify a similar array of sequences in human DNA which, when removed from normal control processes or modified by mutation, result in neoplasia. One approach to this problem will take advantage of the observation that genes related to the transforming region of MC29 are found not only in chickens, but in other avian species and mammals (Sheiness and Bishop 1979). Thus, we can hope to use avian viral probes to identify and isolate regions of human DNA involved in cell transformation.

## Heterogeneity of Endogenous Baboon Proviral DNA

Evidence is accumulating that retrovirus DNA sequences constitute a substantial portion of the mammalian genome. In the best characterized organism, the mouse, at least four different classes of endogenous retrovirus-related sequences are present, accounting for up to 0.35% of the *Mus* genome. In *Mus cervicolor,* this includes approximately six copies of the Gross-type murine leukemia virus genome, six of Woolly monkey—Gibbon ape virus-related genome, up to 25 M432 viral genomes, and at least 25 mammary tumor virus-related type B viral genomes (Todaro et al. 1980; Morris et al. 1977). It also includes the 400–1800 copies of intracisternal A particle sequences detected in the DNA of several strains of mice (Lueders and Kuff 1977). These DNA sequences, which have a complexity of at least 5600 nucleotide pairs, are related to the M432 retrovirus genome of *Mus cervicolor*.

The type A particles have an associated reverse transcriptase activity and their main structural protein is immunologically related to the major M432 virus internal protein (Kuff et al. 1980). Nevertheless, the biological significance of the type A particles remains obscure.

In primates, six different endogenous retroviruses have been detected and characterized. These include owl monkey type C and squirrel monkey type D viruses, both New World monkey retroviruses; and baboon, macaque and colobus type C viruses and the langur monkey type D virus, all Old World monkey retroviruses. In each case, the respective retrovirus is integrated in the host genome in multiple copies (see Todaro et al. 1980).

In the baboon, multiple copies of three different primate retroviruses have been detected thus far. Baboon endogenous virus (BaEV) sequences are reiterated about 100 times (McAllister et al. 1978). The closely related macaque type C retroviruses, MMC-1 and MAC-1, which have limited sequence homology with BaEV, are also highly reiterated in the baboon cell chromosome (Tainsky, manuscript in preparation). Further, the type D retrovirus of the spectacled langur, which is also unrelated to BaEV, is homologous to sequences present in baboon cell DNA (Benveniste and Todaro 1977). Together, these proviruses constitute 0.02–0.04% of the baboon genome.

As an initial step in understanding the complexities of integrated BaEV genomes, we are analyzing these sequences in both virus-producing and in nonvirus-producing baboon cells. We recently reported a detailed restriction enzyme map of the BaEV unintegrated linear DNA that was isolated from freshly infected permissive cells (Cohen et al. 1980). The 5′ to 3′ orientation of the viral RNA genome in the map was determined. As with other well-characterized retroviral DNAs, BaEV unintegrated linear DNA was found to contain a terminal repeat consisting of both 5′ and 3′ end sequences. It is approximately 550 nucleotide pairs in length.

Although the patterns of BaEV fragments observed in Southern blotting experiments of baboon chromosomal DNA are complex, the unintegrated DNA map provided a basis for analysis of these integrated genomes as well. As will be discussed, the reason for this complexity is primarily because the approximately 100 integrated BaEV genomes in baboon DNA contain considerable sequence heterogeneity. This was not unexpected since it was found earlier that baboon DNA is noninfective or poorly infective in transfection experiments. By comparison, DNA isolated from human cells productively infected with BaEV and containing only 5–6 proviral copies is highly infectious by transfection (McCallister et al. 1978). In addition, hybrids formed between baboon cell DNA and labeled BaEV

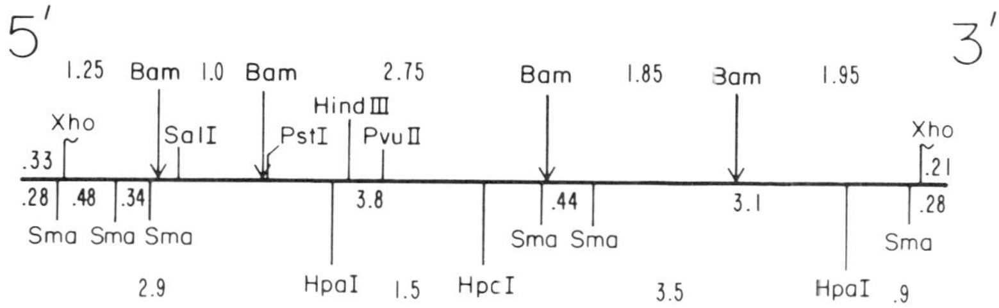


**Figure 15.** Restriction enzyme map of baboon endogenous virus unintegrated viral DNA isolated from freshly infected permissive cells.

complementary DNA was found to have a lower thermal stability and a broader melting profile then hybrids formed between the human producer-cell DNA and the same probe (Rice, unpublished results).

Among the many integrated BaEV genomes, three specific sequence alterations have been detected so far and two of these have been well characterized. The latter heterogeneities include the absence of modification of a Bam HI recognition site 2.25 kb from the 5′ end of the genome and a specific 150 base pair deletion which occurs between the Bam HI recognition sites 1.25 kb and 2.25 kb from the 5′ end of the genome.

From the restriction map (Figure 15), it is clear that the failure of Bam HI to cut a BaEV genome 2.25 kb from the 5′ end would result in the appearance of a new Bam HI fragment of 3.75 kb. This fragment can be seen in Bam Hi digests of DNA from a baboon embryo fibroblast line (BEF-3) that is a BaEV producer cell (Figure 16, lanes G–I). It appears to be present in an equal molar ratio to the other internal Bam HI fragments and indicates that approximately one-half of the BaEV proviruses in BEF-3 cell DNA have this sequence modification.

The faint 3.9 kb band above the 3.75 kb band is the other major heterogeneity. The 3.75 kb fragment is a subset of the 3.9 kb fragment, but with a 150 base pair deletion to the left of the missing (or modified) Bam HI site 2.25 kb from the 5′ end.

It is not only those genomes which are missing the Bam HI site that show the deleted and undeleted fragment variation. When the Bam HI site is present, fragments of 1.18 kb and 1.0 kb are generated and the 1.0 kb fragment is a subset of the faint 1.18 kb fragment but with the approximately 150 base pair deletion.

On the other hand, DNAs from five of six baboon tissues (from three juvenile baboons) digested with Bam HI show the converse of the baboon embryo fibroblast DNA. Their proviruses, while still containing the 2.25 kb Bam HI site heterogeneity, have a preponderance of genomes of the undeleted variety. That is, they have intense 3.9 kb (instead of 3.75 kb) and intense 1.18 kb (instead of 1.0 kb) fragments (Figure 16, lanes A–D, F), DNA from the liver of a fourth juvenile baboon (Figure 16, lane E) was of the BEF-3 Bam HI pattern.

Since it is the deleted form of the proviral genome that is present as a replication

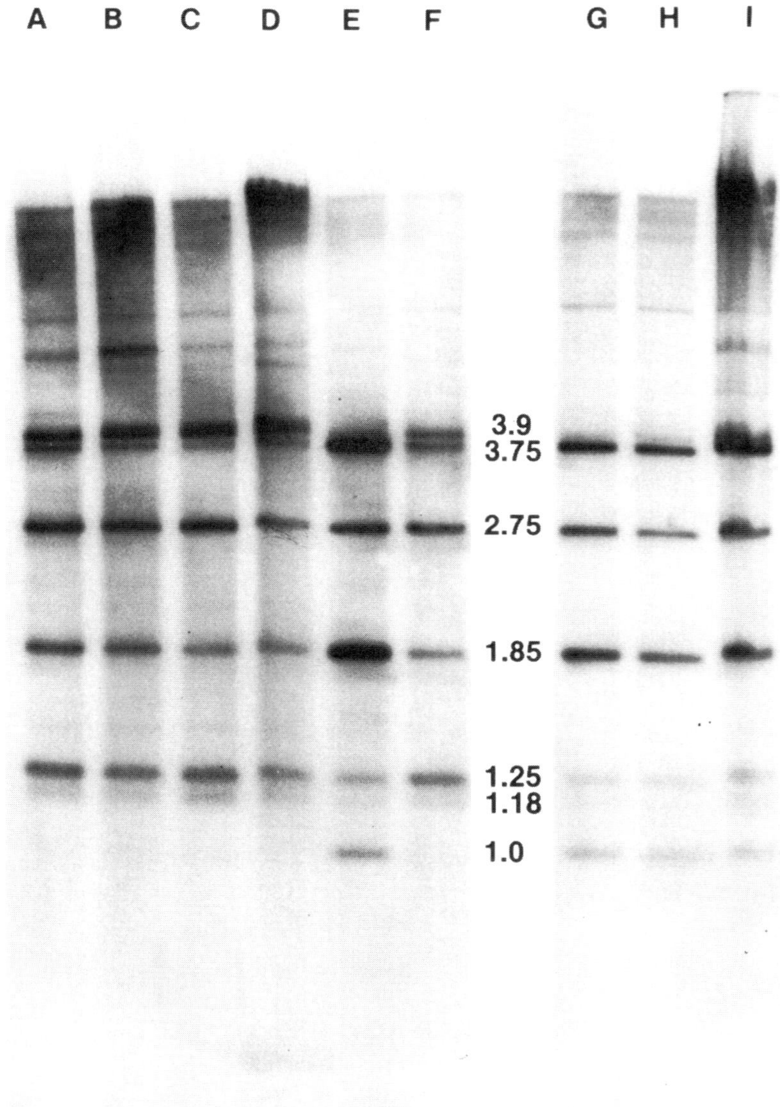


**Figure 16.** Bam HI digests and blots of DNAs from (A) baboon 984 spleen, (B) baboon 984 thymus, (C) baboon 932 spleen, (D) baboon 932 thymus, (E) baboon 658 liver, (F) baboon 495 liver; and BEF-3 cell DNA from (G) passage 36, (H) passage 17, and (I) passage 20.

intermediate in acutely infected permissive cells (Cohen et al. 1980) and it is this form that predominates in a baboon cell line that is producing BaEV (i.e., BEF-3, in contrast to the undeleted predominant DNA form of nonproducer tissues), it is tempting to consider the possibility that a specific deletion coincides with provirus activation. This possibility is currently being pursued both by characterization of λ phage clones of baboon cell DNA and by studying the infectivity and sequence arrangement of proviruses present in the DNA of baboon tumors.

## Heterogeneity of Endogenous Mouse Type C Viruses

### *Genetic Instability of Retroviruses*

It has become clear in recent years that retroviruses exhibit an extraordinary level of genetic instability. Thus, when cell clones are isolated from mouse cell cultures producing murine leukemia virus, as many as 30% of the clones are found to release noninfectious virus particles (Table 1). Several experimental approaches have shown that these clones are, in fact, infected with replication-defective mutants of murine leukemia virus (Rein et al. 1978, 1979b) Attempts to remove these spontaneous mutants from virus stocks by cloning cells infected with single particles of wild type virus were not successful; the progeny virus produced by these cells still contained a high proportion of replication-defective mutants (Shields et al. 1978). Thus, these mutants arise at high frequency during each replicative cycle of the virus. The reason for this is not known; perhaps reverse transcription is more error prone than the other steps in retrovirus replication since this is the step which is unique to the viruses.

The defects can apparently occur in any of the three genes known to be required for viral replication: that for internal structural proteins; that for reverse transcriptase; and that for envelope glycoprotein. Similar high levels of spontaneous replication-defective mutants have been observed in the avian as well as murine retroviruses. The genetic instability of the retroviruses is a serious potential complication to many kinds of experiments, but at the same time the mutants should be useful reagents in the analysis of the viral life cycle.

**Table 1.** Frequency of Isolation of Spontaneous Viral Mutants.[a]

| Virus isolate | Mutants/total |
|---|---|
| Moloney murine leukemia virus | 1/3 |
| B-tropic murine leukemia virus | 7/20 |
| N-tropic murine leukemia virus | 6/30 |

[a]Mouse cell cultures were infected with murine leukemia viruses, and the cells were passaged for several weeks or months. Clones of cells were then isolated from the cultures and tested for the production of infectious murine leukemia virus. Each of the clones listed as "mutant" above was producing little or no wild type virus but mutant virus production could be demonstrated by "virus rescue" experiments (Rein et al. 1979b; Gerwin et al. 1979; Rein and Gisselbrecht, unpublished data).

## *Diversity of Endogenous Viruses*

Endogenous virus expression has been examined in the greatest detail in chickens and mice. Chickens exhibit a number of discrete patterns of virus expression (Robinson 1978) and each of these patterns is associated with one or more Mendelian loci. In turn, each of these loci is a proviral genome.

In mice, it has been known for some time that viral antigens can be expressed in the apparent absence of mature virus (Huebner et al. 1970). This observation could reflect the presence of incomplete proviruses in the genome of the mouse or could be due to noncoordinate expression of viral genes. As murine type C viruses have been characterized more precisely in the last decade, it has become clear that several types of mature virus can be produced, even in the same mouse. For example, three distinct murine leukemia viruses have been isolated from BALB/c mouse tissues or cell cultures: (1) B-tropic, able to multiply well in BALB/c mouse cells; (2) N-tropic, able to multiply well in NIH Swiss mouse cells; and (3) xenotropic, able to multiply in nonmurine cells.

As biochemical and serological techniques have become more sophisticated, the number of different endogenous viral genomes detectable in the mouse has increased dramatically. Thus, there are at least two distinct subclasses of xenotropic murine leukemia virus. Further, nucleic acid hybridization kinetics indicate that there are 10–40 copies of virus-related sequences per haploid mouse genome. This complexity is also demonstrated by Southern gel analysis of mouse DNA which has been cleaved with Eco R1, a restriction endonuclease which does not cut within the genomes of the known murine leukemia viruses. This analysis shows a large number of distinct bands in the mouse genome. In the AKR mouse strain, some of these bands have been identified with known viral genomes previously identified by correlating biological parameters with liquid hybridization measurements (Steffen et al. 1979).

## *Interactions of Endogenous Viruses*

Detailed studies of the murine leukemia viruses produced in mice of the high-leukemic AKR strain have also shown that endogenous viruses of different classes can recombine with each other. Thus, preleukemic thymocytes produce a virus, termed mink cell focus-inducing virus (MCF), which is not an endogenous virus encoded in the germ line, but rather a new virus which arises by recombination between AKR endogenous viruses during the lifetime of each mouse. MCF is of special interest since it may be important in the etiology of AKR lymphomas.

While it is clear that MCFs are recombinants between endogenous viruses, still other viruses have been shown to be produced by AKR lymphoma cells. In one case, single cell clones of AKR lymphoma cells were shown to be releasing two distinct viruses. One of these is an MCF-like virus, while the other is a novel virus of a type not previously observed *in vivo*. This virus is totally unable to replicate itself, thus termed a replication-defective virus, and is only replicated when the host cell is coinfected with a second helper virus which is able to supply the missing replicative functions (Rein et al. 1979a). The replication-defective virus produced

**Table 2.** Virus Production by AKR Leukemia Cell Lines.[a]

| Cell line | CPFU/ml[b] | FIU/ml[c] |
|---|---|---|
| AKRSL1 | $2 \times 10^3$ | $2 \times 10^2$ |
| AKRSL2 | $2 \times 10^3$ | $1 \times 10^3$ |
| AKRSL3 | $2 \times 10^3$ | $3 \times 10^2$ |

[a]Cell lines were derived from AKR leukemic tissue by R. Nowinski and E. Hays and were a kind gift of R. Nowinski. Culture fluids from these cell lines were tested in two infectivity assays: the complementation plaque assay, which detects replication-defective murine leukemia viruses and the $S^+L^-$ focus assay, which detects viruses able to replicate themselves on mouse cells.

[b]Complementation plaque forming units/ml.

[c]Focus-inducing units/ml, as detected in the $S^+L^-$ focus assay.

by the lymphoma cells is detected by its ability to fuse indicator cells in the presence of a complementing virus. Recent studies show that the replication-defective virus codes for an envelope glycoprotein, but no internal structural proteins (Rein et al., unpublished data). As is shown in Table 2, several AKR lymphoma cell lines have now been found to produce two viruses, one a helper virus and the other a replication-defective virus. Experiments are now underway to determine whether the replication-defective virus is a mutant, a recombinant, or a true endogenous virus and whether this newly discovered virus produced by malignant cells plays any role in the disease process.

Recent studies have also shown that endogenous viruses can recombine with exogenous viruses, as well as with each other. This is obviously a major factor which must be considered in the interpretation of a wide variety of experiments. Thus, when any of the well-characterized exogenous viruses, such as Friend, Moloney, or Rauscher murine leukemia virus, is injected into mice, the mice produce replicas of the injected virus, but also recombinants between this virus and an endogenous virus. In the case of Friend murine leukemia virus, two distinct types of recombinants with endogenous viruses have been described. One, termed spleen focus-forming virus, has lost the ability to replicate, but is a highly virulent leukemia virus.

## Discussion

The initial demonstrations that retroviruses could exist as inherited elements within the cell genome led to speculations of their role in the normal development of the host species (Huebner et al. 1970). Examples of interspecies transmission was also seen as a means of enriching the genetic variability of new hosts (Todaro 1980). Such ideas added to the substantial interest in these viruses in addition to their demonstrated oncogenic potential. This general philosophy follows from the classical viewpoint that functionality is required for maintaining inherited elements within the cell genome. Despite the novel appeal of a role in normal development, no substantive evidence for this has appeared and indeed the extent of heterogeneity between and within species makes such ideas rather doubtful. It seems much more logical to approach this family of viruses from a parasite-host standpoint utilizing the new information gained from studies of the structural organization of the genome and new concepts allowing for independent existence of DNA segments which can be summarized as "selfish DNA" (Orgel and Crick 1980; Doolittle and Sapienza 1980). Thus, for the retroviruses whose integrated state has been studied by direct sequence analysis, the analogy to bacterial transposons is quite clear (Figure 1). The presence in certain species of inherited elements reiterated from 100–1000 times can be explained by replication-dependent transposition, the only selection process being for lack of insertion into vital cell genes causing lethal mutations. As the new genome evolved with time, one would expect conservation of the control signals found in the insertion sequence-like elements (LTR) flanking the unique viral structural genes. Variable loss and potential gain of new host sequences within the transposable unit could also occur, accounting for the origin of acute transforming viruses and the occurrence of defective integrated genomes. As described for the baboon endogenous virus, an outbred population would show considerable heterogeneity in number, organization, and function (in terms of making an infectious virus) of its integrated proviruses. If transposition can occur without an infectious cycle, then the only functions which need be retained are those assuring retention and transposition. The final degree of reiteration which can be achieved without detriment to the host may be substantial, as indicated by the A particle genomes in mouse cells which account for at least 0.3% of the cell genome. Even if the concept of a role in normal development for integrated noninfectious proviruses is discarded, their utility for studies of genome function since they are a class of mutants is clearly indicated. While we have some confidence that the transposon model will account for the existence of large numbers of proviral DNA copies in normal cells, the acquisition of genes from the host cell leading to transforming potential requires further consideration. Current evidence indicates that the normal host transforming genes (*sarc* and equivalents) are found in host DNA apart from retroviral elements and in this form are negative in DNA transformation assays (Oskarsson et al. 1980). We assume that they are specifically functional during some phase of differentiation although this remains to be shown. Once spliced appropriately to retroviral elements and containing at least one LTR, the same sequences are active. Since the LTR contains splice signals (mRNAs for *gag* and *env* genes contain these sequences), the generation of transforming viruses would require (1) a splice acceptor sequence adjacent to cellular *sarc* and (2) insertion of a provirus (or LTR) in a configuration which permits formation of a new transposon including *sarc*. While such events may be rare, it seems possible to design experiments which would use the retroviral LTRs in attempts to rescue cellular genes which can be assayed in selective systems. This approach may be the one of choice in searching for human transforming genes analogous to those described above for the acute leukemia and sarcoma viruses.

While we feel increasingly confident in the assessment of what retroviruses are, there is still ample room for speculation on their ultimate origin. Gross (1974) has advanced the law of obligate communicability which states simply that everything we study today has originated elsewhere. Ultimately, however, one must stop and find out where that elsewhere is. We doubt outer space theories, but rather prefer one of inner space. According to this view, retroviruses originated first, by evolution of the 1S-like sequences (i.e., LTRs) to an autonomous state, and second, by the accumulation between two LTRs of host cell sequences which coded for structures which could assemble into virions. This would involve host genes (or functional domains) already specialized for performance of functions required for a replicating unit. Thus, primary sequence homology between a retroviral phosphoprotein and the $NH_2$-terminus of one histone class could be one example of such usurpation of host genes. A conceptual basis for this derives from the organization of DNA as coding regions, exons separated by noncoding regions, introns (Gilbert 1978). Since a gene may have multiple exons separated by introns, one can imagine the accumulation of exons from several genes into a new element of use to an evolving entity on its way to becoming a retrovirus. Current sequence studies of structural proteins and the virion reverse transcriptase should contribute to a critical test of the above hypothesis. Such comparative data has increased our confidence that the retrovirus classification scheme is based upon common ancestry of current members.

The ability to generate multiple variants of a single virus by recombination with related sequences in cell DNA and by rescue of normal elements clearly makes it difficult to evaluate the oncogenic potential of a given isolate. This definition is made even more difficult based on possible indirect mechanisms involving, for example, persistent stimulation of subpopulations of lymphoid cells via viral antigen receptors leading to expanded target cell numbers for spontaneous transformation (Ihle et al. 1980) or introduction of hormone sensitive promotors (as may be the case with the mouse mammary tumor virus) which again expands the susceptible cell population. Conceivably, a totally benign virus capable of integration within the germ line could spawn descendants with a variety of pathogenic potentials. The time scale for such occurrences may be quite extended and impossible to predict. One can accommodate within this view the possibility of virus-free tumors (and species) which have a viral-related etiology and isolation from tumors of viruses which result from disease rather than being etiologic agents. Thus, increased replication of a specific cell population may be responsible for the generation of defective viruses, as found in the AKR leukemic cell lines described here.

In summary, retroviruses provide a variety of interesting and unique features for studies of viral origin, interrelationships, evolution, and pathogenesis. These have relevance to a broad set of problems rather than being strictly limited to interest by virologists.

ACKNOWLEDGMENTS

The work of the authors was supported under Contract NO-1-CO-75380 with the National Cancer Institute, National Institutes of Health, Bethesda, Maryland.

The senior author, Dr. Raymond V. Gilden, is especially grateful to Prof. W.H. Hildemann and Prof. Ray D. Owen for guidance and support during the crucial early phase of his career.

## References


Barbacid, M., Hunter, E., and Aaronson, S.A. 1979. Avian reticuloendotheliosis viruses: Evolutionary linkage with mammalian type C retroviruses. J. Virol. 30:508–514.

Barbacid, M., Long, L.K., and Aaronson, S.A. 1980. Major structural proteins of type B, type C, and type D oncoviruses share interspecies antigenic determinants. Proc. Natl. Acad. Sci. U.S.A. 77:72–76.

Bauer, G. and Temin, H.M. 1979. RNA-directed DNA polymerase from particles released by normal goose cells. J. Virol. 29:1006–1013.

Benveniste, R.E. and Todaro, G.J. 1977. Evolution of primate oncornaviruses: An endogenous virus from langurs *(Presbytis spp.)* with related virogene sequences in other world monkeys. Proc. Natl. Acad. Sci. U.S.A. 74:4557–4561.

Chang, E.H., Maryak, J.M., Wei, C.M., Shih, T.Y., Shober, R., Cheung, H.L., Ellis, R.W., Hager, G.L., Scolnick, E.M., and Lowy, D.R. 1980. Functional organization of the Harvey murine sarcoma virus genome. J. Virol. 35:76–92.

Charman, H.P., Gilden, R.V., and Oroszlan, S. 1979. Reticuloendotheliosis virus: Detection of immunological relationship to mammalian type C retroviruses. J. Virol. 29:1221–1225.

Cohen, M., Nicolson, M.O., McAllister, R.M., Shure, M., Davidson, N., Rice, N.R., and Gilden, R.V. 1980. Baboon endogenous virus genome. I. Restriction enzyme map of the unintegrated DNA genome of a primate retrovirus. J. Virol. 34:28–39.

Crick, F. 1979. Split genes and RNA splicing. Science 204:264–271.

Darnell, J.E., Jr. 1978. Implications of RNA · RNA splicing in evolution of eukaryotic cells. Science 202:1257–1260.

Dayhoff, M.O. 1976. Survey of new data and computer methods of analysis. In Atlas of Protein Sequence and Structure. M.O. Dayhoff, ed. Vol. 5, suppl. 2, pp. 1–8. Washington, D.C.: National Biochemical Research Foundation.

Dhar, R., McClements, W.L., Enquist, L.W., and Vande Woude, G.F. 1980. Terminally repeated sequence (TRS) of integrated Moloney sarcoma provirus: Nucleotide sequence of TRS and its host and viral functions. Proc. Natl. Acad. Sci. U.S.A. 77:3937–3941.

Doolittle, W.F. and Sapienza, C. 1980. Selfish genes, the phenotype paradigm and genome evolution. Nature 284:601–603.

Frankel, A.D., Neubauer, R.L., and Fischinger, P.J. 1976. Fractionation of DNA nucleotide transcripts from Moloney sarcoma virus and isolation of sarcoma virus-specific complementary DNA. J. Virol. 18:481–490.

Franklin, R.B., Maldonado, R.L., and Bose, H.R. 1974. Isolation and characterization of reticulendotheliosis virus transformed bone marrow cells. Intervirology 3:342–352.

Gerwin, B.I., Rein, A., Levin, J.G., Bassin, R.H., Benjers, B.M., Kashmiri, S.V.S., Hopkins, D., and O'Neill, B.J. 1979. Mutant of B-tropic murine leukemia virus synthesizing an altered polymerase molecule. J. Virol. 31:741–751.

Gilbert, W. 1978. Why genes in pieces? Nature 271:501.

Gonda, M.A., Rice, N.R., and Gilden, R.V. 1980. Avian reticulendotheliosis virus: Characterization of the high-molecular weight viral RNA in transforming and helper virus populations. J. Virol. 34:743–751.

Graf, T. and Beng, H. 1978. Avian leukemia viruses interaction with their target cells *in vivo* and *in vitro*. Biochem. Biophys. Acta 516:269–299.

Gross, L. 1974. Facts and theories on viruses causing cancer and leukemia. Proc. Natl. Acad. Sci. U.S.A. 71:2013–2017.

Hanafusa, H. 1978. Cell transformation by RNA tumor viruses. Compr. Virol. 10:401–483.

Harvey, J.J. 1964. An unidentified virus which causes the rapid production of tumors in mice. Nature 204:1104–1105.

Henderson, L.E., Gilden, R.V., and Oroszlan, S. 1979. Amino acid sequence homology between histone H5 and murine leukemia virus phosphoprotein p12. Science 203:1346–1348.

Henderson, L.E., Copeland, T.D., Sowder, R., and Oroszlan, S. 1981. Primary structure of the low-molecular weight nucleic acid binding proteins of murine leukemia. J. Biol. Chem., in press.

Hoelzer, J.D., Franklin, R.B., and Bose, H.R. 1979. Transformation by reticulendotheliosis virus, development of a focus assay and isolation of a nontransforming virus. Virology 93:23–30.

Hozumi, N. and Tonegawa, S. 1976. Evidence for somatic rearrangement of immunoglobulin genes coding for variable and constant regions. Proc. Natl. Acad. Sci. U.S.A. 73:3628–3632.

Hu, S.S.F., Lai, M.M.C., and Vogt, P.K. 1979. Genome of avian myelocytomatosis virus MC29: Analysis by heteroduplex mapping. Proc. Natl. Acad. Sci. U.S.A. 76:1265–1268.

Huebner, R.J., Kelloff, G.J., Sarma, P.S., Lane, W.T., Turner, H.C., Gilden, R.V., Oroszlan, S., Meir, H., Myers, D.D., and Peters, R.L. 1970. Group-specific antigen expression during embryogenesis of the genome of the C-type RNA tumor virus: Implications for ontogenesis and oncogenesis. Proc. Natl. Acad. Sci. U.S.A. 67:366–376.

Hunter, E.S., Brown, A.S., and Bennett, J.C. 1978. Amino-terminal amino acid sequence of the major structural polypeptides of avian retroviruses: Sequence homology between reticuloendotheliosis virus p30 and p30s of mammalian retroviruses. Proc. Natl. Acad. Sci. U.S.A. 75:2708–2712.

Ihle, J.N., Lee, J.C., Enjuanes, L., Cicurel, L., Horak, I., and Peppersack, L. 1980. Chronic immunostimulation as a possible mechanism in C-type viral leukemogenesis. In Viruses and Naturally Occurring Cancer. M. Essex, G. Todaro, and H. zur Hausen, eds. New York: Cold Spring Harbor Laboratory, pp. 1049–1064.

Kang, C.-Y. and Temin, H.M. 1974. Reticuloendotheliosis virus nucleic acid sequences in cellular DNA. J. Virol. 14:1179–1188.

Kirsten, W.H. and Mayer, L.A. 1967. Morphologic response to a murine erythroblastosis virus. J. Natl. Cancer Inst. 39:311.

Kuff, E.L., Callahan, R., and Howk, R.S. 1980. Immunological relationship between the structural proteins of intracisternal A particles of *Mus musculus* and the M432 retrovirus of *Mus cervicolor*. J. Virol. 33:1211–1214.

Lai, M.M.C., Hu, S.S.F., and Vogt, P.K. 1979. Avian erythroblastosis virus: Transformation-specific sequences form a contiguous segment of 3.25 kb located in the middle of the 6 kb genome. Virology 97:366–377.

Lueders, K.K. and Kuff, E.L. 1977. Sequences associated with intracisternal A particles are reiterated in the mouse genome. Cell 12:963–972.

McAllister, R.M., Nicolson, M.O., Heberling, R.L., Charman, H., Rice, N., and Gilden, R.V. 1978. Infectivity of endogenous baboon type-C virus-related genes. In Advances in Comparative Leukemia Research P. Bentvelzen, J. Hilgers, and D.S. Yohn, eds. Amsterdam, New York: Elsevier North Holland Biomedical Press, pp. 135–138.

Misono, K.S., Sharief, F.S., and Leis, J. 1980. Primary structure of Rous sarcoma virus RNA-associated polypeptide pp12. Fed. Proc. 39:1611.

Morris, V.L., Medeiros, E., Ringold, G.M., Bishop, J.M., and Varmus, H.E. 1977. Comparison of mouse mammary tumor virus-specific DNA in inbred, wild and Asian mice, and in tumors and normal organs from inbred mice. J. Mol. Biol. 114:73–91.

Niall, H.D., Sauer, R., and Allen, D.W. 1970. The N-terminal amino acid sequence of two avian leukosis group-specific antigens. Proc. Natl. Acad. Sci. U.S.A. 67:1804–1809.

Orgel, L.C. and Crick, F.G.H.C. 1980. Selfish DNA: The ultimate parasite. Nature 284:601–603.

Oroszlan, S., Copeland, T.D., Summers, M.R., Smythers, G., and Gilden, R.V. 1975. Comparative primary structure analysis of the p30 protein of woolly monkey and gibbon type C viruses. Virology 77:413–417.

Oroszlan, S. and Gilden, R.V. 1978. RNA tumor virus antigens. Scand. J. Immunol. 7 (Suppl. 6):81–96.

Oskarsson, M., McClements, W.L., Blair, D.L., Vande Woude, G.F., and Maizel J.V. 1980. Properties of a normal mouse cell DNA sequence (sarc) homologous to the *src* sequence of Moloney sarcoma virus. Science 207:1222–1224.

Rabin, H., Benton, C.V., Tainsky, M.A., Rice, N.R., and Gilden, R.V. 1979. Isolation and characterization of an endogenous type C virus of rhesus monkeys. Science 204:841–842.

Rasheed, S., Gardner, M.B., and Huebner, R.J. 1978. *In vitro* isolation of stable rat sarcoma viruses. Proc. Natl. Acad. Sci. U.S.A. 75:2972–2976.

Rein, A., Gerwin, B.I., Bassin, R.H., Schwarm, L., and Schidlovsky, G. 1978. A replication-defective variant of Moloney murine leukemia virus. I. Biological characterization. J. Virol. 25:146–156.

Rein, A., Athan, E., Benjers, B.M., Bassin, R.H., Gerwin, B.I., and Slocum, D.R. 1979a. Isolation of a replication-defective murine leukemia virus from cultured AKR leukemia cells. Nature 282:753–754.

Rein, A., Benjers, B.M., Gerwin, B.I., Bassin, R.H., and Slocum, D.R. 1979b. Rescue and transmission of a replication-defective variant of Moloney murine leukemia virus. J. Virol. 29:494–500.

Robinson, H.L. 1978. Inheritance and expression of chicken genes that are related to avian leukosis sarcoma virus genes. Curr. Top. Microbiol. Immunol. 83:1–36.

Roussel, M., Saule, S., Lagrou, C., Rommens, C., Beng, H., Graf, T., and Stehelin, D. 1979. Three new types of viral oncogene of cellular origin specific for hematopoietic cell transformation. Nature 281:452–455.

Rup, B.J., Spence, J.L., Hoelzer, J.D., Lewis, R.B., Carpenter, C.R., Rubin, A.S., and Bose, H.R. 1979. Immunosuppression induced by avian reticuloendotheliosis virus: Mechanism of induction of the suppression cell. J. Immunol. 123:1362–1370.

Scolnick, E.M., Papageorge, A.G., and Shih, T.Y. 1979. Guanine-nucleotide binding activity as an assay for *src* protein of rat-derived murine sarcoma viruses. Proc. Natl. Acad. Sci. U.S.A. 76:5355.

Sheiness, D. and Bishop, J.M. 1979. DNA and RNA from uninfected vertebrate cells contain nucleotide sequences related to the putative transforming gene of avian myelocythomatosis virus. J. Virol. 31:514–521.

Shields, A., Witte, O.N., Rothenberg, E., and Baltimore, D. 1978. High frequency of aberrant expression of Moloney murine leukemia virus in clonal infections. Cell 14:601–610.

Shields, A., Goff, S., Paskind, M., Otto, G., and Baltimore, D. 1979. Structure of the Abelson murine leukemia virus genome. Cell 18:955–962.

Shih, T.Y., Williams, D.R., Weeks, M.O., Maryak, J.M., Vass, W.C., and Scolnick, E.M. 1978. Comparison of the genomic organization of Kirsten and Harvey sarcoma viruses. J. Virol. 27:45–55.

Shih, T.Y., Weeks, M.O., Young, H.A., and Scolnick, E.M. 1979a. Identification of a sarcoma virus coded phosphoprotein in nonproducer cells transformed by Kirsten or Harvey murine sarcoma virus. Virology 96:64–79.

Shih, T.Y., Weeks, M.O., Young, H.A., and Scolnick, E.M. 1979b. p21 of Kirsten murine sarcoma virus is thermolabile in a viral mutant temperature sensitive for the maintenance of transformation. J. Virol. 31:546–556.

Shih, T.Y. and Scolnick, E.M. 1980. The molecular biology of mammalian sarcoma viruses. In Viral Oncology. G. Klein, ed. New York: Raven Press.

Simek, S. and Rice, N.R. 1980. Analysis of the nucleic acid components in reticulendotheliosis virus. J. Virol. 33:320–329.

Steffen, D., Bird, S., Rowe, W.P., and Weinberg, R.A. 1979. Identification of DNA fragments carrying ecotropic proviruses of AKR mice. Proc. Natl. Acad. Sci. U.S.A. 76:4554–4558.

Todaro, G.J., Benveniste, R.E., Sherwin, S.A., and Sherr, C.J. 1978. MAC-1, a new genetically transmitted type C virus of primates: "Low frequency" activation from stumptail monkey cell cultures. Cell 13:775–782.

Todaro, G.J. 1980. Interspecies transmission of mammalian retroviruses. In Molecular Biology of RNA Tumor Viruses. J.R. Stephenson, ed., New York: Academic Press, pp. 47–76.

Todaro, G.J., Callahan, R., Rapp, U.R., and De Larco, J.E. 1980. Genetic transmission of retroviral genes and cellular oncogenes. Brit. J. Cancer 41:663–664.

Van Zaane, D. and Bloemers, H.P.J. 1978 The genome of the mammalian sarcoma virus. Biochem. Biophys. Acta 516:249–258.

Webster, R.G. and Laver, W.G. 1971. Antigenic variation in influenza virus biology and chemistry. Progr. Med. Virol. 13:271–338.

Young, H.A., Shih, T.Y., Scolnick, E.M., Rasheed, S., and Gardner, M.B. 1979. Different rat-derived transforming retroviruses code for an immunologically related intracellular phosphoprotein. Proc. Natl. Acad. Sci. U.S.A. 76:3523–3527.

Hildemann, ed. Frontiers in Immunogenetics

# Immunological Characterization of Human Leukemias

Susan L. Melvin

*Division of Immunology, St. Jude Children's Research Hospital, 332 North Lauderdale, P.O. Box 318, Memphis, Tennessee*

Human leukemias can be distinguished by their cell morphology into myeloid and lymphoid leukemias. Each has acute and chronic forms—terms which originally referred to the relative time courses of the respective disease processes. However, current usage of the terms chronic and acute reflect the more or less differentiated appearance of the malignant cells. In adults both chronic and acute forms of lymphoid and myeloid leukemias are observed. In children the acute forms predominate. Acute lymphocytic leukemia (ALL) is the most frequent form of leukemia in children and is the single most frequent malignancy in individuals under 20 years of age. It strikes approximately one child in 4,000 and is a leading cause of death by disease for this age group (Levin et al. 1974). The following discussion focuses on recent immunological studies of leukemia cells from children with ALL. The purposes of these studies are to further our understanding of the biology of both normal and malignant lymphoid cells and to relate this information to the clinical aspects of the disease as well.

The etiology of ALL is unknown although irradiation, certain chromosomal abnormalities, and immune deficiencies may be predisposing conditions in a very small proportion of the cases (Miller 1976; Miller 1967). In most cases there is no evidence of any predisposing genetic, immunological or environmental factors in spite of any early age of onset and a slight predominance of affected boys. The duration of symptoms prior to diagnosis is short and the symptoms are explainable by an overabundance of malignant, or blast cells. At diagnosis, blasts have generally replaced most of the normal cellular constituents of the bone marrow. Morphologically, these cells appear to be transformed lymphocytes and/or lack any evidence of myelocytic, monocytic, or erythroid differentiation. Blasts are often present in the circulation and organomegaly is frequently observed. Tumor masses are observed infrequently, but their presence is an important adverse prognostic feature. The systemic nature of the disease, the undifferentiated appearance of these malignant cells and, finally, differences in individual patient's responses to therapy raise a number of questions. From the most basic to the applied, these questions are:

What are the biological properties of ALL blasts?

Can the biological properties of the blasts be used to determine the cellular origin of ALL?

Conversely, can these blasts give us any insights into normal differentiation processes?

Can the biological properties of the blast cells be related to the clinical aspects of ALL—either the initial disease or recurrent disease?

## Comparison of Normal Lymphocytes and ALL Blasts

The premise of these immunological investigations is that the ALL blasts share with or retain some properties of normal lymphocytes. The methods for the most part are those used to define normal human lymphocyte subpopulations.

The two major divisions of normal lymphocytes in human as in animals are the T-cell and B-cell lineages. These populations are distinguishable by their ontogenic development, their antigenic properties, and their functional capacities (Table 1). The T-cell population is dependent upon the thymus during ontogeny. Mature T-cells are functionally active as either helper or suppressor cells in antibody responses, responder cells in mixed leukocyte cultures (MLC), cytolytic effector cells in graft rejection and in many antitumor responses. On the other hand, B-cells which differentiate independently of the thymus are the cells which secrete immunoglobulin, or are the immediate precursors of such cells. B-cells may be subject to either helper or suppressor effects of T-cells. They may function as stimulator cells rather than responder cells in mixed leukocyte cultures. They may participate in hyperacute graft rejection or antileukemia responses by producing specific antibodies. Both T-cells and B-cells include antigen-specific cells and cells responsive to appropriate mitogens. Functionally and antigenically discrete subpopulations or maturational stages are recognized in both the T-cell and B-cell lineages.

In some lymphoid malignancies of adults, the malignant cells have functional T- or B-cell properties. When acute lymphocytic leukemia blasts are tested for these same properties, they are strikingly devoid of functional capabilities. The one exception is that they can generally stimulate in mixed leukocyte cultures. This property, although associated with B-cells, is not absolutely specific for B-cells. ALL blasts do not secrete immunoglobulin and only 2% of ALL patients have blasts which bear membrane or surface immunoglobulin. Rare individuals may have blasts which have T-cell function determined by their ability to suppress immunoglobulin production by normal B-cells (Broder et al. 1978). This summary clearly points out that, in general, ALL blasts bear little functional resemblance to mature lymphocytes. In view of those negative results, it is possible that ALL blasts may

**Table 1.** Comparison of Normal Lymphocytes and ALL Blasts.

| Characteristics | Normal lymphocytes T-cells | Normal lymphocytes B-cells | ALL blasts |
|---|---|---|---|
| Thymus dependent | ++ | − | ? |
| Helper cell (for Ig) | + | − | − |
| Suppressor cell (for Ig) | + | − | −[a] |
| MLC responder | + | − | − |
| MLC stimulator[b] | − | + | + |
| Cytolytic effector | + | − | ? |
| Ig producer | − | ++ | −[a] |
| Mitogen responsive | + | + | − |

[a]Rare individuals positive.

[b]Nonlymphoid cells may also stimulate.

resemble immature lymphocytes or are nonfunctional variants of T or B-cells. Evidence which supports the notion that ALL blasts are similar to immature lymphoid cells is the demonstration of terminal deoxynucleotidyl transferase (Tdt) activity in ALL blasts (Greenwood et al. 1977). This enzyme is normally found in thymocytes and in some lymphoid cells within the bone marrow, whereas mature lymphoid cells lack significant Tdt activity.

In the ontogenic development of normal lymphocytes, differentiation stages may be associated with specific anatomical sites. Stem cells or precursor cells are first detected in the yolk sac and later become detectable in fetal liver and finally, in the bone marrow. Some normal cells in the bone marrow show commitment to T-cell or B-cell differentiation. Some marrow cells are responsive to humoral factors from the thymus and are thought to progressively differentiate during passage through the thymus. The more mature T-cells are a minority population in the thymus, but are present in large numbers in the blood, spleen and lymph nodes. Mature B-cells may also be found in the blood, but are most prevalent in the nodes and spleen. They occupy areas in these organs which are generally distinct from those occupied by mature T-cells. Some lymphoid cells may also return to and be stored in the marrow. At each passage to a new anatomic site immature lymphocytes are expected in the circulation. The same cell type might also be found in the organ of origin and the organ which is the cell's destination. One or more of these stages of early lymphocyte differentiation are therefore candidates for the normal counterpart of the ALL blast.

The assumption of a normal counterpart for ALL does not exclude the possibility that the blasts might also have unique features not shared with normal cells. Therefore, the immunological characterization of ALL blasts has been attempted by two complementary approaches. One has been the search for membrane antigens and receptors of normal lymphocyte populations on the blast. The second has been to immunize animals with ALL blasts for the identification of possibly leukemia-associated antigens. Once found, these antigens were, in turn, sought on minor populations of normal lymphoid cells. All leukemia-associated markers which have been sufficiently investigated appear to be normal differentiation markers of T-cells, B-cells, or early lymphoid cells rather than leukemia-specific markers. The two groups of markers will therefore be considered together as differentiation markers.

Human T-cell markers are of two general types, i.e., the formation of spontaneous rosettes with sheep erythrocytes (E-rosettes) and the T-cell membrane antigens. T-cells from the periphery and T-cells from the thymus can be discriminated by both types of markers (Borella and Sen 1975; Mills et al. 1975; Galili and Schlesinger 1976). Mature peripheral T-cells form E-rosettes which dissociate at elevated incubation temperatures. Hence, these are heat-labile rosettes. By contrast, thymocytes form rosettes in similar numbers at high and at low temperatures and are therefore heat stable. Using appropriately absorbed heteroantisera to human T-cells, T-cells from both the peripheral lymphoid organs and the thymus are reactive. Additional adsorptions indicate that there are thymus-specific antigens. With the advent of hybridoma antibodies, it is evident that there are many antigenically distinct subpopulations of human T-cells (Reinherz and Schlossman (1980).

Cells of the B-cell series are distinguished by immunoglobulin synthesis although secretion occurs only at a late stage of differentiation. Mature but nonsecreting B-cells have surface immunoglobulin, receptors for the Fc portion of immunoglobulin and receptors for the third component of complement (C3). The earliest identifiable cells in the B-cell lineage have weak cytoplasmic immunoglobulin but no surface immunoglobulin (Gathings et al. 1977; Pearl et al. 1978).

A less specific marker of B-cells is the *Ia*-like antigen, a membrane antigen analogous to the mouse *Ia* antigen. Allotypic differences in these antigens lead to an MLC response and are probably responsible for the stimulatory activity of ALL blasts in the MLC. It has been described as a leukemia-associated antigen since heteroantisera to the *Ia*-like antigen react with most leukemia blasts, but not with most blood lymphocytes. The antigen is, however, a common determinant on the *Ia*-like molecule and is present on normal B-cells, early myeloid cells, monocytes, and macrophages and on both lymphoid and myeloid leukemias (Billing et al. 1976; Schlossman et al. 1976).

A second leukemia-associated antigen which is more restricted in its cellular distribution than is the *Ia*-like antigen can be detected by heteroantisera to ALL blasts. It is present on most ALL blasts and absent from normal blood lymphocytes, thymocytes, myeloid cells, and most myeloid leukemias (Greaves et al. 1975). A small fraction of normal cells from bone marrow and from fetal liver are also identified by these sera (Brown et al. 1975; Greaves et al. 1977). These observations suggest that this common ALL (cALL) antigen may be a stem cell antigen, although conclusive evidence is still lacking.

When unselected ALL specimens are assayed for these markers, it is immediately clear that different children with the diagnosis of ALL may have blasts with different membrance characteristics. Individual markers identify from as few as 2% of ALL specimens to as many as 68% of specimens. Using a battery consisting of the markers described, it is possible to positively identify ALL blasts from 95% of children with ALL. A closer look at the data from individual patients reveals that these individual markers are not independently expressed. Some markers, like E-rosette formation and the common ALL antigen, appear to be mutually exclusive while other like the common ALL antigen and the *Ia*-like antigen are often coordinately expressed.

## Differentiation of Antigen Marker Patterns

We can simplify the results into four major marker patterns. These patterns are designated as common, T-cell, B-cell, and undifferentiated ALL. The most frequent pattern, the common ALL, is characterized by the presence of both the *Ia*-like antigen and the common ALL antigen. It is observed in 62% of newly diagnosed ALLs. T-cell ALL blasts lack the common ALL pattern although some may bear either *Ia*-like or common ALL antigens. The positive identifying feature of these blasts is the presence of T-cell antigens. One-half of the T-cell specimens will also be E-rosette positive. A minority of ALLS (19%) are T-cell ALL by these criteria. B-cell ALL occurs in only 2% of the patients and is characterized by blasts with both *Ia*-like antigen and surface immunoglobulin. The undifferentiated ALL account for the remaining 17% of new ALLs. They have blasts with fewer detectable surface markers than do the other three groups. They may have either the *Ia*-like antigen or the common ALL antigen, but not both. A few will have no detectable markers. Although there is no overlap among the groups as they are defined, there are occasional intermediate marker patterns or incomplete displays of membrane antigens (Melvin, in press). These less frequent patterns may form the basis for future subgroups of ALL.

Of the four groups, the T-cell specimens are the easiest to relate back to possible stages of normal cell differentiation (Figure 1). All T-cells, with the possible exception of the earliest stem cells, bear some T-cell antigens identifiable by xenogeneic anti-T-cell sera. As suggested earlier, blasts which have T-cell markers are by no means homogenous in their display of membrane antigens and receptors. These differences are used to delineate subgroups of T-ALL which have more or less differentiated blast cell properties. Peripheral, "resting" T-cells are characterized by heat labile rosettes. The *Ia*-like and cALL antigens are absent. Activation of these cells is accompanied by two marker changes—increased stability of rosette formation and acquisition of the *Ia*-like antigen (Gergely et al. 1974; Galili and Schlesinger 1976; Evans et al. 1978). Thymocytes which are also stable rosette formers generally lack the *Ia*-like antigen although activation of these cells might lead to the same "activated" phenotype.

The "activated" phenotype and the "resting" or mature T-cell phenotype are only occasionally observed in ALL. The thymocyte phenotype accounts for approximately one-half of T-ALL specimens. The rest of the T-ALL specimens are E-rosette negative and have one of three marker patterns. The first is absence of all detectable markers except the T-cell antigens. The second is the addition of the

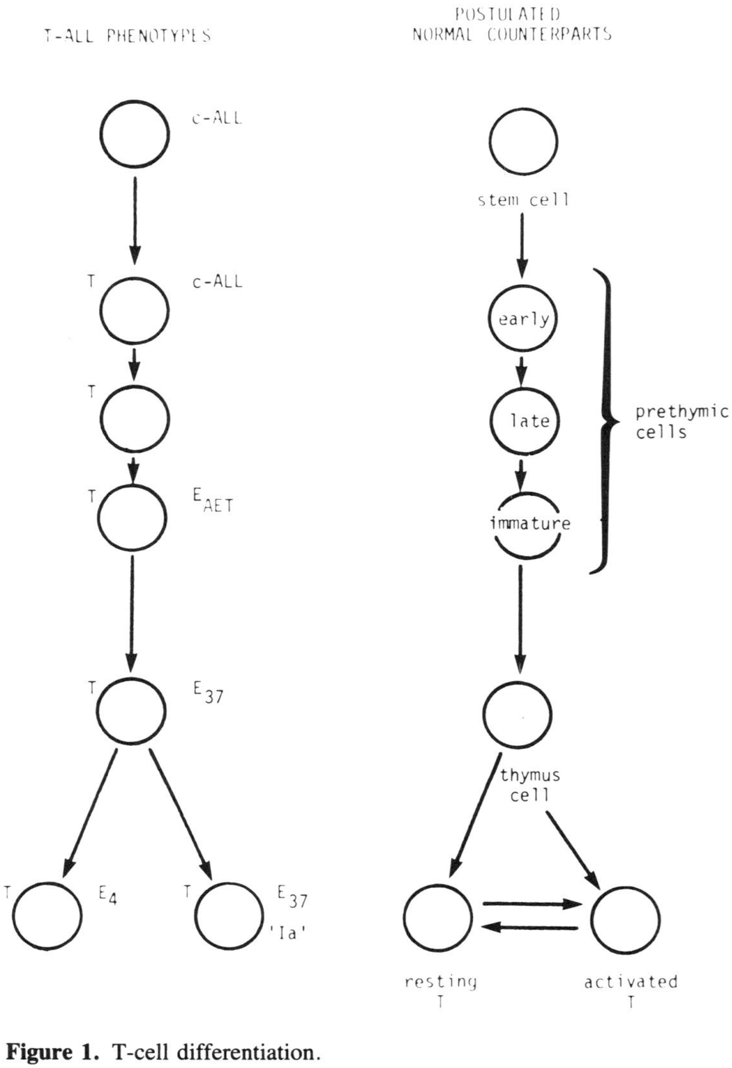


**Figure 1.** T-cell differentiation.
T: T-cell antigens; cALL: common ALL antigen; $E_{AET}$; receptors for 2-aminoethylisothio uronium bromide treated sheep erythrocytes; $E_{37}$: receptors for sheep erythrocytes, stable at 37°C; $E_4$; receptors for sheet erythrocytes, labile at 37°C; 'Ia': human analogue of *Ia* antigen.

common ALL antigen. The third comes closest to the E-positive phenotype in that E-rosette formation becomes possible when the sheep erythrocytes are pretreated so as to enhance rosette formation (Melvin 1979). These may be "immature" rosette-forming cells. Since we lack adequate markers for normal human T-cells that are less differentiated than thymocytes, we can only postulate that these T-cell ALL phenotypes are representative of prethymic stages of T-cell differentiation. The simplest progression of prethymic differentiation suggested by the ALL data is a linear one beginning with an incompletely defined stem cell, which probably bears the common ALL antigen. The first commitment to T-cell differentiation would be acquisition of T-cell antigens, followed by loss of the cALL antigen and later the acquisition of an "immature" rosetting phenotype. Following this sequence are the thymocyte and then the peripheral T-cell phenotypes.

In a somewhat similar fashion, there are other ALL blast specimens with characteristics of early B-cell differentiation. In addition to 2% of ALL specimens which are surface immunoglobulin positive, 15-20% of specimens contain blasts with weak cytoplasmic immunoglobulin (Vogler et al. 1978; Pullen et al. 1981). In normal bone marrow, cells with weak cytoplasmic immunoglobulin and no surface immunoglobulin are called pre-B cells. The pre-B ALL blasts generally have the surface phenotype of the common ALL group. The remaining two-thirds of the common ALL group show no evidence of commitment to either T-cell or B-cell lineages. However, the distribution of the common ALL antigen on ALL specimens with the presumed pre-T-cell or pre-B-cell phenotypes and the presence of antigenic cross-reactivity with some normal cells suggest that the common ALL phenotype identifies a lymphoid stem cell. If the normal counterpart of common ALL is a precursor of both T-cells and B-cells, the schemes of T-cell and B-cell differentiation can be combined into a single scheme. In addition, the heterogeneity of blast phenotypes observed in ALL can be explained by this same unifying differentiation scheme.

The phenotypes of undifferentiated ALL may fit into this differentiation scheme as even earlier precursor cells, cells which branch into a separate line of differentiation or as variants. Since the same surface phenotypes are present in some cases of acute myelogenous leukemia, more positive means of identifying these cells are necessary to discriminate among the various possibilities.

We conclude that ALL is a malignancy in which the blasts are heterogeneous in their expression of membrane antigens and receptors. ALL includes some cases which show evidence of commitment to either T-cell or B-cell differentiation but in all cases the disease is manifest as an accumulation of cells apparently blocked or retarded in early stages of differentiation. This is not to say that cells are necessarily fixed in a state of differentiation at the time of malignant transformation. Clearly, in at least one of the adult leukemias, chronic myelogenous leukemia, abundant evidence indicates that the malignancy although initially manifest by an accumulation of relatively differenitated myeloid cells involves stem cells for the myeloid, platelet, and red cell lines (Fialkow et al. 1967; Rastrick et al. 1968). The block in differentiation in ALL may be coincident with the malignant transformation or may occur after the malignant cells have progressed through at least some differentiation. A third alternative is that ALL blasts are representative of aberrant, disorganized differentiation. Obviously, the differentiation scheme presented must be confirmed in normal lymphoid cells, but meanwhile it provides a convenient conceptual model for understanding the heterogeneity within ALL.

Heterogeneity among ALL specimens is also evident from studies of nonimmunological properties of ALL blasts. Correlations between these properties and surface markers provide evidence of biological heterogeneity among the marker-defined ALL group. Blasts with B-cell, T-cell and non-T/non-B phenotypes have different mean proportions of cells actively synthesizing DNA suggesting different growth kinetics for the respective leukemic cell populations (Tsukimoto et al. 1976; Murphy et al. 1977). These groups also have different mean numbers of receptors for cortisone, one class of agents used in the treatment of ALL (Yarbro et al. 1977). Other observations, primarily from tissue culture lines, indicate that cells with T-cell or B-cell phenotypes have different sensitivities to several of the individual drugs commonly used in the treatment of ALL (Ohnuma et al. 1978). In addition, new experimental antileukemia drugs are being tested clinically and may have a preferential effect on the groups of ALL as defined by surface markers (Smyth, in press). It seems reasonable that the cell surface phenotypes may be markers for differences in such fundamental cell behaviors as growth kinetics of the cell population, cell migratory pathways, and drug sensitivity. These properties, in turn, could have important clinical implications when the cells in question are also malignant.

## Clinical Correlates of ALL Markers

We have compared the clinical features and clinical courses among the four surface marker defined groups of ALL (Bowman et al., in press). It is well established that certain clinical features at diagnosis are related to prognosis in childhood ALL (Miller 1975; Simone et al. 1975). Children with extremely high white cell counts, tumor masses, or central nervous system leukemia are at high risk of relapsing within the first year of therapy. Children who lack these risk features have a 70% chance of long-term survival and possible cure (Aur et al. 1978; George et al. 1979). When the four marker groups are analyzed for the presence of high risk features, the T-cell group has the highest proportion, 82%, of children with one or more of these risk features. The common ALL group and the B-cell group have low representation of high risk features (5% and 0%, respectively). The undifferentiated groups are intermediate with 20% of patients having high risk features. The types of risk features also differ among these groups. The T-cell group includes almost every patient with a mediastinal or thymic enlargement, or with CNS disease. The B-cell group coincides with a group of patients with abdominal tumor masses. High circulating white cell counts are observed in all groups except the B-cell group, but are most prevalent in the T-cell group. The high proportion of T-cell ALLs with high risk features suggests that T-cell ALL is a highly aggressive form of ALL and one which responds poorly to conventional therapy. This strong association makes it difficult to determine if the T-cell markers can be used as independent prognostic indicators or if subsets of T-cell ALL have different prognoses. The E-rosette marker which has been used longer than any of the other T-cell markers is the only one we can currently evaluate in these respects. In our prospective study, E-positivity cannot be accurately predicted on an individual basis from the clinical features. In fact, some children with E-positive blasts have no high risk clinical features. This small group of T-ALLs has a significantly poorer response to therapy than do other children with no high risk features. These data support the concept that the biological properties of the blasts are important in determining the clinical manifestations and the disease course and may be of independent prognostic value. There is no difference in distribution of the clinical risk features between T-ALL patients with E-positive blasts and those with E-negative blasts. Further followup is needed to determine if the smaller groups of T-ALL subsets are of additional prognostic significance.

Although rare, patients who have surface immunoglobulin positive blasts (B-cell ALL) are clinically significant because of abdominal masses at diagnosis, metabolic complications during therapy and the high risk of early treatment failure (Woolf et al. 1976).

In our experience, patients with undifferentiated ALL include an unexpected number of early treatment failures and every patient for whom a change in diagnosis was made after initiation of therapy. The treatment failures include equal numbers of children with and without high risk features. Again, in those patients without high risk features, the blast phenotype may be a significant marker or determinant of clinical response.

Patients of the common ALL group have fewer early relapses as would be anticipated from the low incidence of risk features in this group. The facts that there are still some early relapses and that later relapses are to be anticipated indicate the need for further discriminatory tests in this largest group of patients.

These clinical correlations and the *in vitro* studies cited earlier suggest that the marker defined groups of ALL may have blasts with different growth properties and possibly different susceptibility to chemotherapy. Modern therapy for childhood ALL consists of three phases—remission induction, CNS prophylaxis, and continuation therapy. Combination chemotherapy in induction results in elimination of detectable blasts in approximately 95% of patients within 4–6 weeks. CNS prophylaxis destroys blasts within the CNS which are inaccessible for systemic therapy and which would otherwise terminate remission in over 50% of patients. Systemic treatment consisting of combination chemotherapy with agents other than those used in induction continues for 2-1/2 years, providing the patient remains in remission. For the 50% of patients who complete this phase, all therapy is stopped. It is generally assumed that early detection of relapse might be used to therapeutic advantage. Cell-surface markers as expressions of blocked states of differentiation are potential markers for monitoring disease activity if sufficiently sensitive detection methods can be developed. Implicit in this application of marker studies to clinical studies is the assumption that the marker(s) will be stable throughout the disease. Few direct comparisons of surface markers on blast cells found at original diagnosis and at relapse have been made.

## Antigenic Modulation and Variation

It is well documented in mice that thymus leukemia antigens can undergo a stable but reversible loss *in vivo*. This phenomenon of antigenic modulation and the intense selective pressure exerted through the mutagenic and cytotoxic effects of chemotherapeutic agents require that the assumption of stable antigen expression in human leukemias be documented or refuted.

To this end we have engaged in a systematic study of surface markers, following individual patients from diagnosis through sequential relapses. The results have been rewarding and somewhat surprising. To begin with, changes in marker defined groups occurred in 9 of 33, or more than 25% of our relapse patients (Table 2). The changes were primarily from the good prognosis or common ALL phenotype to the undifferentiated phenotype which in untreated patients was associated with poor response to therapy. Six patients showed this type of change. Two patients whose blasts were undifferentiated ALL prior to treatment had blasts of the common ALL type at relapse. The ninth patient had B-cell ALL at diagnosis. At relapse, the blasts had no detectable immunoglobulin and the patient was therefore classified as undifferentiated ALL.

Since our group assignments are based on the pattern of markers rather than on any individual test, these groupings minimize the changes observed. In fact, 16 of the 33 individual patients (48%) who were tested more than once during the course of their disease show marker changes. The changes are most often the loss of a single marker. The classification of T-ALL specimens was not changed, since no detectable changes occurred in the T-cell antigens. However, we have observed changes in the cALL antigen and the loss of E-receptor activity in some of these T-ALL specimens. Overall the most frequent change is in the common ALL antigen. Both losses and gains in this antigen are observed and are responsible for all but one of the changes in group assignments. Losses are observed more frequently than gains probably because of the large number of patients whose blasts initially have the antigen. Another significant finding is that this antigen may be lost and then regained in sequential relapses of the same patient. Thses observations are consistent with those of other investigators showing that the cALL antigen may be easily

**Table 2.** Sequential Marker Study.

| Group | 1st Test | 2nd test |
|---|---|---|
| T-cell | 11 pt → | 11 pt |
| Common | 16 pt → | 10 pt |
| | | 2 pt |
| | | 6 pt |
| Undifferentiated | 5 pt → | 3 pt |
| | | 1 pt |
| B-cell | 1 pt → | 0 pt |

modulated on the cell surface (Ritz et al., in press). Roberts et al. (1978) have reported changes in the common ALL antigen on nearly 40% of samples from acute leukemia patients including both children and adults. Also consistent with our observations are the reported losses of immunoglobulin isotype, loss of the ability to form E-rosettes, and the aquisition of T-cell antigens in several lymphoid malignancies (Fialkow et al. 1973; Borella et al. 1979).

The usefulness of surface markers in monitoring patients for disease activity is limited by the degree to which normal cells also express the marker in question and the stability of the marker. Although the common ALL antigen is the most specific of the available markers, the sequential studies indicate that this marker is too unstable to be a reliable or useful indicator of recurrent disease. How this instability is related to the type of therapy or its clinical utility in recurrent ALL is unclear at present. It is possible that frequent changes in the cALL antigen occur because the antigen's orientation in the cell membrane makes it highly susceptible to the extracellular environment. To the extent that drug resistance may be a membrane phenomenon, conversion to drug resistance might secondarily affect other membrane molecules including the surface marker.

The marker instability which results in changes in group assignments highlights the interrelatedness of the surface marker-defined groups. Some interrelatedness was suggested earlier from the intermediate surface marker patterns exhibited by some ALL specimens, phenotypic heterogeneity within individual ALL specimens and now by the sequential marker studies. Several *in vitro* observations also support this idea. Phenotypically different cell lines which were derived from a single leukemic individual and which have the same karyotypic markers indicate that blasts with T-cell, B-cell, and common ALL phenotypes can arise from the same leukemia clone (Minowada et al. 1978). Established leukemic cell cultures are phenotypically stable, with the exception of two common-ALL-like lines that developed weak cytoplasmic Ig with no change either in surface phenotype or in karyotype (HurWitz et al. 1979; Minowada et al. 1979). Selection may have been responsible for both of these observations. Since the phenotypes are thought to be expressions of the degree of differentiation achieved, it might also be possible to alter the blast phenotype with appropriate differentiation stimuli. This will be a difficult task to accomplish since the blasts obviously fail to differentiate beyond a certain point *in vivo*.

Studies of the common ALL antigen in another leukemia, chronic myelogenous leukemia, are also suggestive of spontaneous *in vivo* changes in leukemic cell phenotypes. During the initial chronic phase of the disease, the cALL antigen is undetectable. As the disease progresses CML typically develops an acute phase or blast crisis. In a minority of patients in blast crisis the leukemic cells have a lymphoid-like morphology, bear the common ALL antigen and are responsive to an ALL-like induction regimen (Beard et al. 1976; Janossy et al. 1977). Those observations led Janossy et al. (1976) to postulate that in some cases of CML the leukemic stem cell has the common ALL phentype and that its normal counterpart might be a precursor of both lymphoid and myeloid lines. It is this more primitive cell type which becomes the dominant cell in blast crisis. These observations demonstrate the coincidence of changes in disease course and drug responsiveness with changes in leukemic cell surface phenotype in a second human leukemia. How generalizable these observations are to other malignancies is unknown. Such generalization would certainly depend upon the underlying mechanism or mechanisms whereby the malignant cells escape total destruction, express drug resistance and regrow. In the examples presented the blasts with a growth advantage may also be the least differentiated or the least antigenic variants of the original cell population. At present the many alternative explanations for phenotypic shifts in blast phenotype cannot be distinguished. An understanding of the mechanism of unstable blast phenotype might, however, provide a clue to the selective and/or adaptive processes which permit recurrence of leukemia.

ACKNOWLEDGMENTS
The author wishes to express her gratitude to Drs. John Aur, Paul Bowman, Gary Dahl, Gaston Rivera, and other members of the leukemia service at St. Jude Children's Research Hospital for providing leukemia specimens. Skillful technical assistance was provided by Ms. Pamela Watkins and Mr. Robert Greene, Jr. Excellent secretarial assistance was provided by Ms. Linda Wood. This work was supported by Cancer Center Support Grant CA21765-02 from the National Cancer Institute, and by ALSAC.

## References

Aur, R.J.A. et al. 1978. Childhood acute lymphotic leukemia—Study VIII. Blood 42:2123–2134.

Beard, M.E. et al. 1976. Blast crisis of chronic myeloid leukemia (CML). I. Presentation simulating acute lymphoid leukemia (ALL). Br. J. Haematol. 34:167–178.

Billing, R.J. et al. 1976. Human B-lymphocyte antigens expressed by lymphocytic and myelocytic leukemia cells. I. Detection by rabbit antisera. J. Exp. Med. 144:167–178.

Borella, L. and Sen, L. 1975. E receptors on blasts from untreated acute lymphocytic leukemia (ALL): Comparison of temperature dependence of E-rosettes formed by normal and leukemic lymphoid cells. J. Immunol. 114:187–190.

Borella, L. et al. 1979. Shifts in expression of cell membrane phenotypes in childhood lymphoid malignancies at relapse. Blood 54:64–71.

Bowman, W.P. et al. 1981. Cell markers in acute lymphocytic leukemia: A clinical perspective. Cancer Res., in press.

Broder, S. et al. 1978. Characterization of a suppressor-cell leukemia. Evidence for the requirement of an interaction of two T-cells in the development of human suppressor effector cells. N. Engl. J. Med. 298:66–72.

Brown, G. et al. 1975. Leukemia-associated antigens in man. J. Natl. Cancer Inst. 55:1281–1289.

Evans, R.L. et al. 1978. Peripheral human T-cells sensitized in mixed leukocyte culture synthesize and express *I*a-like antigens. J. Exp. Med. 148:1440–1445.

Fialkow, P.J. et al. 1967. Clonal origin of chronic myelocytic leukemia in man. Proc. Natl. Acad. Sci. U.S.A. 58:1468–1471.

Fialkow, P.J. et al. 1973. Immunoglobulin and glucose-6-phosphate dehydrogenase as markers of cellular origin in Burkitt lymphoma. J. Exp. Med. 138:89–102.

Galili, U. and Schlesinger, M. 1976. The formation of stable E-rosettes by human T-lymphocytes activated in mixed lymphocyte reactions. J. Immunol. 117:730–735.

Gathings, W.E. et al. 1977. Immunofluorescent studies of the development of pre-B-cells, B-lymphocytes and immunoglobulin isotype diversity in humans. Eur. J. Immunol. 7:804–810.

George, S.L. et al. 1979. A reappraisal of the results of stopping therapy in childhood leukemia. N. Engl. J. Med. 300:269–273.

Gergely, P. et al. 1974. Spontaneous and PHA-induced rosetting of human blood, tonsil lymphocytes, and MLC blasts with sheep, human, and horse erythrocytes. Clin. Exp. Im unol. 25:23–27.

Greaves, M.F. et al. 1975. Antisera to acute lymphoblastic leukemia cells. Clin. Immunol. Immunopathol. 4:67–84.

Greaves, M.F. et al. 1977. Membrane phenotyping: Diagnosis, monitoring and classification of acute "lymphoid" leukemias. Hematol. Blood Transfus. 20:61–75.

Greenwood, M.F. et al. 1977. Terminal deoxynucleotidyl transferase distribution in neoplastic and hematopoietic cells. J. Clin. Invest. 59:889–899.

Hurwitz, R.L. et al. 1979. Characterization of a leukemic cell line of the pre-B phenotype. Int. J. Cancer 23:174–180.

Janossy, G. et al. 1976. Target cell in chronic lyeloid leukemia and its relationship to acute lymphocytic leukemia. Lancet 2:1058–1061.

Janossy, G. et al. 1977. Comparative analysis of membrane phenotypes in acute lymphoid leukemia and in lymphoid blast crisis of chronic myeloid leukemia. Leukemia Res. 1:289–300.

Levin. D.L. et al. 1974. Cancer rates and risks. U.S. Department of Health, Education and Welfare Bulletin 1:75–691.

Melvin, S.L. 1981. Immunologic definition of leukemic cell surface phenotypes. Cancer Res., in press.

Melvin, S.L. 1979. Comparison of techniques for detecting T-cell acute lymphocytic leukemia. Blood 54:210–215.

Miller, D.R. 1975. Prognostic factors in childhood leukemia. J. Pediatr. 87:672–676.

Miller, R.W. 1967. Persons with exceptionally high risk of leukemia. Cancer Res. 27:2420–2423.

Miller, R.W. 1976. The feature in common among persons at high risk of leukemia. In Biology of Radiation Carcinogenesis. J.M. Yuhas, R.W. Tennant, and J.D. Regan, eds. New York: Raven Press.

Mills, B. et al. 1975. Reactivity of antihuman thymocyte serum with acute leukemia blasts. J. Immunol. 115:1038–1044.

Minowada, J. et al. 1978. Human leukemia cell lines: Evidence for differentiation toward T- and B-cell axis within a leukemia. A.A.R.C. Abstr. 19:109.

Minowada, J. et al. 1979. A Philadelphia chromosome positive human leukaemia cell line (NALM-1) with pre-B characteristics. Leukemia Res. 3:261–266.

Murphy, S.B. et al. 1977. Pretreatment cytokinetic studies in 94 children with acute leukemia. Relationship to other variables at diagnosis and to outcome of standard treatment. Blood 49:683–691.

Ohnuma, T. et al. 1978. Differential chemotherapeutic susceptibility of human T-lymphocytes and B-lymphocytes in culture. J. Natl. Cancer Inst. 60:749–752.

Pearl, E.R. et al. 1978. B-lymphocyte precursers in human bone marrow. J. Immunol. 120:1169–1175.

Pullen, J. et al. 1981. Southwest Oncology Group experience with immunologic phenotyping in acute lymphoblastic leukemia of childhood. Cancer Res., in press.

Rastrick, J.M. et al. 1968. Direct evidence for presence of Ph′ chromosome in erythroid cells. Br. Med. J. 1:96–98.

Reinherz, E.L. and Schlossman, S.F. 1980. The differentiation and function of human T-lymphocytes. Cell 19:821–827.

Ritz, J. et al. 1981. Monoclonal antibodies specific for acute lymphoblastic leukemia cells. Cancer Res., in press.

Roberts, M. et al. 1978. Acute lymphoblastic leukemia (ALL) associated antigen. I. Expression in different hematopoietic malignancies. Leukemia Res. 2:105–114.

Schlossman, S.F. et al. 1976. Distribution of *Ia*-like molecules on the surface of normal and leukemic cells. Proc. Natl. Acad. Sci. U.S.A. 73:1288–1292.

Simone, J.V. et al. 1975. Initial features and prognosis in 363 children with acute lymphocytic leukemia. Cancer 36:2099–2108.

Smyth, J.F. et al. 1981. The clinical pharmacology of the adenosine deaminase inhibitor 2′-deoxycoformycin. Cancer Res., in press.

Tsukimoto, I. et al. 1976. Surface markers and prognostic factors in acute lympholastic leukemia. N. Engl. J. Med. 294:245–248.

Vogler, L.B. et al. 1978. Pre-B cell leukemia. A new phenotype of childhood lymphoblastic leukemia. N. Engl. J. Med. 298:872–878.

Woolf, L.J. et al. 1976. Poor prognosis of children with acute lymphocytic leukemia and increased B-cell markers. J. Pediatr. 89:956–958.

Yarbro, G.S.K. et al. 1977. Glucocorticoid receptors in subpopulations of childhood acute lymphocytic leukemia. Cancer Res. 37:2688–2695.

Hildemann, ed. Frontiers in Immunogenetics

# Epidemiology and Genetics of Insulin Dependent Diabetes Mellitus in the White and Black Population from the Southeastern United States

Ronald T. Acton, Bruce O. Barger, Buris R. Boshell, Rodney C.P. Go, Catherine C. Murphy, Pamela J. Reitnauer, and Jeffrey M. Roseman

*Departments of Microbiology, Public Health, and Medicine, and Immunogenetics Unit of the Diabetes Research and Training Center, University of Alabama in Birmingham, University Station, Birmingham, Alabama*

## Introduction

It is now recognized that idiopathic diabetes mellitus is a genetically determined group of heterogenous disorders which all have glucose intolerance in common (National Diabetes Data Group 1979). The two major clinical types of diabetes are now classified as insulin-dependent diabetes mellitus (IDDM) and non-insulin-dependent diabetes mellitus (NIDDM). IDDM, previously termed juvenile-onset diabetes, is characterized by an abrupt, early age of onset, a lack of stimulated insulin output and a tendency to develop ketoacidosis. NIDDM, which was called maturity-onset diabetes, occurs primiarily in middle or older age groups although it can be found in the young (Fajans, et al. 1976). Although insulin is not required in this type of diabetes to prevent ketosis it may be used to correct fasting hyperglycemia, which can be achieved in many patients with diet and/or use of oral agents. A large percentage of patients with this type of diabetes are obese. In addition to the aforementioned clinical parameters, there is compelling evidence that these two forms of diabetes are genetically distinct disorders Tattersall and Pyke (1972) observed that 50% of monozygotic twin pairs are discordant for IDDM whereas nearly all the twins were concordant for NIDDM. Moreover, MacDonald (1974) observed an equal incidence of NIDDM among ancestors of IDDM subjects and non-diabetics. As will be discussed, HLA is associated with IDDM but not NIDDM and is another means that can be used to distinguish between the two types of diabetes (Nerup et al. 1976). In addition to the evidence for genetic heterogeneity, there is also substantial data pointing to different etiological and pathological mechanisms which contribute to generating various types of diabetes (Acton and Roseman 1978).

At this juncture, much is known about the epidemiological and possible etiological factors contributing to onset of IDDM. For example, the prevalence of IDDM has been estimated in several populations. Gorwitz et al. (1976) as well as Kyllo and Nuttal (1978) estimated the prevalence in Michigan and Minnesota school-age children to be 1.6 to 1.9 cases per thousand. Based on the data reported by Cudworth (1978), Spielman et al. (1980) estimated a prevalence of 2.6/1000. Large scale health surveys have estimated the prevalence of diabetes in individuals up to the age of 45 as 5.9 to 8.1 per thousand (Sayetta and Murphy 1979). These latter data are subject to doubt since all types of diabetes are included. Diabetes registries in Great Britian (Bloom et al. 1975) and Denmark (Christau et al. 1977) have provided data on the incidence of the disease. In Great Britain, the incidence of diabetes under the age of 16 was 7.67/100,000, while in Denmark for diabetes occurring under the age of 30, it was 13.2/100,000. The peak age of onset in Britain was 11 years with a secondary peak near 5 years, while the peak in Denmark was 12 to 14 years. The distribution of IDDM by sex has been observed in most studies to be fairly equal. Age of onset was often found to vary in the British and Denmark registries by sex, with females preceeding males by one to two years. From these registries as well as the report by West et al. (1978), it appears autumn and winter represent the highest seasons of onset. Consistent with the seasonal occurrence of IDDM is the data which reveals a significant positive correlation between the incidence of various virus infections and increased antibody titers to these agents (Craighead 1978). Coxsackie B4 and mumps have often been implicated as the causative agents of IDDM. In fact, Yoon et al. (1979) isolated Coxsackie B4 from the pancreas of a subject who expired after an acute onset of IDDM. Following the onset of IDDM, pancreatic islet cell antibodies and evidence of cell-mediated immunity to these cells can be demonstrated as well (Irvine et al. 1976; Bottazzo et al. 1978; Nerup et al. 1971).

The initial finding by Singal and Blajchmann (1973) that HLA-B15 is associated with IDDM generated enthusiasm for further studies aimed at understanding the genetics. Since these initial findings, the HLA antigens B8, B15, Cw3, Dw3, Dw4, DR3, and DR4 have been found to be significantly associated with IDDM in various white populations, while B7 and Dw2 are significantly decreased (Ryder et al. 1979; Cudworth 1978; Christy et al. 1979; Barbosa et al. 1977; Suciu-Foca et al. 1979; Farid et al. 1979). The HLA specificity associated with IDDM has been found to vary among various racial and ethnic groups. For example, Bw54 and B12 are significantly increased in Japanese IDDM subjects (Nakao et al. 1977; Kawa et al. 1978). In addition, Aw30 has been reported significantly increased in the Italian IDDM population Aw26 in Jewish IDDM patients (Illeni et al. 1977; Gazit et al. 1977).

There have been a number of studies to determine if the IDDM susceptibility gene(s) is linked to the major histocompatibility complex. The most revealing information has come from studies involving multiply affected IDDM families.

Cudworth and Woodrow (1975), Rubinstein et al. (1977), Bengsch et al. (1978), and Barbosa et al. (1977) all found an increased concordance of HLA haplotypes between diabetic sib pairs compared with diabetic/healthy sibs. Both Rubinstein et al. (1977) and Barbosa et al. (1977) state that their data support an autosomal recessive mode of inheritance of the IDDM susceptibility gene(s) with 50% penetrance. The latter investigator found linkage of the IDDM susceptibility gene and the major histocompatibility complex on chromosome 6 at a recombination fraction of 13% and a lod score of 3.98.

Although other genetic markers have been reported associated with IDDM, the data has not been as impressive as for HLA. Many of these studies were conducted before diabetes was grouped into various clinical types. These include studies of the blood group antigens (McConnell et al. 1956; Andersen and Lauritzen 1960; Buckwalter 1964; Berg et al. 1967) and the ability to taste phenylthiocarbamide (PTC) (Terry and Segal 1947; Harris et al. 1949; Terry 1950). Recently Vague et al. (1978) observed that the Lewis negative (Le a – b –) red blood cell phenotype was found 3 times more frequently in diabetics regardless of clinical types than in controls. This data has been disputed by Leslie and Pyke (1979). Lucarelli et al. (1978) investigated the distribution of nine genetic polymorphic systems in IDDM patients and healthy controls. They found a significant decrease of the red cell acid phosphatase; the CB phenotype was found decreased in male IDDM patients while the distribution in females was similar to controls. Moreover, the B phenotype of the ABO blood group in the female IDDM patients and MM homozygotes in male IDDM patients were significantly increased.

We began an investigation of the IDDM white and black patient population in the southeastern United States over 2 years ago. The aim was to correlate the epidemiology, genetics and natural history of the disease in a clinically well defined population. At the initiation of the study, there was a paucity of data on the IDDM population in the United States with regard to the aforementioned parameters. Moreover, little information was available on the black population which was of particular interest, since previous studies had indicated that IDDM in blacks from primitive and developing African areas is rare (Jackson and Huskisson 1965). In the United States, it has been observed that the prevalence of this disease in young black Americans is higher than in the African black population but less than in American whites (Sultz et al. 1972; MacDonald 1975). We now present our findings to date on the epidemiology and association of IDDM with a number of genetic polymorphisms as well as linkage of the IDDM susceptibility gene to the major histocompatibility complex.

## Materials and Methods

### *Sample*

The subjects for this study included 386 unrelated white IDDM patients and 201 healthy controls as well as 87 black IDDM patients and 335 healthy controls. HLA typing was done on 209 white IDDM patients and 195 controls. In the black sample, 75 IDDM patients and 243 controls were HLA typed. There were 30 multiply-affected IDDM white families. Of these, 25 were sib pairs and five parent-child combinations. These multiply-affected families constituted approximately 9% of all the IDDM families examined. The controls did not have first degree relatives with diabetes of any type nor second degree relatives with IDDM. A fasting blood sugar was obtained on all controls and no abnormal results were found. The criteria of IDDM used for inclusion in this study were age of onset less than forty years, insulin dependence, ketosis prone, and non-obese.

The IDDM patients were obtained from the inpatient and outpatient clinics of the Diabetes Research and Training Center (DRTC), Children's Hospital as well as Cooper Green Hospital of the University of Alabama in Birmingham, camps for juvenile-onset diabetics sponsored by the Alabama and Louisiana Affiliates of the American Diabetes Association (ADA), and the Alabama State Registry of IDDM. A retrospective medical record review of the DRTC identified several of the IDDM patients used in this study. The multiply affected families were also identified this way.

### *Tissue Typing*

A microdroplet lymphocyte cytotoxicity test, as described by Mittal et al. (1968) with modifications by Terasaki et al. (1978) was utilized for HLA-A and -B typing. Antisera obtained from our own screening program, Dr. Paul Terasaki, and NIH were utilized for HLA typing. This allowed for the use of at least 2 different antisera for each antigen tested. The antigens tested were A1, 2, 3, 11, w23, w24, 25, 26, 28, 29, w30, w31, w32, w33, w34, w36, B7, 8, 13, 14, 15, 17, 18, 27, w35, 37 w38, w39, 40, w41, w42, w44, w45, w49, w50, w51, and w52. For DR typing, B-lymphocytes were isolated by nylon wool column extraction. The antigens tested were DR1, 2, 3, 4, 5, and 7. The typings for 30 of the black patients as well as 36 controls and 11 multiply-affected white families were verified with antisera series w13, w14, w15, w16, and w17 from the Eighth International Histocompatibility Workshop.

To insure reliability of HLA typing, several controls were used. Within each tray, there were positive and negative controls used as references for that individual tray. The processing and typing was checked internally by submitting known samples for reevaluation. An external check came from participation in the International Cell Exchange (Bernoco et al. 1978). Cells for HLA typing were received from the cell exchange for typing and the results sent back and checked for accuracy.

Each lot of complement used in the assays was checked for cytotoxicity. This was done by plating the complement, anti-lymphocyte serum, and cells to check for reactions. The highest dilution of complement which gave a positive reaction (usually in the range 1:1 to 1:8) was used.

### *Blood Group Typing*

The red blood cell assays were conducted using the standard procedures described in the Technical Manual of the American Association of Blood Banks (Miller 1977). The antigens of the ABO and Lewis systems were detected using the direct assay methods. The reagent vendor was Gamma Biologic, Inc.

### *PTC Taste Response*

The taste response to PTC was performed by a modification of the procedure described by Harris and Kalmus (1950). A saturated stock solution at 18°C was made and dilutions carried out to give the concentrations described by Hartmann (1939). A threshold value of 4 was chosen which, as described by Hartmann, is at the lower limit for detecting tasters and at the border where one expects to find a few tasters scoring as non-tasters. Subjects were asked to swirl a few milliliters of either deionized $H_2O$ or PTC from coded cups around in their mouths and their taste response registered by a trained interviewer.

### *Statistical Analysis*

The HLA phenotype frequencies for the IDDM patients and controls were analyzed by a maximum likelihood method as described by Mittal (1976). The comparisons of HLA frequencies between IDDM patients and controls were made by the likelihood ratio asymptotic chi square. The relative risks were estimated by Woolf's (1955) method. Some investigators have multiplied the p-values by the number of antigens tested, Bonferroni inequality, to minimize the possibility of an antigen showing an altered frequency by chance. This approach may be too conservative, so it has been suggested that results be compared with other published studies or that a second series of cases be investigated (Rahi 1979; Svejgaard 1976). We therefore chose not to multiply the p-value by the number of antigens tested.

The IDDM patients were analyzed for sex, season of onset, and age of onset using the chi square test for discrete variables and the Student's t-test for continuous variables. The chi square test was used for all discrete variable analysis of HLA antigens by the epidemiologic features (age, sex, season, age of onset).

The frequencies for concordance of haplotypes between sib pairs was determined by chi square analysis. The Student's t-test was used in the analysis of season of onset and age of onset differences between haploidentical and HLA identical sib pairs, as well as parent-child IDDM's.

Linkage analysis was performed using the computer program GENPED (Elston and Kaplan) which uses the Elston and Stewart (1973) algorithm for two linked loci. The method of Elston and Stewart (1973) was used to calculate the likelihood of two genetic models, autosomal recessive and autosomal dominant. In the likelihood analysis, a disease prevalence of 0.0026 was used and the penetrance varied from 0.2–0.6. The same parameter estimates were used in calculating the lod scores as suggested by Spielman et al. (1980).

## Results

### *Epidemiology*

Table 1 compares the characteristics of the IDDM patients and control subjects that were sampled for the population analysis (Murphy et al. 1980a; Reitnauer et al. 1980). A total of 87 black and 386 white IDDM patients were analyzed. The proportion of males to females in both races were equivalent and approximately

**Table 1.** Characteristics of Subjects Sampled from the Southeastern United States.

| | Controls | | IDDM patients | |
|---|---|---|---|---|
| | White | Black | White | Black |
| No. of subjects | 335 | 271 | 87 | 386 |
| Sex | | | | |
| Male | 38% | 46% | 60% | 45% |
| Female | 62% | 54% | 40% | 55% |
| Age, years | | | | |
| Mean ± SEM | 25.6 ± 0.4 | 26.7 ± 0.5 | 21.6 ± 1.2 | 20.4 ± 0.63 |
| Range | 14.1 − 54.5 | 9.9 − 56.3 | 4.5 − 45.4 | 2.5 − 81.6 |
| Age at onset, years | | | | |
| Mean ± SEM | | | 15.2 ± 1.1 | 12.5 ± 0.38 |
| Range | | | 0.25 + 38.7 | 0.75 ± 39 |
| Peak months of onset | | | April, May | Jan., June, July |

50%. The mean age of both black and white IDDM patients was approximately the same although the range of age was not quite as broad in the black patients sampled. The mean age of onset of disease was approximately 3 years greater in the black as compared with the white patients. However, the range was nearly the same in both groups. Using date of appearance of first symptoms as date of onset, the peak onset was found to be April and May for the black patient population as compared with January for the white patients. In the white patient population, there was a slightly smaller peak in June and July as well. The season of onset was not found to vary significantly by age of onset.

### *HLA Associations*

The frequencies of those HLA antigens which were found to significantly deviate between the patient and control populations are listed in Table 2 (Murphy et al. 1980a; Reitnauer et al. 1980). B8, B15, and B18 were all found to be increased in the white IDDM patients sampled. However, the increase in B18 was not found to be statistically significant. The estimated relative risks for IDDM in white individuals who possess B8, B15, and B18 were 2.4, 1.9, and 1.8, respectively. B7 and B14 were found significantly decreased in this population of IDDM subjects compared to bealthy controls. The strongest associations with IDDM were found for the DR antigens. Of the 104 IDDM white patients that were HLA typed, DR3 and DR4 were found to be significantly increased while DR2 and DR7 were decreased. DR2 was not found in the patient population sampled. The strongest association was with DR4 with a relative risk of 12.2. In the black IDDM patients, B8, B13, and B15 were found significantly increased as compared with healthy controls. The relative risks for B8, B13, and B15 were calculated as 2.4, 2.8, and 5.7, respectively. B14 was not found in any of the 75 patients, but in 4.9% of the control population. Also, in the black patient population, DR3, DR4, as well as DR7 were found to be increased. Again, the stronger association was with DR4 with a relative risk of 4.9. DR2 and DR5 were both significantly decreased in this

**Table 2.** Frequencies (%) of HLA Antigens Found to Significantly Deviate Between IDDM Patients and Controls.

| | Whites | | | | Blacks | | | |
|---|---|---|---|---|---|---|---|---|
| HLA antigen | PF[a] IDDM (N = 209) | PF controls (N = 195) | RR[b] | P[c] | PF IDDM (N = 75) | PF controls (N = 243) | RR | P |
| B8 | 36.4 | 19.0 | 2.4 | <0.0001 | 16.0 | 7.4 | 2.4 | <0.03 |
| B13 | — | — | — | — | 5.3 | 0.8 | 6.8 | <0.02 |
| B15 | 25.4 | 15.4 | 1.9 | <0.01 | 10.7 | 2.1 | 5.7 | <0.002 |
| B18 | 16.8 | 10.3 | 1.8 | <0.06 | — | — | — | — |
| B7 | 13.4 | 21.0 | 0.6 | <0.04 | — | — | — | — |
| B14 | 1.4 | 9.7 | 0.1 | <0.0001 | 0 | 4.9 | — | <0.01 |
| | (N = 104) | (N = 79) | | | (N = 57) | (N = 104) | | |
| DR3 | 57.7 | 32.9 | 2.6 | <0.0008 | 52.6 | 26.9 | 3.0 | <0.0012 |
| DR4 | 66.4 | 13.9 | 12.2 | <0.0001 | 31.6 | 8.7 | 4.9 | <0.0003 |
| DR7 | 4.8 | 26.6 | 0.1 | <0.0001 | 28.1 | 12.5 | 2.7 | <0.02 |
| DR2 | 0.0 | 34.2 | — | <0.0001 | 1.8 | 37.5 | 0.03 | <0.0001 |
| DR5 | — | — | — | — | 3.5 | 26.9 | 0.10 | <0.0001 |

[a]PF = Phenotype frequencies.

[b]RR = Relative risk computed by Woolf's, 1955 method.

[c]P = Level of statistical significance.

**Table 3.** Relative Risks of IDDM for White Individuals Possessing Various HLA-B and -DR Phenotypes.

| HLA phenotype | Relative risk | Chi square | P |
|---|---|---|---|
| B8,BX | 1.5 | 2.59 | NS |
| B8,B8 | 10.6 | 7.69 | <0.01 |
| B15,BX | 1.1 | 0.22 | NS |
| B15,B15 | 3.1 | 2.10 | NS |
| B8,B15 | 15.2 | 11.92 | <0.001 |
| DR3,DRX | 0.4 | 5.00 | <0.05 |
| DR3,DR3 | 4.7 | 4.60 | <0.05 |
| DR4,DRX | 1.2 | 0.99 | NS |
| DR4,DR4 | 13.5 | 9.19 | <0.01 |
| DR3,DR4 | 20.7 | 28.84 | <0.001 |

NS = Not significant; P value greater than 0.05.

patient population. Thus, B8, B15, DR3, and DR4 were increased significantly while DR2 was decreased in both the white and black IDDM population.

Some interesting associations were found when the relative risks of IDDM were assessed in white individuals possessing various HLA-B and -DR phenotypes. As can be seen in Table 3, a white individual homozygous for B8 or possessing B8 and B15 is at a much greater risk for developing IDDM than one possessing B8 or B15 in combination with other *B* locus antigens or a *B* locus blank. Of the individuals who were typed B8/Blank or B15/Blank, it was estimated from the gene frequencies in our population the number which would be homozygotes or heterozygotes. It is interesting to note that a white individual homozygous for either DR3 or DR4 is also at an increased risk for IDDM as opposed to possessing either DR3 or DR4 alone. A white individual possessing both DR3 and DR4 is at a significantly greater risk (RR = 20.7) for developing IDDM than for any other of the phenotype combinations. A sufficient number of black IDDM patients were not available to conduct a similar analysis.

Table 4 is a compilation of four 2 × 2 contingency tables, illustrating that B15 alone does not appear to be significantly associated with IDDM in our white patient population. B8 and DR3 are in linkage disequilibrium in our white control as well as IDDM patient population with a delta value of 0.0145, whereas B15 and DR4 are not. Therefore, as seen in this table, when the presence or absence of B15 is held constant and the presence or absence of DR4 in the white IDDM patient population is compared versus the healthy controls, the latter antigen is always found to be significantly associated with the disease. At the present there are not enough black IDDM patients in our sample to conduct a similar analysis.

## *PTC Taste Response Associations*

Data published more than 30 years ago suggest that the inability to taste PTC is associated with diabetes (Terry and Segall 1947; Terry 1950). Due to the fact that these observations were made before diabetes was separated into various clinical

**Table 4.** Stratified Association of HLA-B15 and -DR4 with IDDM in the White Population.

| | HLA-B15⁺ | | | | HLA-B15⁻ | | | |
|---|---|---|---|---|---|---|---|---|
| | IDDM | Controls | RR | P | IDDM | Controls | RR | P |
| $DR4^+$ | 20 | 3 | 6.7 | <0.01 | 49 | 8 | 7.4 | <0.0001 |
| $DR4^-$ | 7 | 7 | | | 54 | 65 | | |
| | **$DR4^+$** | | | | **$DR4^-$** | | | |
| $B15^+$ | 20 | 3 | 1.1 | NS | 7 | 7 | 0.9 | NS |
| $B15^-$ | 49 | 8 | | | 96 | 66 | | |

subtypes, we decided to reinvestigate this possibility (Acton et al., unpublished observations). As can be seen in Table 5, a significant association was observed between the ability to taste PTC and IDDM in our black population. Therefore, black individuals who can taste PTC have a 2.7 fold greater risk for developing IDDM over those who cannot taste this substance.

Other investigators have reported an association between ABO as well as Lewis blood group antigens and diabetes (McConnell et al. 1956; Andersen and Lauritzen 1960; Buckwalter 1964; Berg et al. 1967; Lucarelli et al. 1978; Vague et al. 1978; Leslie and Pyke 1979). We therefore conducted a study which included 160 white and 50 black IDDM subjects in order to compare the frequency of ABO and Lewis blood group antigens with data obtained from 78 white and 137 black healthy controls. No statistically significant associations between these blood group antigens and IDDM in the two patient populations were found.

### *Linkage Analysis*

The next series of investigations were aimed at establishing the mode of inheritance of IDDM and to determine if the susceptibility gene(s) was linked to the major histocompatibility complex. To date we have only been able to obtain a sufficient number of white families where more than one individual is affected with IDDM for these analyses (Murphy et al. 1980b). Twenty-five sib-sib and 5 parent-child

**Table 5.** The Frequency (%) of PTC[a] Taster State in IDDM Patients and Controls.

| | White | | | Black | | |
|---|---|---|---|---|---|---|
| PTC | Controls (N = 113) | IDDM (N = 312) | P | Controls (N = 207) | IDDM (N = 61) | P |
| + | 42.2 | 42.6 | | 23.7 | 45.9 | |
| − | 57.8 | 56.4 | NS | 76.3 | 54.1 | <0.001 |

[a]PTC—phenylthiocarbamide.

**Table 6.** Haplotype Concordance for (24) Diabetic Sib Pairs.

| | 2 Haplotypes | 1 Haplotype | 0 Haplotype |
|---|---|---|---|
| Observed | 12 (50%) | 12 (50%) | 0 (0%) |
| Expected | 6 (25%) | 12 (50%) | 6 (25%) |

$X^2 = 12$; df = 2; $p < 0.01$.

families which contained a total of 62 IDDM individuals and 98 unaffected subjects have been investigated. The observed and expected haplotype concordance among 24 affected sib pairs is shown in Table 6. One family was not included due to the observation of a cross-over in one of the sib pairs. Twelve of these 24 sib pairs were found to share 2 haplotypes and 12 shared 1 haplotype. None of the affected sib pairs were discordant for both haplotypes. These findings were significantly different from the expected values of 25%, 50%, and 25% for the sharing of 2, 1, and 0 haplotypes, respectively (Mattiuz et al. 1970). As can be seen in Table 7, when the haplotypes were compared between the IDDM proband and healthy sibs, there was no significant difference in the haplotype segregation observed from that expected.

The data from all 30 families were next analyzed for linkage. These data are summarized in Table 8. As can be seen, a prevalence for IDDM of 0.0026 was assumed. When the lod scores were summed over the 30 pedigrees, the total lod score was found to be at a maximum of 2.46 at ($\Theta_M = \Theta_F$) = 0.0 for an autosomal dominant model where gene frequency (q) = 0.0029 and penetrance (f) = 0.39. The stability of the lod score calculated under the dominant model was further studied by varying the gene frequencies used in the calculations from 0.003 to 0.033 (f = 0.4). This gave a maximum variation of only 4.6% at $\Theta = 0.0$. When penetrance was varied from 0.2 to 0.6, an inverse relationship with the lod score was observed. Of the 30 families used in these analyses, 5 had a parent and child affected with IDDM. A negative lod score of −0.63 was calculated for these families alone. However, a lod score of 3.09 was calculated when only the data from families with at least a sib pair affected with IDDM were utilized. When calculations were performed to compare the likelihoods of a recessive mode versus

**Table 7.** Haplotype Concordance for Diabetic:Healthy Sibs from (25) Families.

| | 2 Haplotypes | 1 Haplotype | 0 Haplotype |
|---|---|---|---|
| Observed | 13 (34.2%) | 19 (50%) | 6 (15.8%) |
| Expected | 9.5 (25%) | 19 (50%) | 9.5 (25%) |

$X^2 = 2.61$; df = 2; p = not significant.

**Table 8.** Maximum Likelihood Parameter Estimates and Lod Scores Obtained for Linkage Between the Gene for Susceptibility to IDDM and HLA (30 Families).

| | Recessive | | Dominant | |
|---|---|---|---|---|
| Prevalence | 0.0026[a] | 0.0026[a] | 0.0026[a] | 0.0026[a] |
| $\theta_M = \theta_F$ | 0.5[a] | 0.217 | 0.5[a] | 0.0 |
| q | 0.0525 | 0.0541 | 0.0033 | 0.0029 |
| $f_{AA}$ | 0.9419 | 0.8886 | 0.4431 | 0.3942 |
| $f_{Aa}$ | 0.0 | 0.0 | 0.4431 | 0.3942 |
| $f_{aa}$ | 0.0 | 0.0 | 0.0 | 0.0 |
| Log likelihood | −239.158 | −237.706 | −236.268 | −233.810 |
| Lod score | | 1.45 | | 2.46 |

[a]Parameters fixed at these values.
q = gene frequency; f = penetrance; $\theta$ = recombination fraction.

a dominant mode of inheritance for the IDDM susceptibility gene(s), the dominant mode was found 7879 times more likely if linkage was assumed. If free recombination between HLA and the IDDM susceptibility gene(s) was assumed, the dominant mode of inheritance was 779 times more likely than the recessive mode.

## Discussion

This report represents the first detailed analysis of the epidemiology and genetic features of IDDM in the white and black population of the southeastern United States.

The epidemiologic data obtained in this sample differs somewhat from that reported for other populations. The peak age of onset of 9 years observed in our white sample is younger than two other studies of IDDM subjects in the U.S. Fleegler et al. (1979) reported a peak age of onset of 12 years whereas White and Graham (1971) observed 11 years. This difference may result from the fact that we obtained a large portion of the sample from summer camps for juvenile diabetics, which resulted in a selection bias toward younger subjects. The females in our study had an earlier age of onset (peak 8–9 years) than the males (peak 10 years) which agrees with the findings of others in the U.S., Britain, Denmark, and Canada (White and Graham 1971; Christau et al. 1977; West et al. 1979; Bloom et al. 1975). There was a larger number of males in the 0–4 year age group as reported by Bloom et al. (1975) in Britain and West et al. (1979) in Montreal. We were unable to find in the current literature age of onset data for black IDDM subjects.

The season of onset data obtained by us for white IDDM subjects is similar to that for the Southern as well as Northern Hemisphere reported by others (Bloom et al. 1975; Christau et al. 1977; Gamble and Taylor 1969; MacMillan et al. 1977; Fleeger et al. 1979; West et al. 1979). Throughout the world, the incidence of onset of IDDM is highest during the fall and winter months. Although there are no reports by others to compare with our black season of onset data, the spring peak months of onset (April, May) are different than that for white IDDM subjects. At present we have no explanation for this difference.

The association of B8 and B15 with IDDM in our white subjects agrees with the findings of others in a number of different countries (see Christy et al. 1979 and Ryder et al. 1979 for review). This includes Austria, Australia, Britain, Canada, Denmark, Finland, Germany, Ireland, Israel, Italy, and the U.S. (Ludwig et al. 1977; Zimmet et al. 1979; Farid et al. 1978; Nerup et al. 1974; Koivisto et al. 1977; Ilonen et al. 1980; Bengsch et al. 1978; Singal and Blajchmann 1973; Solow et al. 1978; Fitzgerald and Drury 1978; Gazit et al. 1977; Illeni et al. 1977; Barbosa et al. 1978; Suciu-Foca et al. 1977). Although other antigens have been shown to be positively associated with IDDM in various white populations and ethnic groups, B8 and B15 are most consistently found. B7 has also been shown to be negatively associated with the disease in many of these studies. In our black IDDM sample, B8 and B15 as well as B13 were found positively associated with the disease. Briggs et al. (1980) did not find an increase of B8 and B15 in IDDM subjects from a southern African black tribe (Xhosa). DR3 and DR4 were both significantly increased in our white and black IDDM subjects. The results of HLA association studies of several racial and ethnic groups as part of the Eighth International Histocompatibility Workshop demonstrated this same association, with the exception that DR3 and DR4 in the Japanese IDDM population was not increased but DRw8 was instead (Svejgaard et al. 1980). Moreover, while DR4 was increased in African black patients, DR3 was not. Maeda et al. (1980) have recently reported that DR3 is significantly increased in Chinese IDDM patients. The workshop report also agreed with our findings that the highest risk for IDDM is found in subjects possessing the DR3,4 phenotype. In our white IDDM sample, B8 and DR3 are both independently associated with the disease. The workshop report found the B8 association to be entirely secondary to the increase of DR3. However, our data agrees with the workshop report that the increase of B15 is secondary to increases of DR4 in this disease.

Our findings of an association of the ability to taste PTC and IDDM in negroid subjects is interesting in light of previous data. Kitchin et al. (1959) and Farid et al. (1977) have shown an association with the PTC taster state and autoimmune thyroid disease. The latter group of investigators found that persons who are PTC tasters and possess B8 have an increased risk of developing the disease. Terry and Segall (1947), in a small sample of 11 black diabetics, found all could taste PTC, while 20.4% of the controls were taste blind. Harris et al. (1949) found no difference between the taste response of 103 black diabetics and healthy controls. Terry (1950), in a study of 13 black negroid diabetics, found all could taste PTC. In addition to the small sample sizes these studies were conducted before diabetes was grouped into various disorders. We have not found a significant difference between black NIDDM and healthy subjects with respect to the PTC taste response.

We failed to confirm reports that various ABO and Lewis blood groups are associated with IDDM in either of the races sampled (McConnell et al. 1956; Andersen and Lauritzen 1960; Buckwalter 1964; Berg et al. 1967; Vague et al.

1978; Lucarelli et al. 1978). Again this is perhaps due to a lack of strict ascertainment of the subjects to be studied with regard to type of diabetes, or differences in these particular samples of patients.

Our linkage data is in agreement with those of others and the Eighth International Workshop report that the IDDM susceptibility gene(s) segregates with the HLA region of chromosome 6 (Cudworth and Woodrow 1975; Barbosa et al. 1977; Falk et al. 1978; Rubinstein et al. 1977; Bengsch et al. 1978; Svejgaard et al. 1980). Barbosa et al. (1978) in their linkage analysis assumed a recessive mode of inheritance. In our analysis of 30 pedigrees, either a dominant or a recessive mode of inheritance was assumed (Murphy et al. 1980b). However, linkage between the IDDM susceptibility gene(s) and the HLA region of chromosome 6 is stronger for a dominant model utilizing the same population prevalence. This supports the conclusion of Spielman et al. (1979). Barbosa et al. (1978) chose not to include a parent-child affected family and one where there was an IDDM subject in the third generation. Since inclusion of these types of families increases the likelihood of autosomal recessive inheritance, we chose to use sib-sib as well as parent-child IDDM affected families so as not to bias the analysis toward one form of inheritance. We find, as well as did Barbosa et al. (1980), that there is less evidence for linkage of the IDDM susceptibility gene to HLA in parent-child affected IDDM families. Another aspect of our data which differs is the finding of a maximum lod score of 2.46 at a recombination fraction of 0.0, assuming a dominant mode of inheritance as opposed to 0.13–0.20 for other studies. Since IDDM might be caused by a virus and has the features of an autoimmune disease one could speculate that the susceptibility gene is a gene modulating the immune response in affected subjects.

There are two features of our data, and in certain instances, those of others which provide direction for future studies. First, it is likely that IDDM is in itself a heterogeneous disorder. This could explain the different findings in both the population and linkage studies. Therefore, large homogeneous populations of IDDM subjects that have been critically ascertained should be investigated further. These studies should particularly include families where sib-sib, partent-child as well as relatives from 2 and possibly 3 generations affected with the disease. Such studies coupled with an evaluation of immune parameters such as pancreatic islet-cell antibodies, cell-mediated immunity to islet cells, and antibodies to exogenous insulin might very well reveal additional forms of IDDM. Secondly, one could speculate that the increased prevalence of IDDM in American as compared with African blacks is attributable to admixing of a white gene(s) predisposing them to IDDM. In order to test this hypothesis, additional genetic polymorphisms will need to be assessed in black and white caucasoid IDDM and healthy control subjects from the same geographical location. In preliminary studies, we have determined that the gene frequencies of *ABO, Rh, Duffy, MNS,* and *Hb* in black IDDM patients are more like healthy white controls than negroid healthy controls (Reitnauer et al., unpublished observations). The frequency of other genetic markers are currently being evaluated in order to calculate genetic distance between these groups. Although much knowledge has been gained since the observations by Singal and

Blajchmann (1973) that B15 is associated with IDDM, the genetics of this disease has not been fully elucidated. Provided the aforementioned studies can be conducted on large patient populations the genetics of IDDM should be unraveled in the near future.

ACKNOWLEDGMENTS

We would like to express appreciation to the entire clinical staff of the Diabetes Research and Education Hospital, Outpatient Clinics and Children's Hospital, University of Alabama in Birmingham, as well as the staff of Camp Seale Harris and Camp Whispering Pines sponsored by the American Diabetes Association, Alabama and Louisiana affiliates, respectively for access to diabetic patients. The assistance of Dr. Russell Cunningham, Dr. Sam Eichold, Faye Smedley, Letha Wells, Jayne Roberson, James Shoaf, Linda Baker, Susan Snead and Mary Estock is gratefully acknowledged. Supported in part by grants from the Juvenile Diabetes Foundation (78R144), the Appalachian Regional Commission (ARC-78-156 AL6350-78-I-302-0613) and the Diabetes Trust Fund.

## References

Acton, R.T. and Roseman, J.M. 1978. New vistas in the etiology, genetics, pathogenesis and natural history of juvenile-onset diabetes. J. Med. Assn. State Ala. 48:25–39.

Andersen, J. and Lauritzen, E. 1960.Blood groups and diabetes mellitus. Diabetes 9:20–24.

Barbosa, J., King, R., Noreen, H., and Yunis, E.J. 1977. The histocompatibility system in juvenile, insulin-dependent diabetes multiplex kindreds. J. Clin. Invest. 60:989–998.

Barbosa, J., Cheva, M.M., Noreen, H., and Anderson, V.E. 1978. Analysis of linkage between the major histocompatibility system and juvenile, insulin-dependent diabetes in multiplex families. Reanalysis of data. J. Clin. Invest. 62:492–495.

Barbosa, J., Cheva, M.M., Anderson, V.E., Noreen, H., Johnson, S., Reinsmoen, N., McCarty, R., King, R., and Greenberg, L. 1980. Linkage analysis between the major histocompatibility system and insulin-dependent diabetes in families with patients in two consecutive generations. J. Clin. Invest. 45:592–601.

Bengsch, N., Köbberling, J. Eckert, G., and Willms, B. 1978. HLA-typing in juvenile diabetes with and without positive family history and in families with one and two diabetic siblings. Diabetologia 15:447–451.

Berg, K., Aarseth, S., Lundevall, J., and Reinskou, T. 1967. Blood groups and genetic serum types in diabetes mellitus. Diabetologia 3:30–34.

Bernoco, D., Perdue, S., Terasaki, P.J., Loon, J., and Park, M.S. 1978. International cell exchange. In Clinical Histocompatibility Testing, Vol. 3. C.B. Carpenter, ed. New York: Grune & Stratton, pp. 29–32.

Bloom, A., Hayes, T., and Gamble, D. 1975. Register of newly diagnosed diabetic children. Br. Med. J. 3:580–583.

Botazzo, G.F., Mann, J.I., Thorogood, M., Baum, F.D., and Doniach, P. 1978. Autoimmunity in juvenile diabetics and their families. Br. Med. J. 2:165–168.

Briggs, B.R., Jackson, W.P.V., DuToit, E.D., and Botha, M.C. 1980. The histocompatibility antigen distribution in diabetes in Southern African blacks (Xhosa). Diabetes 29:68–70.

Buckwalter, J.A. 1964. Diabetes mellitus and the blood groups. Diabetes 13:164–168.

Christau, B., Kromann, H., Ortved Anderson, O., Christy, M., Buschard, K., Arming, K., Højland Kristensen, I., Peitersen, B., Steinrud, J., and Nerup, J. 1977. Incidence, seasonal and geographical patterns of juvenile-onset insulin-dependent diabetes mellitus in Denmark. Diabetologia 13:281–284.

Christy, M., Green, A., Christau, B., Kromann, H., Nerup, J., Platz, P., Thomsen, M., Ryder, L.P., and Svejgaard, A. 1979. Studies of the system and insulin-dependent diabetes mellitus. Diabetes Care 2:209–214.

Craighead, J.E. 1978. Current views on the etiology of insulin-dependent diabetes mellitus. N. Engl. J. Med. 299:1439–1445.

Cudworth, A.G. 1978. Type I diabetes mellitus. Diabetologia 14:281–291.

Cudworth, A.G. and Woodrow, J.C. 1975. Evidence for HLA linked genes in juvenile diabetes mellitus. Br. Med. J. 3:133–135.

Elston, R. and Stewart, J. 1973. The analysis of quantitative traits for simple genetic models from $F_1$ and backcross data. Genetics 73:695–711.

Elston, R. and Kaplan, E. GENPED, General Pedigree Analysis Program—A Fortran Program. Cbapel Hill, North Carolina: University of North Carolina, Department of Biostatistics.

Fajans, S.S., Floyd, J.C., Jr., Tattersall, R.B., Williamson, J.R., Pek, S., and Taylor, C.I. 1976. The various faces of diabetes in the young. Arch. Intern. Med. 136:194–202.

Falk, C.T., Suciu-Foca, N., and Rubinstein, P. 1978. Possible localization of the gene(s) for juvenile diabetes mellitus (JDM) to the HLA region of chromosome 6. Cytogenet. Cell Genet. 22:298–300.

Farid, N.R., Barnard, J.M., and Bryant, D.G. 1977. HLA and phenylthiocarbamide (PTC) tasting in autoimmune thyroid disease. Tissue Antigens. 10:414–416.

Farid, N.R., Barnard, J.M., Pepper, B., Noel, E.P., Kelly, F., Davis, A.J., Hobeika, C., and Marsball, W.N. 1978. The association of HLA with juvenile diabetes mellitus in Newfoundland. Tissue Antigens 12:215–222.

Farid, N.R., Sampson, L., Noel, P., Barnard, J.M., Davis, A J., and Hillman, D.A. 1979. HLA-D-related (DRw) antigens in juvenile diabetes mellitus. Diabetes 28:552–557.

Fitzgerald, G.A. and Drury, M.I. 1978. HLA identity in juvenile onset diabetes. Irish J. Med. Sci. 147:430–434.

Fleegler, F., Rogers, K., Drash, A., Rosenbloom, A., Travis, L., and Court, J. 1979. Age, sex, and season of onset of juvenile diabetes in different areas. Pediatrics 63:374–379.

Gamble, P., and Taylor, K. 1969. Seasonal incidence of daibetes mellitus. Br. Med. J. 3:631–633.

Gazit, E., Sartani, A., Mizrachi, Y., and Ravid, M. 1977. HLA antigen in Jewish patients with juvenile-onset diabetes mellitus. Diabet. Metab. 3:55–58.

Gorwitz, K., Howen, G., and Thompson, T. 1976. Prevalence of diabetes in Michigan school-age children. Diabetes. 25:122–127.

Harris, H., Kalman, H., and Trotter, W.R. 1949. Taste sensitivity to phenylthiourea in goiter and diabetes. Lancet 2:1038–1039.

Harris, H. and Kalmus, H. 1950. The measurement of taste sensitivity to phenylthiocarbamide (PTC). Ann. Eugenet. (Lond.) 15:24–31.

Hartmann, G. 1939. Application of individual taste differences toward phenylthiocarbamide in genetic investigations. Eugenics 9:123–135.

Illeni, M.T., Pellegris, G., DelGuercio, M.J., Tarantino, A., Busetto, F., DiPietro, C., Clerici, E., Gavatta, G., and Chiumello, G. 1977. HLA antigens in diabetic children. Diabetes 26:870–873.

Ilonen, J., Herva, E., Tülikainen, A., ÅAkerblom, H.K., Mustonen, A., Koivukangas, T., and Kouvalainen, K. 1980. HLA genetics of insulin-dependent juvenile-onset diabetes mellitus in northern Finland. Tissue Antigens 15:381–388.

Irvine, W.J., McCallum, C.J., Campbell, C.J., Ducan, L.J.P., Farquhar, J.W., Vaughan, H., and Morris, P.J. 1976. Pancreatic islet-cell antibodies in diabetes mellitus correlated with the duration and type of diabetes co-existent autoimmune disease and HLA type. Diabetes 26:138–147.

Jackson, W.P.U. and Huskisson, J. 1965. Diabetes Interracial Comparisons. South African Med. J. 39:526–531.

Kawa, A., Nakazawa, M., Kono, Y., Sakaguchi, S., Nakamura, S., and Kanehisa, T. 1978. HLA-Bw54 and B5 in Japanese diabetes with juvenile-onset and insulin-dependency. Experientia 34:669.

Kitchin, F.D., Howel-Evans, W., Clarke, C.A., McConnel, R.B., and Sheppard, P.M. 1959. PTC taste response and thyroid disease. Br. Med. J. 1:1069–1074.

Koivisto, V.A., Kuitunen, P., Tülikainen, A., and Åkerblum, H.R. 1977. HLA antigens in patients with juvenile diabetes mellitus, coeliac disease and both of the diseases. Diabet. Metab. 3:49–53.

Kyllo, C. and Nuttal, F. 1978. Prevalence of diabetes mellitus in school-age children in Minnesota. Diabetes. 27:57–60.

Leslie, R.D.G. and Pyke, D.A. 1979. Letter to the editor. Diabetologia 16:139.

Lucarelli, P., Scacchi, R., Corbo, R.M., Palmarino, R., Orsini, M., Campea, L., Carapella, E., and Pascone, R. 1978. Genetic polymorphisms in juvenile-onset diabetes. Hum. Hered. 28:89–95.

Ludwig, H., Schernthaner, G., and Mayr, W.R. 1977. The importance of HLA genes to susceptibility in the development of juvenile diabetes mellitus. Diabet. Metab. 3:43–48.

MacDonald, M.J. 1974. Equal incidence of adult onset diabetes among ancestors of juvenile diabetics and non-diabetics. Diabetologia 10:767–773.

MacDonald, M.J. 1975. Lower frequency of diabetes among hospitalized Negro than white children: Theoretical implications. Acta Genet. Med. Gemellol. 24:118–126.

MacMillan, D.R., Kotovan, M., Zeidner, D., and Hofezi, B. 1977. Seasonal variation in the onset of diabetes in children. Pediatrics 59:113–115.

Maeda, H., Taneuchi, F., Juji, T., Akanuwa, Y., Kasuga, M., Lee, Y.S., Kosaka, K., and Tsai, S.H. 1980. HLA-DRw3 in juvenile onset diabetes mellitus in Chinese. Tissue Antigens 15:173–176.

Mattiuz, P., Ihde, D., Piazza, A., Capellini, R., and Bodmer, W. 1970. New approaches to the population genetics and segregation analysis of the HLA system. In Histocompatibility Testing 1970. P.I. Terasaki, ed. Copenhagen: Munksgaard, pp. 193–205.

McConnell, R.B., Pyke, D.A., and Roberts, J.A.F. 1956. Blood groups in diabetes mellitus. Br. Med. J. 1:772–776.

Miller, W.V. (ed.) 1977. Technical Manual of the American Association of Blood Banks (seventh edition). Philadelphia: J.B. Lippincott, pp. 83–127.

Mittal, K.K., Mickey, M.R., Singal, D.P., and Terasaki, P.I. 1968. Serotyping for non-transplantation XVIII. Refinement of microdroplet lymphocyte cytotoxicity test. Transplantation 6:913–927.

Mittal, K.K. 1976. The HLA polymorphism and susceptibility to disease. Vox Sang. 31:161–173.

Murphy, C.C., Acton, R.T., Barger, B.O., Roseman, J.M., and Go, R.C.P. 1980a. Genetics of diabetes mellitus. I. Evidence from linkage analysis of IDDM to HLA within multiply affected families suggests a dominant mode of inheritance of susceptibility. (Submitted for publication).

Murphy, C., Acton, R., Barger, B., Kirk, K., Reitnauer, P., and Roseman, J. 1980b. Epidemiologic and HLA features of insulin-dependent diabetes mellitus. (Submitted for publication).

Nakao, Y., Fukunishi, T., Koide, M., Akasawa, K., Ikeda, M., Yohata, M., and Imura, H. 1977. HLA antigens in Japanese patients with diabetes mellitus. Diabetes 26:736–739.

National Diabetes Data Group. 1979. Classification and diagnosis of diabetes mellitus and other categories of glucose intolerance Diabetes. 28:1039–1057.

Nerup, J., Ortved Andersen, O., and Bendixen, G. 1971. Antipancreatic cellular hypersensitivity in diabetes mellitus. Diabetes 20:424–427.

Nerup, J., Platz, P., Ortved Andersen, O., Christy, M., Lyngsøe, J., Poulsen, J.E., Ryder, L.P., Staub-Nielsen, L., Thomsen, M., and Svejgaard, A. 1974. Lancet 2:864–866.

Nerup, J., Ortved Andersen, O., Christy, M., Platz, P., Ryder, L., Thomsen, M., and Svejgaard, A. 1976. HLA autoimmunity, virus and the pathogenesis of juvenile diabetes mellitus. Acta Endocrinol. (suppl. 205) 83:167–175.

Rahi, A. 1979. HLA and eye disease. Br. J. Opthalmol. 68:283–292.

Reitnauer, P., Acton, R., Barger, B., Budowle, B., Murphy, C., Roseman, J., and Go, R. 1981. A population genetics study of insulin-dependent diabetes mellitus in young black Americans. Tissue Antigens, in press.

Rubinstein, P., Suciu-Foca, N., and Nicholson, J.F. 1977. Genetics of juvenile diabetes mellitus. A recessive gene closely linked to HLA-D and with 50 percent penetrance. N. Engl. J. Med. 297:1036–1040.

Ryder, L.P., Andersen, E., and Svejgaard, A. 1979. HLA and Disease Registry, Third Report. Copenhagen: Munksgaard.

Sayetta, R. and Murphy, R. 1979. Summary of current diabetes-related data from the National Center for Health Statistics. Diabetes Care 2:105–119.

Singal, D.P. and Blajchmann, M.A. 1973. Histocompatibility (HLA) antigens, lymphocytic antibodies, and tissue antibodies in patients with diabetes mellitus. Diabetes 22:429–432.

Solow, N., Hidalgo, R., and Singal, D.P. 1978. Juvenile-onset diabetes: HLA-A, -B, -B, and -DR alloantigens. Diabetes 28:1–4.

Spielman, R., Baker, L., and Zmijewski, C. 1980. Inheritance of susceptibility to juvenile-onset diabetes. In Genetic Analysis of Common Diseases: Application to Predictive Factors in Coronary Heart Disease. C. Sing and M. Skolnick, eds. New York: Alan R. Liss, pp 567–585.

Suciu-Foca, N., Nicholson, J.F., Reemstma, K., et al. 1977. The HLA system and the genetics of juvenile diabetes mellitus (J.D.M.). Daibet. Metab. 3:193–198.

Suciu-Foca, N., Rubinstein, P., Nicholson, J., Susinno, E., Weiner, J., Godfrey, M., Hardy, M., Rayfield, E., and Reemstma, K. 1979. Juvenile diabetes mellitus and the HLA system. Transplant. Proc. 11:1309–1313.

Sultz, H.A., Schlesinger, E.R., Mosher, W.E., and Feldman, J.G. 1972. Childhood diabetes mellitus. In Long-term Childhood Illness. Pittsburgh: Pittsburgh Press, pp. 223–248.

Svejgaard, A. 1976. HLA and Disease. In Manual of Clinical Immunology. N. Rose and H. Freedman, eds. Washington, D.C.: American Society of Microbiology, pp. 841–850.

Svejgaard, A., Platz, P., and Ryder, L.P. 1980. Insulin-dependent diabetes mellitus. In Histocompatibility Testing 1980. P. Terasaki, ed. Los Angeles: UCLA Tissue Typing Laboratory, pp. 638–656.

Tattersall, R.B. and Pyke, D.A. 1972. Diabetes in identical twins. Lancet 2:1120–1122.

Terasaki, P.I., Bernoco, D., Park, M.S., Ozturk, G., and Iwaki, Y. 1978. Microdroplet testing for HLA-A, -B, -C, and -D Antigens. Am. J. Clin. Pathol. 69:103–120.

Terry, M.C. and Segall, G.G. 1947. The association of diabetes and taste-blindness. J. Hered. 38:135–137.

Terry, M.C. 1950. Taste-blindness and diabetes in the colored population of Jamaica. J. Hered. 41:306–307.

Vague, Ph., Melis, C., Mercier, P., Vialettes, B., and Lassmann, V. 1978. The increased frequency of the Lewis negative blood group in a diabetic population. Diabetologia 15:33–36.

West, R., Belmonte, M., Colle, E., Crepeau, M., Wilkins, J., and Pointer, R. 1979. Epidemiologic survey of juvenile-onset diabetes in Montreal. Diabetes 28:690–693.

White, P. and Graham, C. 1971. The child with diabetes. In Joslin's Diabetes Mellitus, ed. 11. A Marble, P. White, et al. eds. Philadelphia: Lea and Febinger, pp. 339–360.

Woolf, B. 1955. On estimating the relation between blood groups and diseases. Ann. Hum. Genet. 19:251–253.

Yoon, J.W., Austin, M., Takashi, O., and Notkins, A.L. 1979. Virus-induced diabetes mellitus: Isolation of a virus from the pancreas of a child with diabetic ketoacidosis. N. Engl. J. Med. 300:1173–1179.

Zimmet, P., Kiely, P., Cross, R., Court, J., and Bornstein, J. 1979. HLA patterns in Australian patients with insulin dependent diabetes mellitus. Austal. N. Z. J. Med. 9:633–636.

Hildemann, ed. Frontiers in Immunogenetics

# The Role of Dogma in the Immune Response

Jeffrey A. Frelinger and Brian Shigekawa

*Department of Microbiology, University of Southern California School of Medicine, 2025 Zonal Avenue, Los Angeles, California*

In Ray Owen's laboratory, one of the concepts firmly entrenched in our minds during conversations around the table in the coffee room was the idea that models were put forward to be challenged, not confirmed. Dogma was useful only as long as it continued to explain all of the observations; the observations must not be bent to fit the dogma. All of us felt the need to do experiments not to confirm current prejudices, but rather to test them critically. Any flaws in the dogma should then appear, and a new hypothesis could be put forward to explain the data. We have been motivated primarily by the idea of testing, in the most rigorous way possible, the predictions made on current immunological and immunogenetic dogma.

Part of my motivation for beginning the study of *Ia* antigens was the dogmatic assertion by Bach and colleagues that there were two discrete classes of cell surface molecules associated with the major histocompatability complex: One could be defined by antibodies, and the other was distinguishable by the fact it was not definable by antibodies, but could only be defined by lymphocyte responses. One of these two classes of molecules was the K/D molecule which was classically determined by serology and expressed on all cells. The other was *I* region coded and was responsible for the ability to stimulate mixed lymphocyte culture (Bach et al. 1972). This testing was quite productive when the results of my work with Chella David and Don Shreffler showed that *I* region molecules can be detected quite easily with antibody (David, Shreffler, and Frelinger, 1973).

With this background, I would like to briefly review the status of the understanding of the role of Ly alloantigens for the definition of lymphocyte subsets when we began our work on the use of Ly antisera to define lymphocyte populations responding to discrete subregions of the *H-2* complex. I will briefly mention the work of others which comes to much the same conclusions as we have. I will also describe another system which we have recently been testing rigorously for its adherence to dogma. We had begun our studies on *beige* mice earlier, using these animals to examine the pleiomorphic effects of single gene mutations on the immune system. Later reports by Roder have suggested that *beige* mice have a selective deficit in the natural killer cell population, but are otherwise immunologically normal.

## Definition of Ly Phenotypes in Alloresponding T-cells

Since their description by Boyse and Old (1969), the lymphocyte alloantigens Ly-1 and Ly-2 have been extraordinarily useful. They have been shown to be expressed only on a subpopulation of thymus-derived lymphocytes, and not on other cells. In the classic work of Cantor and Boyse (1975a,b), they were able to show that cells responding in mixed lymphocyte cultures by proliferation to whole *H-2* differences were expressing predominantly the Ly-1 alloantigen, but not the Ly-2 alloantigen. This was shown by selective depletion with anti-Ly-1 of the lymphocyte alloantigen response. Similarly, the cytotoxic effector cells themselves were predominantly of the class Ly-$1^-2^+$. This coupled with work by other groups suggested that the major proliferating cell in the mixed lympocyte culture was an Ly-1-bearing lymphocyte which responded to *Ia* alloantigens, and provided a helper signal to Ly-2,3-bearing lymphocytes (cytotoxic T-lymphocyte precursors) which responded to K/D alloantigens. The Ly-2,3 cells and the Ly-1 cells interacted to generate cytotoxic cells which had the Ly-2,3 phenotype. From these kinds of analyses, it appeared that Ly-$1^+2^+$ pool had little effector function. Similarly, adoptive transfer experiments showed that the Ly-$1^+$ and Ly-$2^+3^+$ phenotypes were relatively stable *in vivo,* while the Ly-$1^+2^+3^+$ phenotype gave rise to cells of all three phenotypes (David et al., 1973). Thus, the following dogma arose: Ly-1 cells were helper cells, Ly-2,3 cells were cytotoxic cells, and Ly-1,2,3 cells acted solely as precursers.

From the start there were several reasons to believe this as the whole story. The Ly-1, and Ly-2,3 population could account for only about 50% of the post-thymic T-lymphocytes. It seemed unlikely that the other 50% of the cells functioned solely as precursors of these two populations. However, there was no evidence to suggest any function. Peter Wettstein and I began our studies of this problem reasoning that if we studied *H-2* mutants, which give both strong proliferative responses and cytotoxic responses, it might be possible to see a proliferative response of Ly-2,3 cells or cytotoxic responsive Ly-1 cells.

It soon became clear that we could eliminate the ability of peripheral T-lymphocytes to respond to *H-2* mutant differences by treatment with either anti-Ly-1 or anti-Ly-2 (Figure 1). Surprisingly, we could never reconstitute the proliferative response by adding back mixtures of Ly-$1^+$ cells and Ly-$2^+$ cells. This demonstrates that proliferating cells are neither Ly-$1^+2^-$ nor Ly-$1^-2^+$ cells, but are in fact Ly-$1^+2^+$ cells (Kelly, 1957).

At about the same time, it became clear in other systems that Ly-1,2 cells were also involved. Pang and his colleagues reported an interaction between an Ly-$1^+2^+$ cell and an Ly-$2^+3^+$ cell for the generation of virus-specific cytotoxic cells

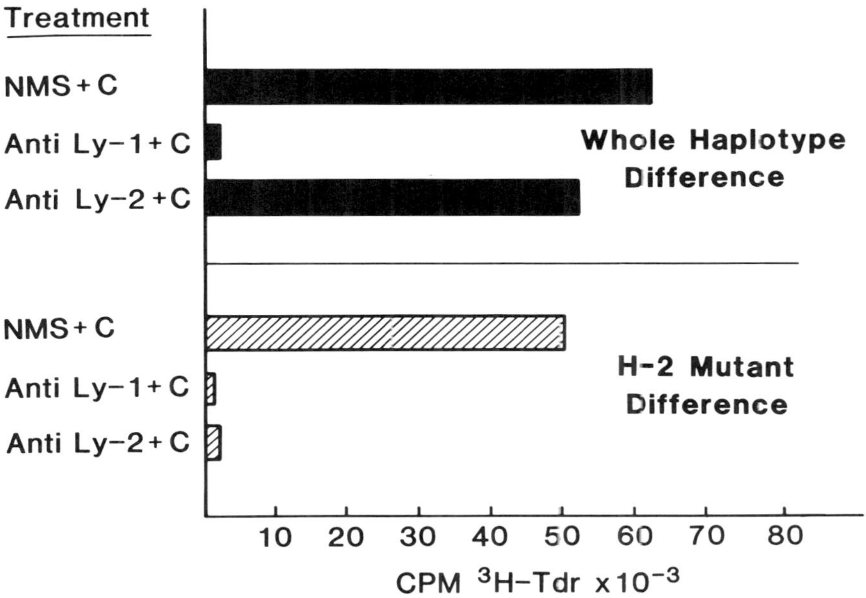


**Figure 1.** Effect of treatment of T-cell with anti-Ly sera + C on mixed lymphocyte reactions. Top panel shows response of B10 cells to C3H.Q stimulators. Bottom panel shows the response of B6 to B6.C-$H$-$2^{bm1}$ stimulators.

(Pang et al. 1976). Similarly, there were indications in this response to mammary tumor virus that there was involvement of Ly-$1^+2^+$ cells in the generation and expansion of the Ly-2,3 population of cytotoxic effectors (Pang et al., 1976).

We began similar experiments to examine the Ly phenotype of the cytotoxic effectors specific for *H-2* mutants. In contrast to those generated by whole haplotype differences, which are normally refractory to treatment by anti-Ly-$1^+$ complement, the effectors were almost completely sensitive to treatment with either anti-Ly-1 + complement, or anti-Ly-2 + complement (Figure 2). Mixtures of Ly-$1^+$ and Ly-$2^+$ cells failed to reconstitute the cytotoxic response demonstrating that the effector itself was an Ly-$1^+2^+$ cell. Interactions were effectively ruled out by the use of the short-term chromium release assay which made it impossible for interactions to occur. Thus the involvement of Ly-$1^+2^+$ cells as amplifier cells is unlikely (Roder et al., 1979).

Other reports of functions of the Ly-1,2 population began to appear. Swain et al. (1979) showed that the Ly-$1^+2^+$ cells produced helper factor in response to H-2K differences. Old and his colleagues showed that there was an Ly-$1^+2^+$ killer involved in cytotoxicity against some syngeneic tumors (Swain et al., 1979). Interestingly, different tumors appear to have different kinds of effectors. Peter Wettstein and I have shown a similar point using antigens to generate cytotoxic effectors.

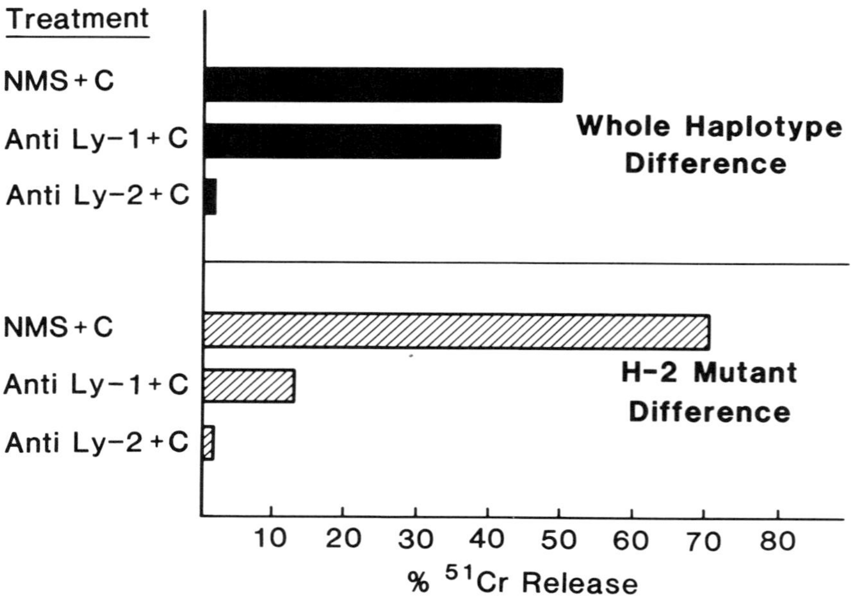


**Figure 2.** Effect of treatment of cytotoxic effector cells with anti-Ly sera + C. Top panel shows cytotoxicity of B10 cells treated after MLR with B10.A stimulation and tested on B10.A(4R) targets. Bottom panel shows identical experiment of B6 cells assayed on B6.C-$H$-$2^{bm1}$.

Here the Ly phenotype of the effector depends on the antigenic difference. Finally, just to complete the confusion, Swain et al. (1980) have recently shown that a cell line, following disparate *I* region stimulation and showing cytotoxic activity for *I-A* region antigen, has the Ly phenotype Ly-$1^+2^-$. Thus, apparently almost any phenotype can occur with any effector function.

The conclusion that we reached from these studies is not that any of the data was incorrect, or that the interpretations were wrong, but rather that Ly antigens are extraordinarily useful for the definition of lymphocyte subpopulations. However, utility rests not only on the precise specificity of the antisera in the experiments, but also on the assays chosen. Thus, there is no universal membrane marker to define a particular function as killing or helpful. The results we have now represent the same kinds of refinements experienced with anti-Thy-1 sera following their introduction.

## The Immunobiology of Beige Mice

Mice with the coat color marker, *beige,* were first described in 1957 (Wettstein et al., 1978). They originally attracted interest as a possible animal model for Chediak-Higashi syndrome. This syndrome, which involves lysosomal granules, has been extensively studied in these animals. More recently, the reports by Roder and his colleagues (1979) showed that *beige* mice were deficient in natural killer cell (NK) activity compared to their congenic B6 partners. Because of the great interest in NK cells and their possible role in tumor immunity, we decided to make a critical evaluation of the immune capacity of *beige* mice in several relevant *in vitro* systems. Although many of these systems were originally tested by Roder, we studied these traits with a rigor not attempted previously. A series of experiments were performed to examine the proliferative and cytotoxic responses of *beige* mice to individual regions of the mouse *H-2* complex. In every case, K alone, K + I, or whole *H-2,* the response of *beige* mice was comparable to those of their congenic partners. Since there was some evidence to believe that *beige* mice might be deficient in their macrophage-like cells because of reduced antibody-dependent cellular cytotoxicity towards tumors, we examined their ability to function as stimulator cells in mixed lymphocyte culture reactions and cell-mediated lymphocytotoxicity. As in the case of their ability to respond to single regions of *H-2*, their ability to stimulate allogeneic cells was intact.

We also studied the ability of *beige* mice to respond to a minor histocompatibility antigen, H-Y. In this case, we could examine the ability of B6-*bg* mice to prime, boost, and function as targets for cytotoxic effector cells, as well as to respond themselves. Thus, if *beige* mice had specific defects in addition to or concomitant with their lack of NK cells, we might be able to determine it in one or all of these steps. In contrast to the results with whole *H-2* differences, the ability of B6-*bg* female cells to respond to male cells was effectively ablated. Thus, *beige* females, primed and boosted *in vitro* with *beige* male cells, were unable to mount a cytotoxic response. These cells were not cytotoxic when tested on either *beige* male or B6 male targets (Figure 3). This result is not solely a defect of the *beige* female, since *beige* females primed and boosted with wild type male cells make cytotoxic effectors capable of lysing either *beige* male or B6 male cells. B6 females respond equally well, or nearly so, to *beige* and/or B6 males. Thus, only when *beige* females are primed *in vivo* with *beige* males can the deficiency be observed. When B6-*bg* females, primed with B6-*bg* male cells *in vivo,* are boosted *in vitro* with either B6 or B6-*bg* male cells, they fail to generate significant cytotoxic responses.

Because of the localization to the priming step *in vivo*, we performed male to female skin grafts. B6 or B6-*bg* females were skin grafted using Bailey's tail-to-tail technique with either B6 or B6-*bg* male skin. Only when *beige* females were grafted with *beige* male skin was there a significant prolongation of skin graft survival. B6-*bg* male grafts survived 29 days versus 25 days for the other combination. While this is not a spectacular difference in MST, it is highly significant, ($p = .01$), and is clearly prolonged. Thus the defect in priming of B6-*bg* females for H-Y antigen on B6-*bg* males cells is apparent both *in vivo* and *in vitro*.

Much emphasis was placed on Roder's result that B6-*bg* mice respond more poorly to tumors and have an increased incidence of metastasis. This observation has been used as evidence that NK cells are implicated in tumor immunity and that NK cells play a vital role in the suppression of metastasis. Our results suggest that

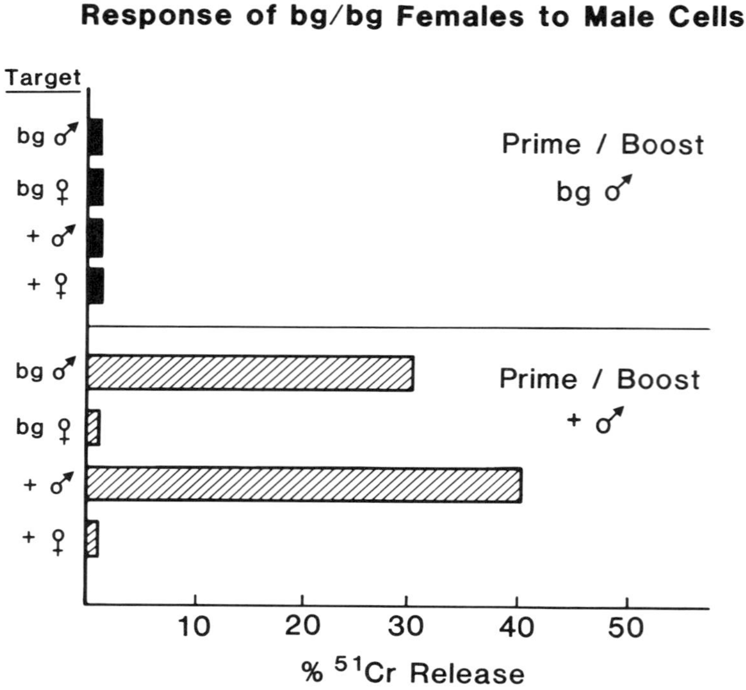


**Figure 3.** Response of B6-*beige* females to male cells. Top panel shows the CML response of *bg* female cells primed *in vivo* and boosted *in vitro* with *bg* male cells. Bottom shows the response against +/+ male cells.

perhaps more important is the inability of T-cells to respond to minor antigen determinants on the surface of cells. Presumably, responses to tumor antigens are much like anti-H-Y responses, and these results suggest that there might be also defects in the ability of *beige* cells to prime for effective cytotoxic responses in *bg* mice.

From these studies then we are left with two possible conclusions: If we accept the dogma, i.e., that *beige* mice represent a singular defect in NK cells, then of course NK cells must be involved in the response to H-Y antigens. On the surface, this seems unlikely. We believe a more plausible explanation is that the effects of the *beige* mutation are more pleiotropic than already believed. Thus the *beige* mutation affects not only cells in the NK lineage, but also cells in the T-cell lineage (or the antigen presenting cell family). Presumably, the response of other single minor *H* antigens should be affected. Roder and his colleagues (1979) reported one skin grafting experiment with multiple non-*H-2* differences, A.BY grafted onto B6, and/or B6-*bg* animals. In this case, they found statistically insignificant prolongation of skin graft survival. This could be attributed to the difficulty of measuring small differences in survival times. Whereas normal wild type cells reject skin grafts from A.BY's in 10-11 days, the response of a single determinant, H-Y, in our hands shows a graft rejection time of about 25 days. Thus a slight difference of less than a day at 10-12 days magnifies into a difference of several days at 25. If we were to pick other *H* antigens leading to longer median survival times, we might see even more striking prolongation.

## Conclusion

Ray Owen instilled the desire to test dogmatic assertions rigorously. Accordingly, we began these studies to critically examine certain current dogmas in immunobiology. We have presented data from two distinct systems which show in a concrete way real limitations in the dogma. With respect to the Ly phenotypes of cells responding to *H-2* differences, separate functions are clearly not as simply defined as they first appeared. In the case of *beige* mice, the defect in NK cells is only one reflection of a complex phenotype caused by a single gene mutation. The latter is, of course, not surprising in view of the fact that single gene mutations can have multiple effects. A classic example of such problems is in adenosine phosphoribosyl transferase deficiency. This deficiency of an enzyme in the purine salvage pathway causes not only multiple disorders in purine metabolism but also immunodeficiency of T-cell lineage in particular. This is not a result of something wrong with the T-cells themselves, but the fact that T-cells turn out to be particularly sensitive to high levels of purines. This is essentially an accident of metabolism.

Our hope and desire from our studies is that our fellow immunogeneticists will remember their genetics.

ACKNOWLEDGMENTS

Supported by NIH Grant CA 22662. JAF is recipient of American Cancer Society Faculty Research Award 179. BS is recipient of American Cancer Society Postdocdoral Fellowship PF-1624.

## References

Bach, F.G., Widmer, M.B., Bach, M.L., and Klein, J. 1972. Serologically defined and lymphocyte-defined components of the major histocompatibility complex in the mouse. J. Exp. Med. 136:1430.

Boyse, E.A. and Old, L.J. 1969. Some aspects of normal and abnormal cell-surface genetics. Ann. Rev. Genet. 3:269.

Cantor, H. and Boyse, E.A. 1975a. Functional subclasses of T-lymphocytes bearing different Ly antigens. I. The generation of functionally distinct T-cell subclasses in a differentiative process independent of antigen. J. Exp. Med. 141:1376.

Cantor, H. and Boyse, E.A. 1975b. Functional subclasses of T-lymphocytes bearing different Ly antigens. II. Cooperation between subclasses of Ly$^+$ cells in the generation of killer activity. J. Exp. Med. 141:1390.

Cantor, H. and Boyse, E.A. 1976. Regulation of cellular and humoral immune responses by T-cell subclasses. Cold Spring Harbor Symp. Quant. Biol. 41:23.

David, C.S., Shreffer, D.C., and Frelinger, J.A. 1973. New lymphocyte antigen system (Lna) controlled by the *Ir* region of the mouse *H-2* complex. Proc. Natl. Acad. Sci. U.S.A. 70:2059.

Kelley, E.M. 1957. Mouse News Letter. 16:36.

Nakayama, E., Shiku, H., Stockert, E., Oettgen, H.I., and Old, L.J. 1979. Cytotoxic T-cells: Ly phenotype and blocking of killing activity by Lyt antisera. Proc. Natl. Acad. Sci. U.S.A. 76:1977.

Pang, T., McKenzie, F.C., and Blanden, R.V. 1976. Cooperation between mouse T-cell subpopulations in the cell-mediated response to a natural poxvirus pathogen. Cell Immunol. 26:153.

Roder, J.C., Lohmann-Matthes, M.-L., Domzig, W., and Wigzell, H. 1979. The beige mutation in the mouse. II. Selectivity of the natural killer (NK) cell defect. J. Immunol. 123:2174.

Stutman, O., Shen, F.-W., and Boyse, E.A. 1977. Ly phenotype of T-cells cytotoxic for syngeneic mouse mammary tumors: Evidence for T-cell interactions. Proc. Natl. Acad. Sci. U.S.A. 74:5667.

Swain, S., Bakke, A., English, M., and Dutton, R.W. 1979. Ly phenotypes and MHC recognition: The allohelper that recognizes K or D is a mature Ly-123 cell. J. Immunol. 123:2716.

Swain, S.C., Dennert, G., Wormsley, S., and Dutton, R.W. 1980. The Lyt phenotype of a long-term allospecific T-cell line. Both helper and killer activities to I-A are mediated by Ly-1 cells. J. Exp. Med. 151.

Wettstein, P.J., Bailey, D.W., Mobraaten, L.E., Klein, J., and Frelinger, J.A. 1978. T-lymphocyte response to *H-2* mutants. I. Proliferation is dependent on Ly-$1^{+}2^{+}$ cells. J. Exp. Med. 147:1395.

Wettstein, P.J., Bailey, D.W., Mobraaten, L.E., Klein, J., and Frelinger, J.A. 1979. T-lymphocyte response to *H-2* mutants: Cytotoxic effects are Ly-$1^{+}2^{+}$. Proc. Natl. Acad. Sci. U.S.A. 76:3455.

# Index